PATHOLOGY OF EMERGING INFECTIONS

Pathology of Emerging Infections

EDITED BY

C. Robert Horsburgh, Jr.
Ann Marie Nelson

ASM PRESS • WASHINGTON, DC

Pathology of emerging infections / editors, C. Robert Horsburgh, Jr.
and Ann Marie Nelson.
        p.   cm.
    Includes bibliographical references and index.
    ISBN 1-55581-120-5
    1. Communicable diseases.   2. Communicable diseases—Pathophysiology.
I. Horsburgh, C. Robert.   II. Nelson, Ann Marie.
    [DNLM: 1. Communicable Diseases—pathology.   2. Communicable Diseases—
epidemiology. WC 100 P296 1997]
RC111.P39   1997
616.9′047—DC21
DNLM/DLC
for Library of Congress   97-13857
                                                                                                          CIP

Contents

Contributors

David G. Addiss
Division of Parasitic Diseases, National Center for Infectious Diseases, Centers for Disease Control and Prevention, 4770 Buford Highway, Mailstop F-22, Atlanta, GA 30341

Ruth Berkelman
National Center for Infectious Diseases, Centers for Disease Control and Prevention, 1600 Clifton Road, N.E., Mailstop C-12, Atlanta, GA 30333

Ralph T. Bryan
National Center for Infectious Diseases, Centers for Disease Control and Prevention, Atlanta, GA 30333

Francis W. Chandler
Department of Pathology, Medical College of Georgia, Augusta, GA 30912

Jacqueline E. Dawson
Viral and Rickettsial Zoonoses Branch, Division of Viral and Rickettsial Diseases, National Center for Infectious Diseases, Centers for Disease Control and Prevention, 1600 Clifton Road, N.E., Mailstop G-13, Atlanta, GA 30333

Carlos del Rio
Division of Infectious Diseases, Emory University School of Medicine, 69 Butler Street, S.E., Atlanta, GA 30303

David T. Dennis
Bacterial Zoonoses Branch, Division of Vector-Borne Infectious Diseases, National Center for Infectious Diseases, Centers for Disease Control and Prevention, Fort Collins, CO 80522

Paul H. Duray
Department of Pathology, National Cancer Institute, National Institutes of Health, 9000 Rockville Pike, Bethesda, MD 20201

Molly Eaton
Division of Infectious Diseases, Emory University School of Medicine, 69 Butler Street, S.E., Atlanta, GA 30303

Monica M. Farley
Division of Infectious Diseases, Emory University School of Medicine, 69 Butler Street, S.E., Atlanta, GA 30303

Sarah S. Frankel
Division of AIDS and Emerging Infectious Disease Pathology, Armed Forces Institute of Pathology, Washington, DC 20306, and Department of Vaccine Research, Division of Retrovirology, Walter Reed Army Institute of Research, 13 Taft Court, Suite 200, Rockville, MD 20850

Benjamin D. Gold
Division of Pediatric Gastroenterology and Nutrition, Department of Pediatrics, Emory University School of Medicine, 2040 Ridgewood Drive, N.E., Atlanta, GA 30322

Scott R. Granter
Brigham and Women's Hospital, Harvard Medical School, Boston, MA 02115

C. Robert Horsburgh, Jr.
Emory University School of Medicine, 69 Butler Street, S.E., Atlanta, GA 30303

Kamal G. Ishak
Department of Hepatic and Gastrointestinal Pathology, Armed Forces Institute of Pathology, Washington, DC 20306-6000

Nancy K. Jaax
Pathology Division, U.S. Army Medical Research Institute of Infectious Diseases, 1425 Porter Street, Fort Detrick, MD 21702-5011

Harold W. Jaffe
Division of AIDS, STD and TB Laboratory Research, National Center for Infectious Diseases, Centers for Disease Control and Prevention, 1600 Clifton Road, N.E., Mailstop A-12, Atlanta, GA 30333

Dennis D. Juranek
Division of Parasitic Diseases, National Center for Infectious Diseases, Centers for Disease Control and Prevention, 4770 Buford Highway, Mailstop F-22, Atlanta, GA 30341

Leo Kaufman
Immunodiagnostic Laboratory, Emerging Bacterial and Mycotic Diseases Branch, National Center for Infectious Diseases, Centers for Disease Control and Prevention, 1600 Clifton Road, N.E., Atlanta, GA 30333

Peter H. Kilmarx
Epidemic Intelligence Service, Epidemiology Program Office, and Epidemiology and Surveillance Branch, Division of STD Prevention, National Center for HIV, STD, and TB Prevention, Centers for Disease Control and Prevention, Atlanta, GA 30333, and The HIV/AIDS Collaboration, P.O. Box 8 Lanna Station, Chiang Rai 57001, Thailand

A. Julio Martinez
Neuropathology Section, Room 586, Presbyterian University Hospital and University of Pittsburgh, Pittsburgh, PA 15213

Aileen M. Marty
Infectious Disease Pathology Branch, Geographic Pathology Division, Department of
Infectious and Parasitic Disease Pathology, Armed Forces Institute of Pathology,
Washington, DC 20306-6000

Eric E. Mast
Hepatitis Branch, Division of Viral and Rickettsial Diseases, National Center for Infectious
Diseases, Centers for Disease Control and Prevention, 1600 Clifton Road, N.E., Mailstop
G-37, Atlanta, GA 30333

Michael M. McNeil
Division of Bacterial and Mycotic Diseases, National Center for Infectious Diseases,
Centers for Disease Control and Prevention, 1600 Clifton Road, N.E., Mailstop C-09,
Atlanta, GA 30333

Frederick A. Meier
Clinical and Anatomic Pathology, Department of Pathology, Alfred I. Dupont Institute,
Children's Hospital, Wilmington, Delaware

Wayne M. Meyers
Mycobacteriology Branch, Division of Microbiology, Department of Infectious and Parasitic
Disease Pathology, Armed Forces Institute of Pathology, Washington, DC 20306-6000

Ronald C. Neafie
Parasitic Disease Pathology Branch, Geographic Pathology Division, Department of
Infectious and Parasitic Disease Pathology, Armed Forces Institute of Pathology,
Washington, DC 20306-6000

Ann Marie Nelson
Division of AIDS Pathology, Department of Infectious and Parasitic Disease Pathology,
Armed Forces Institute of Pathology, Washington, DC 20306-6000

Clarence J. Peters
Special Pathogens Branch, Centers for Disease Control and Prevention, 1600 Clifton
Road, N.E., Mailstop A-26, Atlanta, GA 30333

David A. Schwartz
Department of Pathology and Division of Infectious Diseases, Emory University School of
Medicine, Atlanta, GA 30303, and National Center for Infectious Diseases, Centers for
Disease Control and Prevention, Atlanta, GA 30333

Craig N. Shapiro
Hepatitis Branch, Division of Viral and Rickettsial Diseases, National Center for Infectious
Diseases, Centers for Disease Control and Prevention, 1600 Clifton Road, N.E., Mailstop
G-37, Atlanta, GA 30333

Govinda S. Visvesvara
Host/Parasite Biology Section, Biology and Diagnostics Branch, Division of Parasitic
Diseases, Mailstop F-13, National Center for Infectious Diseases, Centers for Disease
Control and Prevention, 4770 Buford Highway, N.E., Atlanta, GA 30341-3724

Sherif R. Zaki
Infectious Disease Pathology Activity, Division of Viral and Rickettsial Diseases, National
Center for Infectious Diseases, Centers for Disease Control and Prevention, 1600 Clifton
Road, N.E., Mailstop G-32, Atlanta, GA 30333

Acknowledgments

The editors are grateful for the encouragement and support of Florabel G. Mullick, Director, Center for Advanced Pathology, Armed Forces Institute of Pathology (AFIP); Douglas J. Wear, Chairman, Department of Infectious and Parasitic Diseases Pathology, AFIP; and James M. Hughes, Director, National Center for Infectious Diseases, Centers for Disease Control and Prevention. The editors also thank Sunny Walton for excellent secretarial assistance.

Introduction

Ruth L. Berkelman

The world is witnessing the emergence and reemergence of infectious diseases as a significant threat to public health (2, 3). In contrast to predictions earlier in this century, infectious diseases remain the leading cause of death worldwide and have been increasing as a cause of death in the United States since 1980 (6). Many complex factors contribute to this growing threat and to the broader array of recognized pathogens.

Emerging infections, as defined in a report by the Institute of Medicine in 1992, include diseases whose incidence has increased within the past 20 years or whose incidence threatens to increase in the near future (2). The term includes infections caused by new agents, reemerging pathogens whose incidence had previously declined, and organisms that are developing antimicrobial resistance. Established diseases with a recently discovered infectious origin (e.g., peptic ulcer disease caused by *Helicobacter pylori*) are also included in this definition.

The world's population has been increasing explosively and currently exceeds 5 billion individuals. Population is projected to double by the year 2050, with the most marked rise in population occurring in Asia and Africa.

Ruth Berkelman, National Center for Infectious Diseases, Centers for Disease Control and Prevention, 1600 Clifton Road, N.E., Mailstop C-12, Atlanta, GA 30333.

Pathology of Emerging Infections
Edited by C. Robert Horsburgh, Jr., and Ann Marie Nelson
© 1997 American Society for Microbiology, Washington, DC 20005-4171

Concomitantly, the trend towards urbanization is continuing in both the developed and the developing world, and cities marked by poverty and overcrowding favor the spread of many diseases, including tuberculosis. Lack of adequate sanitation and rodent control fosters the spread of cholera and plague, respectively. Lack of adequate infection control practices aids the spread of Ebola virus and other pathogens in impoverished nations in Africa.

Demographic and social changes have contributed to the emergence of infectious diseases. Changes in sexual behavior have promoted the spread of human immunodeficiency virus (HIV) and other sexually transmitted diseases. The use of illicit injection drugs has contributed to the rapid spread of HIV as well as to the spread of hepatitis C and other blood-borne infectious agents.

The dramatic increase in the number of women entering the workplace has resulted in greater numbers of young children in day care. These children are more likely to be exposed to and to acquire respiratory and diarrheal infections; in addition, the high rates of antibiotic use by children attending child care facilities may contribute to the development of antibiotic resistance, particularly in *Streptococcus pneumoniae* and other common community-acquired bacterial pathogens.

Changes in technology also create new niches for microorganisms. The use of newly developed superabsorbent tampons has been associated with toxic shock syndrome, and air conditioning systems have been associated with outbreaks of Legionnaires' disease. Changes in food processing methods (e.g., mass production of hamburger patties or ice cream) have allowed small amounts of food contaminated with pathogens such as *Escherichia coli* O157:H7 and *Salmonella* to contaminate large amounts of a final product.

The widespread use of invasive medical devices has been accompanied by an increased incidence of bloodstream and other infections. Many microorganisms, such as microsporidia and cryptosporidia, are being recognized as significant pathogens of the growing population of patients who are immunosuppressed as a result of chemotherapy, organ transplantation, or HIV infection. As xenotransplantation becomes a more likely therapeutic option, concerns have been raised regarding the risk of transplant recipients acquiring xenozoonoses caused by organisms such as retroviruses that have not previously infected or caused disease in humans.

Changes in land use also affect the incidence and geographic distribution of infectious disease. The emergence of Lyme disease in the eastern United States, for example, coincided with an explosive increase in the deer population, as land previously used for farming was reforested and suburban communities were established. The emergence of other tick-borne diseases, such as human monocytic ehrlichiosis and human granulocytic ehrlichiosis, may also relate to the changing vector-host ecology. Climate changes may affect the emergence or reemergence of disease; drought followed by heavy rains in the Four Corners area in the southwestern United States led to an explosion in the rodent population, which in turn contributed to the outbreak of hantavirus pulmonary syndrome in 1993. The impact of global warming on infectious diseases, particularly vector-borne diseases, is uncertain and warrants further study.

International travel and commerce are increasing at an astounding pace, and both play a significant role in the spread of disease. In the mid-1990s, more than 500 million international trips on commercial airlines were recorded per year; these flights carried persons with drug-resistant tuberculosis, cholera, malaria, and other diseases from one country to another in a few hours. The importation of reptiles carrying *Salmonella* and the shipment of fresh fruits and vegetables contaminated with enteric pathogens from one geographic region to another are examples of international commerce that have resulted in outbreaks of disease. Ebola virus has spread from the Philippines to the United States via the transport of infected nonhuman primates and from Gabon to South Africa via travel of an infected person. The global mixing of pathogens will continue, and disease will emerge if circumstances in the new environment allow survival and proliferation of the introduced pathogen.

The Centers for Disease Control and Prevention, the World Health Organization, and other agencies and organizations have published documents which outline the steps required to respond effectively to microbial threats (1, 5, 7). Priority areas include enhancing disease surveillance, conducting needed epidemiologic and laboratory research, and implementing effective prevention and control programs. Strengthening the capacity to diagnose infectious pathogens is considered a critical step in addressing each of these areas, and laboratory diagnosis of an infectious disease often depends on contributions from many fields. Development and availability of inexpensive and practical diagnostic tests for field use are particularly emphasized. In addition, understanding the pathogenesis of the disease may help in the prevention of the disease as well as its treatment; a research agenda for emerging infectious diseases developed by the National Institutes of Health includes better understanding of the pathogenesis of and host susceptibility to emerging pathogens as a goal (4).

This book illustrates the enormous contribution that pathologists can make, in collaboration with colleagues from other areas such as epidemiology, clinical care, veterinary medicine, and microbiology, to the diagnosis of infectious agents, as well as to the elucidation of the pathogenic mechanisms, which is vital to research of emerging pathogens. Frequently, the responsible pathogen is demonstrated in specimens and then isolated through culture techniques. Since some infectious agents, such as many of the fungi, are morphologically distinct, they can be accurately identified by direct microscopic examination. Various histologic stains are helpful for the diagnosis of such infections as plague and Buruli ulcer; a modification of the acid-fast stain has been helpful in the diagnosis of cryptosporidiosis from stool specimens.

New molecular techniques such as polymerase chain reaction and in situ hybridization have emerged as major technologies, and both of these techniques have been applied to the field of infectious disease pathology. Immunohistochemistry has extended the contributions of pathologists beyond

Priority areas include enhancing disease surveillance, conducting needed epidemiologic and laboratory research, and implementing effective prevention and control programs.

conventional histopathology and has provided new avenues for the detection of specific microbial pathogenic agents, from filoviruses to *Leptospira*. Not only are these techniques helpful in diagnosis, they have also been extremely useful in elucidating the pathogenesis of newly recognized diseases, such as hantavirus pulmonary syndrome and Ebola hemorrhagic fever. Their potential as species-specific diagnostic techniques for diseases such as microsporidiosis is also recognized.

New techniques in pathology such as immunohistochemical examination may allow for more practical means of surveillance for pathogens such as filoviruses. Formalin-fixed biopsy specimens are not infectious, may be transported without special precautions or refrigeration, and may be taken in the most basic field conditions. This technique is being used for surveillance of Ebola hemorrhagic fever in Zaire.

As illustrated in the following chapters, the field of pathology in conjunction with epidemiologic and other expertise is contributing enormously to the prevention and control of both newly recognized and resurgent infectious diseases. Further research and training in infectious disease pathology will be a critical component in the worldwide efforts to address emerging microbial threats.

References

1. **Centers for Disease Control and Prevention.** 1994. *Addressing Emerging Infectious Disease Threats: a Prevention Strategy for the United States.* U.S. Department of Health and Human Services, Public Health Service, Atlanta, Ga.

2. **Institute of Medicine.** 1992. *Emerging Infections: Microbial Threats to Health in the United States.* National Academy of Sciences, Washington, D.C.

3. **Lederberg, J.** 1988. Medical science, infectious disease, and the unity of humankind. JAMA **260:**684–685.

4. **National Institutes of Health.** 1996. *The NIAID Research Agenda for Emerging Infectious Diseases.* U.S. Department of Health and Human Services, Public Health Service, Bethesda, Md.

5. **National Science and Technology Council Committee on International Science and Technology.** 1995. *Infectious Diseases—a Global Health Threat.* Report of the Working Group on Emerging and Reemerging Infectious Diseases. Publication no. 400–451/40284. U.S. Government Printing Office, Washington, D.C.

6. **Pinner, R. W., S. M. Teutsch, L. Simonsen, L. A. Klug, J. M. Graber, M. J. Clarke, and R. L. Berkelman.** 1996. Trends in infectious diseases mortality in the United States. JAMA **275:**189–193.

7. **World Health Organization.** 1994. Emerging infectious diseases. *Weekly Epidemiol. Rec.* **31:**234–236.

chapter 1

Morphology to Molecular Biology: Approaches to the Pathologic Diagnosis of Infectious Diseases

Francis W. Chandler

In the practice of pathology, conventional morphologic methods complemented by specific immunohistologic and molecular biologic studies of tissue specimens can be invaluable for the diagnosis of infectious diseases (5, 20). Correlation of these pathologic approaches with traditional microbiologic culture is desirable but not always possible. Cultures sometimes are not taken or they may fail to yield an isolate, and the only means of confirming a diagnosis is by detecting and identifying an invasive microorganism in clinical specimens. Even when cultures are taken, isolation and characterization of certain agents can take days to weeks. In the pathology laboratory, infection is often not even suspected until the initial histopathologic examination is completed. At that time, it is too late for cultural studies because usually only fixed tissues are available. In all of these situations, the pathologist should follow a systematic approach to detect and identify an unknown pathogen in formalin-fixed, routinely processed tissue specimens. Application of highly sensitive and specific antibodies and molecular probes to identify a causal microorganism or components of an organism in such specimens can often result in a rapid etiologic diagnosis and thus guide the clinician in specific treatment and better patient manage-

Francis W. Chandler, Department of Pathology, Medical College of Georgia, Augusta, GA 30912-3605.

Pathology of Emerging Infections
Edited by C. Robert Horsburgh, Jr., and Ann Marie Nelson
© 1997 American Society for Microbiology, Washington, DC 20005-4171

ment. When immunologic reagents and molecular probes are not available, a presumptive or specific etiologic diagnosis can sometimes be made quickly, inexpensively, and accurately by using conventional morphologic methods. Direct demonstration of infectious agents in tissue sections has other attractive features. For immunodeficient patients, histologic studies provide immediate and indisputable evidence of coexisting infections and of tissue invasion by opportunistic agents, which are often suspected of being environmental contaminants or members of the endogenous microflora when isolated in culture. Histologic studies also can be important in determining whether the host reaction is in response to an invading microorganism or is purely allergic, e.g., invasive versus allergic pulmonary aspergillosis. Lastly, histopathologic methods can detect and identify pathogens that cannot be cultivated, e.g., *Pneumocystis carinii* and *Rhinosporidium seeberi*. Although certain patterns of host reaction can suggest that infection exists, there are no absolute histologic criteria that will establish a presumptive or definitive diagnosis; only detection and identification of the causative agent or its components can do so.

With certain infections, particularly those caused by viruses and bacteria, it may not be possible to specifically identify an infectious agent by conventional morphologic methods. Nevertheless, it can usually be presumed that a particular type of microbe is present, which can then be identified. Immunohistochemistry (3, 4), in situ hybridization (ISH) (17), and, when needed, the polymerase chain reaction (PCR) (6, 7, 11) can be performed on properly fixed, paraffin-embedded tissue specimens to enhance diagnostic specificity and sensitivity. When indicated, transmission electron microscopy also can be a useful diagnostic tool, especially for viral infections (2, 10). Because the geographic distribution of certain pathogens is limited, knowledge of the patient's travels can help resolve the differential diagnosis.

Special histologic stains can be used to effectively demonstrate and study invasive microorganisms in tissue sections (4, 14, 18). The two most important stains for initial screening are one of the silver impregnation procedures for bacteria and a methenamine silver stain for fungi and related pathogens. Silver impregnation procedures, e.g., Steiner, Dieterle, and Warthin-Starry, blacken all bacteria nonselectively and are necessary to demonstrate spirochetes and other non-Gram-stain-reactive bacteria in tissue, e.g., *Treponema pallidum*, *Borrelia burgdorferi*, *Leptospira* spp., *Bartonella* spp., and *Calymmatobacterium granulomatis* (Fig. 1.1). Silver impregnation procedures also effectively demonstrate bacteria that are weakly gram negative in tissue sections, e.g., *Legionella* spp., *Francisella tularensis*, *Helicobacter pylori*, and *Burkholderia pseudomallei* (Fig. 1.2). Bacteria become readily visible when silver is reduced to its metallic state; the black coating of silver makes organisms appear larger and much more distinct and demarcated than with other stains, but it may also distort their morphology. Compared with Gram stains, silver impregnation procedures provide much greater sensitivity, which is important when only small numbers of bacteria are present. Once bacteria are detected, modified Gram stains, such as the Brown and Brenn, Brown-Hopps, and MacCallum-Goodpasture procedures, can be applied to additional tissue sections to distinguish gram-positive from gram-negative bacteria and to demonstrate the gram-positive, filamentous actinomycetes associated with actinomycosis and nocardiosis (Fig. 1.3). The Brown and Brenn procedure is best for demonstrating gram-positive bacteria, and the Brown-Hopps procedure is superior for gram-negative bacteria and rickettsiae. The depth of staining of gram-negative organisms in tissue sections can be intensified by increasing the concentration of basic fuchsin from 0.1% to 1% in the formulation. Generally, rickettsiae are weakly gram negative, but they also can be demonstrated with Giemsa and silver impregnation procedures.

In addition to being acid fast with conventional stains, such as the Ziehl-Neelsen stain, most *Mycobacterium* spp. also are Gomori's methenamine silver (GMS) positive, periodic acid-Schiff (PAS) positive, and weakly gram positive in formalin-fixed, paraffin-embedded tissue sections. *Nocardia* spp., *Legionella micdadei*, *Legionella pneumophila* (rarely), *Rhodococcus equi*, and *Mycobacterium leprae* are less acid resistant (weakly or partially acid fast and non-alcohol fast). Modified acid-fast stains that use an aqueous solution of a weak acid as decolorizer, such as the Fite, Fite-Faraco, and Kinyoun stains, are required to stain these bacteria (Fig. 1.4). The auramine-rhodamine (Truant's) fluorescence procedure for *Mycobacterium* spp. is superior in sensitivity to conventional acid-fast stains for rare organisms, but it requires a fluorescence microscope (Fig. 1.5).

The GMS procedure, or one of its more rapid variants, is the best stain for demonstrating fungi in tissue sections because it provides excellent contrast for screening and usually blackens degenerated and fragmented organisms that are often refractory to the PAS reaction and Gridley procedures. When a counterstain such as 0.2% light green is used, the GMS method reduces nonspecific background staining of normal tissue components and necrotic debris, whereas the PAS and Gridley procedures do not. Most importantly, GMS is superior in sensitivity, because it blackens certain non-fungal pathogens, e.g., actinomycetes causing actinomycosis and nocardiosis, *Mycobacterium* spp., nonfilamentous bacteria with polysaccharide capsules (e.g., *Streptococcus pneumoniae*, *Klebsiella pneumoniae*, and *Haemophilus influenzae*), cyst walls of *P. carinii* and free-living soil amebas (*Acanthamoeba* spp. and *Balamuthia mandrillaris*), algal cells (*Prototheca* spp. and *Chlorella* spp.), spores of certain microsporidians, and cytoplasmic granular inclusion bodies of cytomegalovirus (Fig. 1.6). Although it has low specificity, the GMS stain is extremely helpful for rapid screening of tissue sections from patients with AIDS, who are often infected by multiple pathogens. For retrospective studies of unexplained lesions, tissue sections previously stained by using Giemsa, modified Gram, PAS, and Gridley procedures can be decolorized in acid-alcohol after the coverslip has been removed and can then be restained with GMS. A major limitation of the GMS stain is that it does not allow adequate study of the host reaction to microbial invasion. To circumvent this, tissue sections stained with GMS can be counterstained with hematoxylin and eosin (H&E) for simultaneous demonstration of a microbe and the associated tissue response (Fig. 1.7). Such a stain combination also conserves tissue sections, and it is ideal for teaching and photomicrography.

The GMS procedure, or one of its more rapid variants, is the best stain for demonstrating fungi in tissue sections

Stains for mucin, such as those used in alcian blue and mucicarmine procedures, readily demonstrate the mucopolysaccharide capsule of *Cryptococcus neoformans*. This staining reaction is a convenient diagnostic marker and usually differentiates typical cryptococci from nonencapsulated yeast-form pathogens of similar size and appearance (4). In rare cases, however, capsule-deficient cryptococci may not stain positively for mucin. In addition, mucin stains are not specific for *C. neoformans*, because the cell walls of *Blastomyces dermatitidis* and *Rhinosporidium seeberi* also are variably colored with these stains. Because these last two fungi are nonencapsulated and morphologically distinctive, ordinarily they would not be mistaken for *C. neoformans*. Mucin stains are not routinely used for their identification.

The stain of choice for demonstrating most protozoans in tissue sections is H&E. Giemsa, iron-hematoxylin, PAS, and Masson's trichrome stains also are useful for studying amebae and certain other protozoans in tissue sections and smears, but these procedures sometimes lack contrast and offer little or no advantage if the organisms cannot be initially seen with H&E. Weber's trichrome stain is useful for demonstrating microsporidial spores, and Wilder's reticulum procedure readily stains kinetoplasts of leishmanias and amastigotes of *Trypanosoma cruzi*. The Russell-Movat pentachrome procedure is excellent for demonstrating morphologic components of nematodes, cestodes, and trematodes. Oocysts of *Cryptosporidium parvum* are acid fast in fecal smears, but their acid fastness is lost during fixation and processing of tissues for paraffin embedment.

Several histologic stains for demonstrating viral inclusion bodies have been described, including Shorr's and Lendrum's phloxine-tartrazine procedures and Bosch's and Schleifstein's methods for Negri bodies (4). However, there is no instance in which these inclusion body stains offer more uniformity of quality or better delineation of internal details than is seen with tissue sections properly fixed and optimally stained with H&E (Fig. 1.8). Thus, the routine H&E stain is of practical value for diagnosis of viral infections because it enables the pathologist to evaluate the tissue response and to visualize viral inclusion bodies when present.

Immunohistochemistry is a practical tool with wide applications in infectious disease pathology. When sensitive and specific monoclonal antibodies or polyclonal antisera are available, immunoenzymatic or immunofluorescence labeling of pathogens in smears or formalin-fixed, deparaffinized tissue sections can be routinely used to improve the diagnostic capability of conventional histopathology (3, 4). Immunohistologic methods are invaluable (i) for confirming a presumptive diagnosis, especially when only fixed tissues are available; (ii) for confirming coexisting infections; and (iii) for identifying a pathogen in contaminated specimens. Before selecting immunoreagents, special histologic stains should be routinely performed to formulate a differential diagnosis, to establish a presumptive diagnosis, and, if detected, to localize the etiologic agent. This preliminary step also enables the pathologist to be more cost-effective, by selecting only those immunologic reagents that are needed. For suspected viral infections, immunohistochemistry is particularly helpful when inclusion bodies are not detected with conventional stains or when inclusion

The stain of choice for demonstrating most protozoans in tissue sections is H&E

bodies are detected but atypical. To enhance immunolabeling of viral antigens, tissue sections can be predigested with a proteolytic enzyme, such as a weak trypsin or pepsin solution, to "unmask" immunoreactive sites by freeing cross-linked antigens (3, 4). Antigen retrieval by heating immersed tissue sections mounted on glass slides in a pressure cooker or microwave oven also can enhance immunoreactivity of certain infectious agents, especially viruses (3). Because formalin fixation and paraffin embedment do not appreciably affect the antigenicity of bacteria, fungi, and protozoans, enzymatic digestion or antigen retrieval of tissue sections containing these microorganisms may not be necessary before immunohistologic labeling (4).

Immunoenzyme (IE) methods, e.g., use of immunoperoxidase and immunoalkaline phosphatase, have several advantages over immunofluorescence: (i) IE-stained tissue sections can be counterstained with hematoxylin and evaluated with a standard light microscope, (ii) morphologic detail of the hematoxylin-stained background tissue response can be more easily evaluated in relation to areas of specific IE staining, (iii) unlike with immunofluorescence, interference in microbial fluorescence or contrast by contiguous autofluorescent tissue components is not a problem, (iv) IE-labeled antigen (the colored reaction product) does not fade or quench after prolonged examination, and (v) IE-labeled sections usually can be coverslipped, hermetically sealed, and stored along with conventional histologic sections for permanent record and future study. Experience in our laboratory has shown that the major disadvantage of immunoperoxidase labeling is lack of contrast when only minute amounts of microbial antigens are present, i.e., minute amounts of the colored reaction product can be difficult to detect by light microscopy, even at high magnification. In addition, various endogenous or exogenous pigments encountered in a tissue section can sometimes be mistaken for the colored reaction product with the immunoperoxidase technique, resulting in a false-positive reading. Examples of the diagnostic applications of immunohistochemistry in infectious disease pathology are illustrated in Fig. 1.9–1.11.

The need for rapid and specific diagnoses of infectious diseases has stimulated the development of novel molecular biologic tests. Of these, PCR and ISH have emerged as major technologies for detecting and identifying specific microbial genes and their transcripts in tissue specimens. PCR is an exquisitely sensitive in vitro technique that involves bidirectional, enzymatic synthesis and amplification of a defined DNA sequence by repeated, automated cycles of heat denaturation, primer annealing, and thermostable DNA polymerase-mediated primer extension (6, 11). Amplification results in an exponential increase in the number of target (microbial) DNA sequences. Typically, PCR begins with picogram quantities of template DNA and yields nanogram quantities that can then be detected by conventional methods. PCR can be used to detect virtually any pathogen for which even limited DNA or RNA sequence information is known when fresh or optimally fixed, paraffinized, infected tissue is available (Fig. 1.12). When amplification and identification of viral RNA sequences are attempted, the enzyme reverse transcriptase can be incorporated into the initial PCR cycle (RT-PCR). Applications of PCR in infectious disease pathology include (i)

The major disadvantage of immunoperoxidase labeling is lack of contrast when only minute amounts of microbial antigens are present rapid detection of unique microbial nucleic acid sequences in minute quantities, (ii) detection of microbial pathogens that cannot be cultivated, (iii) detection of hazardous (highly pathogenic) microbes, (iv) detection of microbial nucleic acid sequences in samples from patients with latent infections, (v) strain typing of various microorganisms, (vi) detection of virulence and antimicrobial resistance determinants, (vii) determination of molecular phylogeny of previously uncharacterized pathogens (e.g., *Bartonella henselae* and *Trophyrema whippelii*), and (viii) determination of viral load, by quantitative PCR, for monitoring disease progression and effects of antiviral therapy (6, 7, 15). Because many samples can be analyzed simultaneously, PCR is also useful in epidemiologic investigations and in experimental studies of pathogenesis. Continued refinement of PCR technology, particularly multiplex PCR-based assays, should further advance the accuracy, speed, and screening potential of molecular diagnostic procedures. The main disadvantage of PCR is that it cannot determine tissue localization of microbial nucleic acids. Also, because of the exquisite sensitivity of PCR, false-positive reactions can result from "carryover" of previously amplified DNA (amplicon) or from contamination by true-positive specimens within the laboratory. The applications of in vitro molecular methods as diagnostic tools in infectious disease pathology are reviewed by Podzorski and Persing (13).

ISH enables the pathologist to directly observe molecular information at the level of defined nucleic acid sequences in intact, routinely processed tissue sections (12, 17). The tremendous selectivity and specificity of this technique result from complementary base pairing of single-stranded probe and target nucleic acid sequences to form a stable, double-stranded molecule. ISH has proven to be particularly useful for typing of human papillomaviruses in lesions of the genital tract and for detecting and localizing nucleic acid sequences of viruses that are difficult or impossible to culture, that produce latent infections, or that do not produce characteristic cytopathic effect (Fig. 1.13). In contrast to other hybridization techniques, e.g., Southern and dot blot hybridizations, ISH enables the pathologist to directly identify the exact cell that contains the microbial DNA or RNA of interest in either frozen or fixed, deparaffinized tissue sections by using conventional light microscopy. In addition to the hybridization reaction (signal), the tissue morphology can simultaneously be evaluated by using appropriate counterstains to provide contrast. The advantages of colorimetric methods (e.g., biotinylated probes) to detect hybridization include speed, simplicity, improved tissue localization of the signal, better preservation of tissue morphology, elimination of hazardous radioisotopes, and potential for automation (16, 17). More recently, PCR amplification of microbial nucleic acid sequences in intact, deparaffinized tissue sections mounted on glass slides and subsequent detection of the amplified sequences by colorimetric ISH (PCR-ISH) has increased the sensitivity of ISH and further extended the diagnostic and research applications of these technologies in infectious disease pathology (1, 8, 9).

In conclusion, pathologists can play important roles in recognizing infectious diseases, in detecting emerging and reemerging infections, and in perceiving new patterns of disease caused by diverse pathogens (5, 19). The experienced pathologist can effectively and rapidly diagnose most infectious diseases by using a battery of special histologic stains and, when needed, specific immunohistochemical and molecular biologic techniques. Formalin-fixed, paraffin-embedded tissues are adequate for these studies, but each specimen must contain the suspected agent. Histopathologic findings should be confirmed by cultural and other ancillary studies whenever possible.

Figure 1.1 Congenital syphilis. Numerous treponemes are demonstrated in the thymus gland by the Steiner silver impregnation stain. Steiner and other silver impregnation procedures blacken all bacteria nonselectively, including those that are non-Gram-stain reactive in tissue. Magnification, ×250.

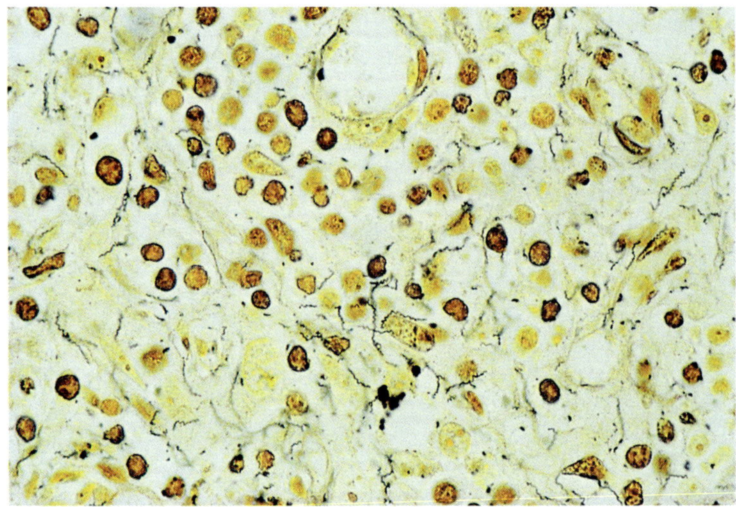

Figure 1.2 Pulmonary legionellosis caused by *L. pneumophila*. Minute bacterial bacilli, blackened with the Steiner silver impregnation stain, tend to cluster within macrophages in a respiratory bronchiole. The black coating of silver, reduced to its metallic state, makes bacteria appear larger and much more distinct and demarcated. Magnification, ×160.

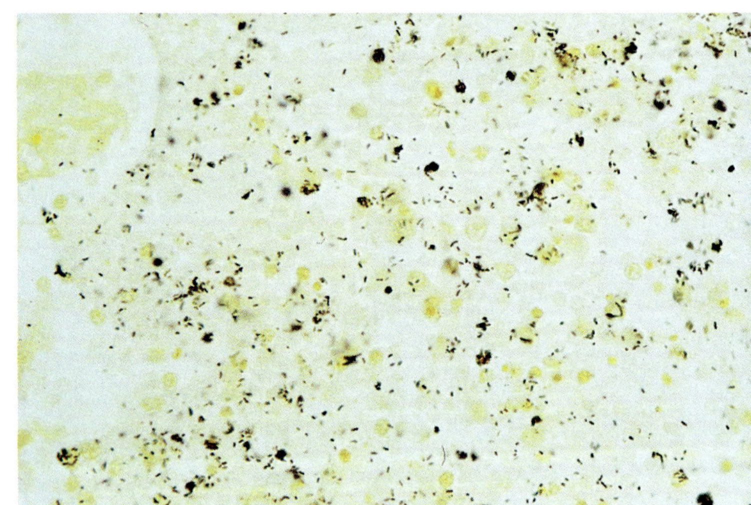

Figure 1.3 Disseminated nocardiosis. Delicate, branched, gram-positive filaments of *Nocardia asteroides* occupy the center of a cerebral abscess. The routinely processed brain section was stained with the Brown and Brenn modified Gram procedure. Brown and Brenn is the stain of choice to demonstrate gram-positive bacteria in histologic sections. Magnification, ×250.

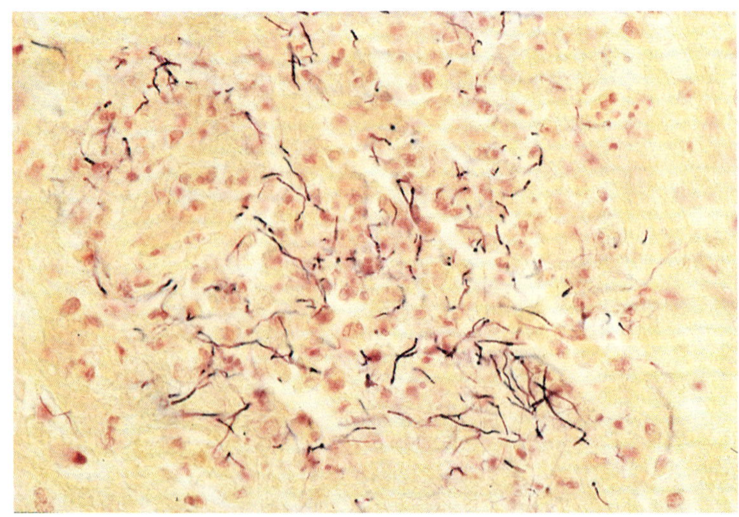

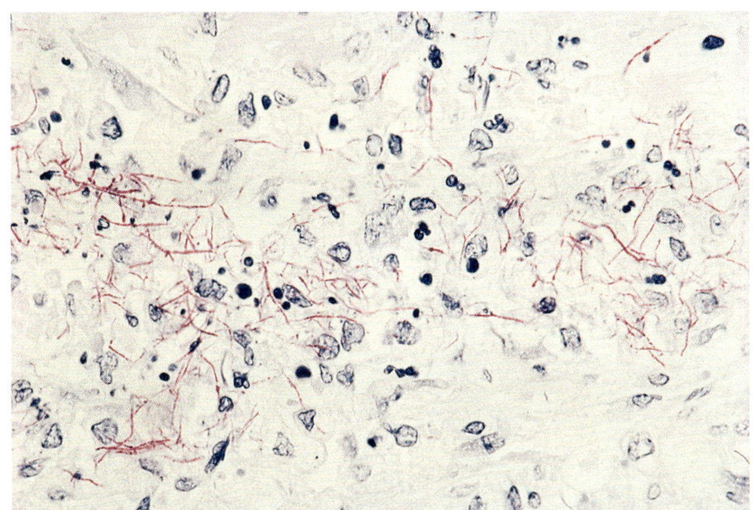

Figure 1.4   Disseminated nocardiosis. A microabscess contains numerous, randomly oriented filaments of *N. asteroides* that are weakly acid fast. Modified acid-fast procedures that use an aqueous solution of a weak acid as decolorizer are required to stain *Nocardia* spp. and M. *leprae* because these organisms are less acid resistant. Fite's acid fast stain was used. Magnification, ×160.

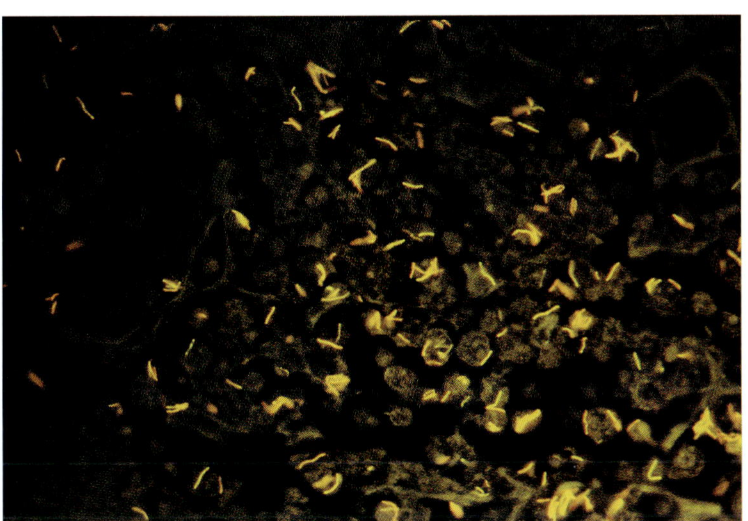

Figure 1.5   Disseminated mycobacteriosis caused by *Mycobacterium avium* complex in an AIDS patient. Myriad elongated bacilli in a cervical lymph node are brightly fluorescent when stained using Truant's auramine-rhodamine procedure. Magnification, ×250.

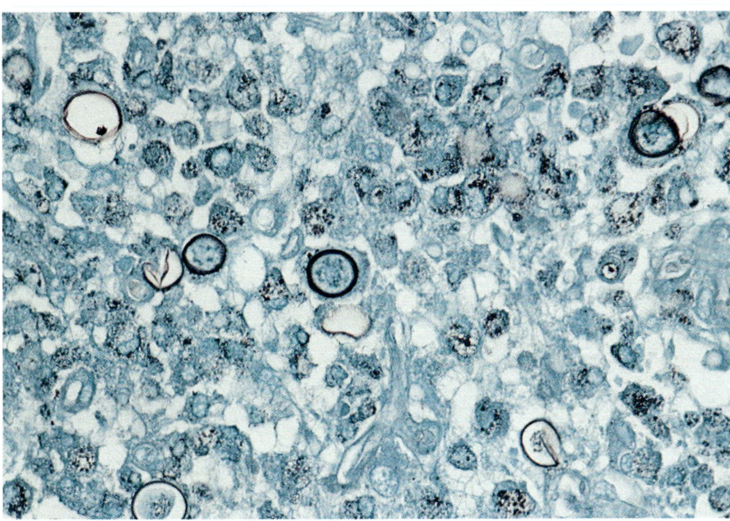

Figure 1.6   Granulomatous amebic encephalitis caused by an *Acanthamoeba* sp. The thick walls of amebic cysts are blackened when stained with Gomori's methenamine silver procedure. This traditional stain for fungi colors all polysaccharide-rich microorganisms. Magnification, ×160.

Figure 1.7 Disseminated histoplasmosis capsulati in an AIDS patient. Extracellular aggregates ("yeast lakes") of proliferating histoplasma cells partially efface the bone marrow. When tissue sections are stained with Gomori's methenamine silver and then counterstained with H&E, fungal morphology and the host reaction can be evaluated simultaneously. Magnification, ×100.

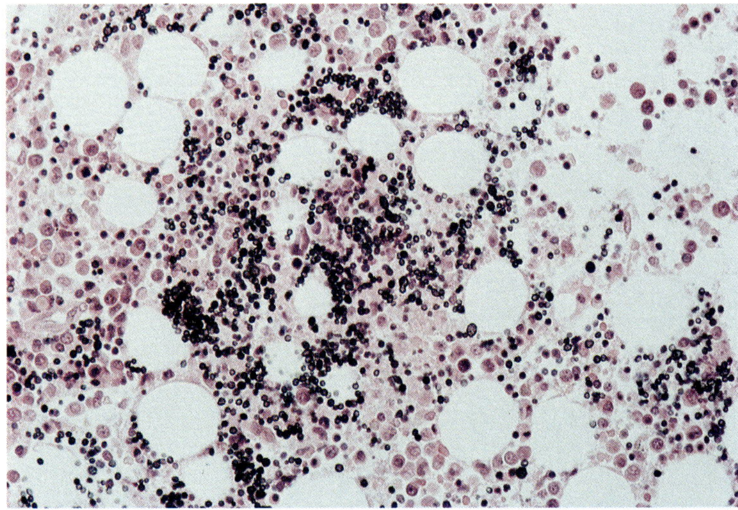

Figure 1.8 Cytomegalovirus pneumonitis in a bone marrow transplant recipient. Isolated alveolar lining cells contain single intranuclear and multiple granular intracytoplasmic inclusions characteristic of this virus. The routine H&E stain enables pathologists to evaluate the host reaction and to visualize viral inclusion bodies when present. Magnification, ×160.

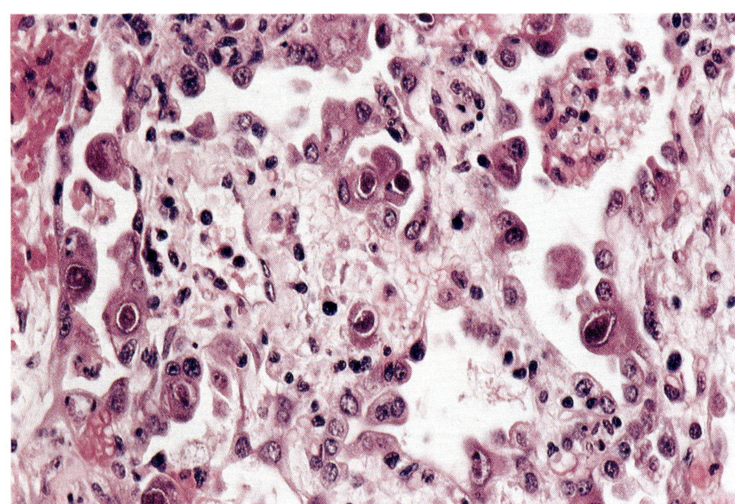

Figure 1.9 Immunoperoxidase localization of herpes simplex virus at the margin of a genital ulcer. Note strong intranuclear and weak intracytoplasmic labeling of viral antigen within epidermal cells in this formalin-fixed, deparaffinized skin section. Magnification, ×160.

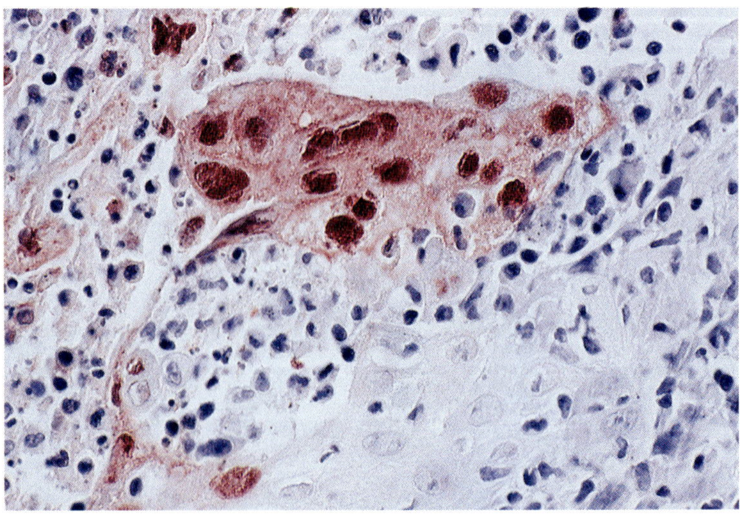

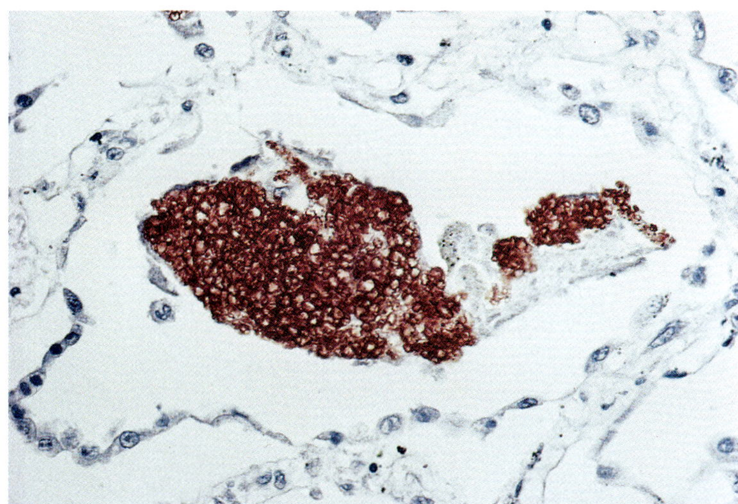

Figure 1.10 Immunoperoxidase labeling of *P. carinii*. Cysts and trophozoites of this organism are readily identified in this routinely processed lung section stained with a commercially available monoclonal antibody (2G2). Magnification, ×160.

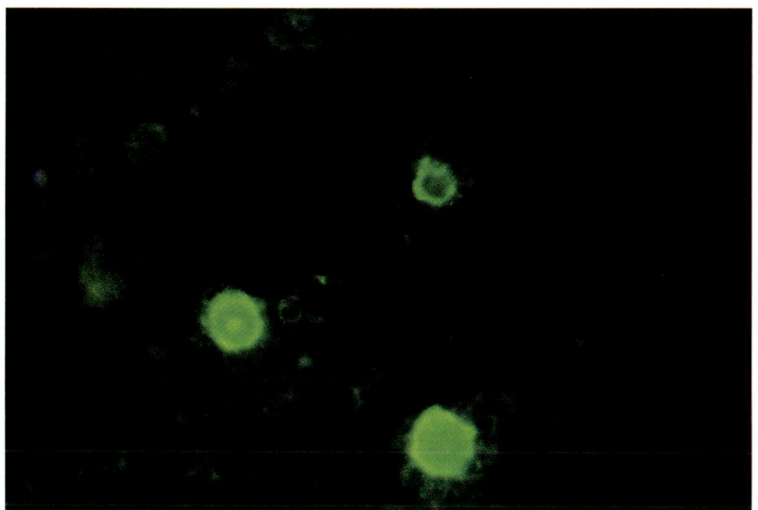

Figure 1.11 Cryptococcal pneumonitis. Brightly fluorescent yeast forms of *C. neoformans* are demonstrated in a pulmonary granuloma. The formalin-fixed, deparaffinized lung section was stained with fluorescein-labeled antiglobulins specific for capsular polysaccharide antigens of this fungus. Magnification, ×400.

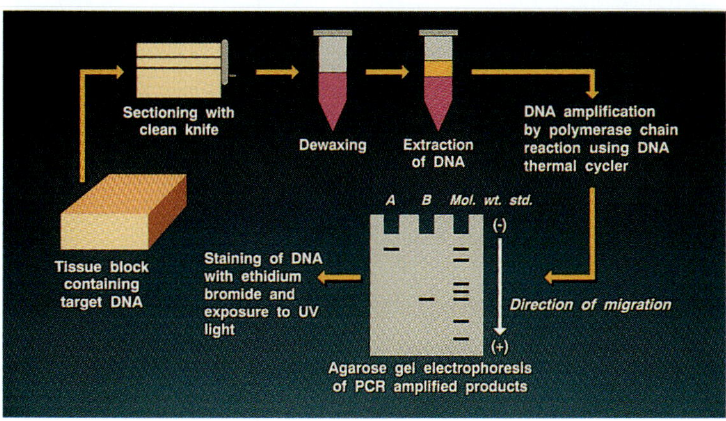

Figure 1.12 Schematic depicting the polymerase chain reaction-based assay for specific microbial DNA sequences in formalin-fixed, paraffin-embedded infected tissues.

Figure 1.13 Detection of human papillomavirus 6/11 in condyloma acuminatum by in situ hybridization using biotinylated probes. Bluish purple signal (hybridization reaction) is observed over nuclei of isolated epithelial cells in this formalin-fixed, deparaffinized tissue section. Nuclear fast red counterstain; magnification, ×50.

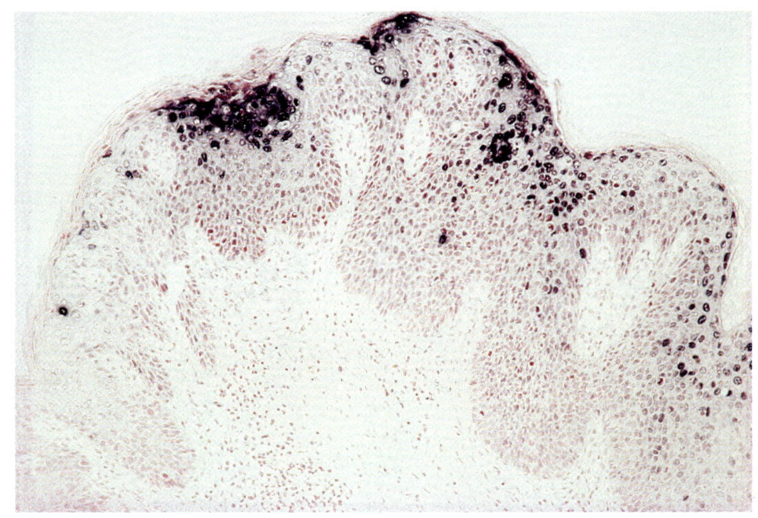

References

1. **Bagasra, O., S. P. Hauptman, H. W. Lischner, M. Sachs, and R. J. Pomerantz.** 1992. Detection of HIV-1 provirus in mononuclear cells by in situ polymerase chain reaction. *N. Engl. J. Med.* **326:**1385–1391.

2. **Burns, W. A.** 1980. Microorganisms, p. 1-35. *In* B. F. Trump and R. T. Jones (ed.), *Diagnostic Electron Microscopy*, vol. 3. John Wiley and Sons, New York.

3. **Cartun, R. W.** 1994. Infectious disease, p. 401-415. *In* C. R. Taylor and R. J. Cote (ed.), *Immunomicroscopy: a Diagnostic Tool for the Surgical Pathologist*, 2nd ed. W. B. Saunders, Philadelphia.

4. **Chandler, F. W.** 1987. Invasive microorganisms, p. 77-102. *In* S. S. Spicer (ed.), *Histochemistry in Pathologic Diagnosis*. Marcel Dekker, New York.

5. **Chandler, F. W.** 1995. Infectious disease pathology: morphologic and molecular approaches to diagnosis (editorial overview). *J. Histotechnol.* **18:**183–186.

6. **Ehrlich, G. D., and S. J. Greenberg.** 1994. *PCR-Based Diagnostics in Infectious Disease*. Blackwell Scientific Publications, Boston.

7. **Figueroa, M. E., and S. Rasheed.** 1991. Molecular pathology and diagnosis of infectious diseases. *Am. J. Clin. Pathol.* **95**(Suppl. 1)**:**S8–S21.

8. **Nuovo, G. J.** 1995. Current concepts in pathologic diagnosis: viral diseases. *J. Histotechnol.* **18:**233–240.

9. **Nuovo, G. J.** 1997. *PCR In Situ Hybridization. Protocols and Applications*, 3rd ed. Raven Press, New York.

10. **Orenstein, J. M.** 1995. The role of electron microscopy in infectious disease diagnosis. *J. Histotechnol.* **18:**211–224.

11. **Persing, D. H., T. F. Smith, F. C. Tenover, and T. J. White.** 1993. *Diagnostic Molecular Microbiology: Principles and Applications*. ASM Press, Washington, D.C.

12. **Piper, M. A., and E. R. Unger.** 1989. *Nucleic Acid Probes: a Primer for Pathologists*. ASCP Press, Chicago.

13. **Podzorski, R. P., and D. H. Persing.** 1995. Molecular methods for the detection and identification of viral pathogens. *J. Histotechnol.* **18:**225–232.

14. **Prophet, E. B., B. Mills, J. B. Arrington, and L. H. Sobin.** 1992. *Laboratory Methods in Histotechnology*. American Registry of Pathology, Armed Forces Institute of Pathology, Washington, D.C.

15. **Relman, D. A., and S. Falkow.** 1992. Identification of uncultured microorganisms: expanding the spectrum of characterized microbial pathogens. *Infect. Agents Dis.* **1:**245–253.

16. **Unger, E. R., F. W. Chandler, M. L. Chenggis, C. Y. Ou, and D. T. Warfield.** 1989. Demonstration of human immunodeficiency virus by colorimetric in situ hybridization: a rapid technique for formalin-fixed paraffin-embedded material. *Mod. Pathol.* **2:**200–204.

17. **Unger, E. R., and D. R. Lee.** 1995. In situ hybridization: principles and diagnostic applications in infection. *J. Histotechnol.* **18:**203–209.

18. **Vacca, L. L.** 1985. *Laboratory Manual of Histochemistry*. Raven Press, New York.

19. **Watts, J. C.** 1994. Surgical pathology and the diagnosis of infectious diseases. *Am. J. Clin. Pathol.* **102:**711–712.

20. **Watts, J. C., and F. W. Chandler.** 1995. The surgical pathologist's role in the diagnosis of infectious diseases. *J. Histotechnol.* **18:**191–193.

chapter 2

Plague

David T. Dennis and Frederick A. Meier

Introduction

Definition

Plague in humans is an acute febrile illness caused by infection with *Yersinia pestis*. It is notorious as a repeated cause of cataclysmic epidemics. *Y. pestis* is maintained in nature as an infection of rodents and their fleas in scattered locations over wide areas of Asia, Africa, and the Americas and only incidentally infects humans and other nonrodent mammals. Humans most often become infected by the bite of rodent fleas; less often, they are infected by handling or ingesting infective animal tissues and rarely are infected by direct airborne spread. The principal clinical forms of plague are lymphadenitic (bubonic), septicemic, and pneumonic plague. All forms are curable if diagnosed and treated early with appropriate antibiotics. However, septicemic and pneumonic plague may be fulminant and fatal despite aggressive therapy. Although there is always a potential for epidemics with plague, the disease can be prevented and con-

David T. Dennis, Bacterial Zoonoses Branch, Division of Vector-Borne Infectious Diseases, National Center for Infectious Diseases, Centers for Disease Control and Prevention, Fort Collins, CO 80522. **Frederick A. Meier,** Clinical and Anatomic Pathology, Department of Pathology, Alfred I. Dupont Institute, Children's Hospital, Wilmington, DE.

Pathology of Emerging Infections
Edited by C. Robert Horsburgh, Jr., and Ann Marie Nelson
© 1997 American Society for Microbiology, Washington, DC 20005-4171

trolled by using standard public health measures of surveillance, early detection, treatment and containment of cases, and sanitation.

History

There have been three well-recognized plague pandemics. The first pandemic (ca. 542 to 767 A.D.) began in northern Africa, killed tens of millions of persons in Europe and Asia Minor, and ushered in the Dark Ages. The second pandemic is thought to have begun in central Asia in the early 14th century; it invaded China and India and spread through Asia Minor to the Mediterranean region. Plague entered Italy in 1347 and repeatedly swept through Europe and the British Isles, where it killed a quarter or more of the affected populations and came to be known as the "Black Death" before eventually dying out in the 18th century. The last great spread of plague, the third (modern) pandemic, is thought to have started in southwestern China in the late 19th century; it struck Hong Kong in 1894 and spread over the next decade by rat-infested steamships to major port cities throughout the world. This last pandemic eventually resulted in an estimated 26 million plague cases and more than 12 million deaths, the overwhelming majority of which occurred in India (32).

The plague bacillus was first isolated by Alexandre Yersin in 1894 in Hong Kong (8). In 1898, Paul-Louis Simond, working in Bombay, conducted experiments with rats and proposed that the plague bacillus was transmitted from rat to rat and from rats to humans by rat fleas (32).

After 1900, the international spread of plague was largely halted by sanitary regulations; however, plague had become newly established in many rodent populations in Eurasia, Africa, and the Americas. In the United States, large outbreaks of rat-borne plague occurred in San Francisco, and by 1908, plague was epizootic in native ground squirrels in counties surrounding the city (27). Plague subsequently spread to various wild rodent populations throughout the western third of the United States. The last notable urban plague outbreak in the United States occurred in Los Angeles, Calif., from 1924 to 1925, and it was complicated by person-to-person pneumonic spread.

Since 1950, plague epidemics around the world have, with few exceptions, been sporadic and relatively quickly contained by using standard infectious disease control measures. Despite modern means to treat and control plague, reports of bubonic and pneumonic plague outbreaks in India in 1994 evoked local panic and exaggerated international responses (10, 17, 39).

Since 1950, plague epidemics around the world have been sporadic and relatively quickly contained

Etiologic Agent

General Microbiology

Y. pestis is a nonmotile, nonsporulating, microaerophilic, gram-negative coccobacillus belonging to the family *Enterobacteriaceae* (30). It grows slowly but well on a wide variety of common microbiologic media (e.g., brain heart infusion broth, sheep blood agar, and MacConkey agar). It grows optimally at 28°C and at a pH of 7.4. *Y. pestis* is surrounded by a diffusable envelope that contains the unique fraction 1 (F1) antigen.

Although it is highly adapted to maintain its complex life cycle in rodent hosts and their fleas, the plague bacillus does not survive as a saprophyte, and it is rapidly killed in nature by temperatures above 40°C and by desiccation.

Y. pestis Virulence Factors

Y. pestis is unique in that it possesses a variety of virulence factors important for its infectivity and survival in selected mammalian and flea hosts (6, 30). The genes encoding these virulence factors reside primarily on three plasmids. The smallest (9.5 kb) of these plasmids is the pesticin or *Pst* plasmid, whose genes encode a plasminogen activator (Pla) and a bacteriocin (pesticin).

The 70-kb low-calcium-response plasmid (*Lcr*) encodes gene products that are responsible for activating a group of virulence factors under low calcium conditions; these factors include outer surface proteins (Yops) and a soluble V antigen. V antigen is believed to be essential for *Y. pestis* survival in macrophages. *Lcr*-positive strains are able to inhibit host production of gamma interferon and tumor necrosis factor alpha. Conversely, *Lcr*-negative strains are avirulent and do not inhibit cytokine production in infected laboratory animals.

The *pFra* plasmid (110 kb) contains genes encoding the F1 envelope antigen and a murine toxin. F1 antigen is produced only by organisms growing at 33°C and above. *Y. pestis* strains expressing the F1 antigen are resistant to phagocytosis in the absence of opsonizing antibodies.

Chromosomal genes encode several other virulence factors, including those associated with lipopolysaccharide endotoxin and with pigment production when *Y. pestis* is grown on some media containing Congo red. Strains that do not produce pigment are usually avirulent to mammals and are unable to induce "blocking" of the flea gut (see "Epizootic Plague," below).

Y. pestis Biotypes

Three biotypes of *Y. pestis*, defined on the basis of their various abilities to ferment glycerol and reduce nitrate, have been associated with the three major plague pandemics of history (19). These are named the antiqua, mediaevalis, and orientalis biotypes. The antiqua biotype is found in parts of Africa, southeastern Russia, and central Asia; the mediaevalis biotype is found around the Caspian Sea; and the orientalis biotype predominates in Asia and is the sole biotype in the Western Hemisphere. Ribotyping studies support the biotype distinctions. In general, wild-type *Y. pestis* strains have an extremely conserved genetic complement and demonstrate similar virulence throughout the world.

Y. pestis Life Cycle

Y. pestis is a zootic infection involving rodents and their fleas in both wild rodent and domestic rodent populations (Fig. 2.1). Infection in humans is incidental, resulting from intrusion by persons into the natural wild cycle or from exposure to plague in commensal rodents and their fleas. Person to person plague occurs as a result of close and direct respiratory exposure to persons with pneumonic (pulmonary) plague and, very rarely, by direct skin or mucous membrane contact with a patient's infectious secretions or exudates. The transmission of infection from person to person by human-biting fleas is possible but has not been definitively described.

Ecology

Introduction

Zootic plague foci and associated endemic areas of human plague are found scattered throughout most of the world (Fig. 2.2). A knowledge of the major ecologic factors supporting the life cycle of Y. pestis in its particular biotopes is vital to understanding the epidemiology of plague and its control and prevention (5, 23, 33). Although more than 200 species of mammals and 150 species of fleas have been found to be naturally infected with Y. pestis, relatively few are important in supporting enzootic or epizootic cycles and fewer still pose a significant public health risk.

Enzootic Plague

In its natural reservoir state, the plague bacillus is found in often inapparent, "silent" enzootic cycles involving relatively resistant wild rodents and their fleas in mostly remote, sparsely populated areas of Asia, Africa, and the Americas (5, 23, 34). Although some of these rodents may sicken and die, most tolerate the infection and population die off does not occur. Nonrodent mammals, although occasionally infected, are incidental hosts and do not contribute to the maintenance of these natural cycles. Cycles of enzootic transmission place humans at small direct risk, and cases that arise from enzootic exposures typically are infrequent and isolated (sporadic) occurrences. Although these enzootic cycles are often referred to as "sylvatic" plague, they most often occur in semiarid or arid grassland sites, such as the steppes of central Asia and the savannas of eastern Africa. Enzootic foci around the world have distinct ecologic profiles with their own characteristic rodent and flea host combinations.

Epizootic Plague

In epizootic plague, infection is spread rapidly in susceptible rodent populations by efficient flea vectors that are often abundant on their hosts. In this circumstance, both rodents and their fleas amplify Y. pestis (5, 23, 33). Epizootics sometimes result in widespread depopulation of affected rodents, and the consequent dispersal of fleas in search of new hosts potentiates Y. pestis spread to contiguous rodent populations, including those living in commensal association with humans. Historically, urban epidemics and pandemics of plague have been associated with epizootics involving the common commensal species, *Rattus rattus* and *Rattus norvegicus*. The smaller, domestic roof, or black, rat (*R. rattus*) is considered the most dangerous host. This ubiquitous rodent lives in intimate domestic association with humans in most areas of the world. It readily travels with cargo and baggage, and along with its companion, the oriental rat flea (*Xenopsylla cheopis*), it has been the most important factor in the noncontiguous spread of plague.

A knowledge of the major ecologic factors supporting the life cycle of Y. pestis in its particular biotopes is vital to understanding the epidemiology of plague and its control and prevention

The Norway rat has not been as important in epidemic urban plague as the black rat. *R. norvegicus* is larger and more aggressive than *R. rattus*; it is a burrowing rodent that typically lives peridomestically and frequents cellars, drains, sewers, alleyways, and refuse dumps.

Although these commensal rats are the principal sources of infected fleas in human plague epidemics, reintroductions of wild strains of *Y. pestis* may be needed to sustain prolonged epizootics. Wild rodent plague may spread directly into populations of rodents that live commensally with humans, or it may spread indirectly through intermediary rodent populations. For example, recent investigations of bubonic plague in Maharashtra State, in west-central India, substantiated previously described sylvatic populations of gerbils (*Tatera indica*) as the probable reservoir source of plague (18, 36) and suggested that *Y. pestis* infection may have been transmitted by fleas to domestic *R. rattus* through intermediary populations of bandicoot rats (*Bandicota bengalensis*) that were numerous in croplands closely surrounding rural villages.

The widely distributed oriental rat flea and the related species *Xenopsylla braziliensis* are the most efficient vectors of plague between rats and between rats and humans (23, 33). At temperatures of 28°C and below, *Y. pestis* multiplies in the gut of these and some other flea species until a clotted bolus is formed that blocks passage of further feedings at the level of the foregut (proventriculus). The starved flea avidly seeks a blood meal, and because of its blockage, the flea regurgitates into the bite wound as it feeds, thus enhancing transmission of the plague bacillus. The ability of *Y. pestis* to produce blockage has recently been shown to be plasmid mediated.

The widely distributed oriental rat flea and the related species Xenopsylla braziliensis are the most efficient vectors of plague between rats and between rats and humans

Incidental Plague

A diverse range of mammals, including humans, can become incidentally infected with *Y. pestis*, either by the bite of an infective flea or by direct contact with infectious tissues, secretions, or exudates. Carnivores, especially felids, canids, and mustellids, are at greatest risk for infection since they prey on rodents. Infected felids, in contrast to canids, often become diseased and have become important potential sources of human plague in the United States. Lagomorphs (e.g., rabbits and hares) occasionally become infected and place hunters at risk for plague (11, 31). Ungulates, including antelope, deer, camels, and goats, can sicken and die from *Y. pestis* infection and can also be sources of human plague (13, 32).

North American Plague Foci

Zootic plague has been found in all states of the United States west of the 100th meridian and has also been found in some areas of Canada and Mexico adjacent to United States plague foci (5, 20, 23). The major United States plague foci include the southwestern focus (comprising northeastern Arizona, most of New Mexico, southern Utah, and southern Colorado), the Pacific coastal focus (comprising California and southern Oregon), the Great Basin focus (encompassing parts of Utah, Nevada, and southern Idaho), and the Rocky Mountain and northern focus (comprising mostly northern Colorado, Wyoming, and Montana).

The principal rodent hosts in the southwestern focus are various burrowing ground squirrels, especially rock squirrels, prairie dogs, wood rats, antelope ground squirrels, deer mice, and related species (5, 26). The major rodent hosts in the various niches of the Pacific Coast focus include California ground squirrels and golden-manteled ground squirrels, chipmunks, deer mice, and voles. Zootic cycles involve various other species of ground squirrels in the Rocky Mountain and Great Basin regions and the black-tailed prairie dog in the Great Plains region. Epizootics of plague have recently occurred in urban tree squirrel populations in cities and towns along the eastern foothills of the Colorado Rocky Mountains, but they pose a small public health risk because tree squirrel fleas do not readily feed on humans (5).

In the past several decades, *Y. pestis*-infected rats occasionally have been found in some United States cities (e.g., Tacoma, Wash.; San Francisco, Calif.; Los Angeles, Calif.; and Dallas, Tex.). However, no widespread epizootics or human plague cases have resulted, possibly because the rats have been infested with only small numbers of fleas or with flea species that are inefficient vectors of *Y. pestis*.

The principal fleas transmitting plague among wild rodent epizootic hosts in the United States include various ground squirrel fleas (especially *Oropsylla montana*), prairie dog fleas (*Opisocrostis* spp.), wood rat fleas (*Orchopeas* spp.), and chipmunk fleas (*Eumolpianus eumolpi*) (5, 20, 23, 26). *O. montana* is the most dangerous vector to persons in the United States, since it is a competent vector that has promiscuous feeding habits and readily bites humans.

South American Plague Foci

In South America, active zootic plague foci exist in Brazil, Bolivia, Peru, and Ecuador, and plague foci in Paraguay, Argentina, and Venezuela have been described previously. *Y. pestis* infection in these foci has been variously found in commensal rats (*Rattus* spp.), cotton rats, rice rats, field mice, cane mice, wild cavies, and domesticated guinea pigs (32). Guinea pigs are reared in homes for food in the Andean region and have been considered a potential commensal risk of infection to humans. *R. rattus* is considered the most important commensal host. The fleas that serve as principal vectors in South American foci are *X. cheopis* on *Rattus* spp. and *Polygenis* and *Pleochaetis* spp. on wild rodents. *Pulex irritans*, the human flea, also parasitizes domesticated guinea pigs and has been suspected as a secondary vector of infection to humans in some Andean outbreaks.

African Plague Foci

Widely scattered active plague foci exist in eastern and southern Africa, including Zaire, Uganda, Kenya, Tanzania, Zambia, Zimbabwe, Mozambique, Botswana, South Africa, Namibia, and Angola and on the Indian Ocean island of Madagascar (23, 32). Less active foci occur in some north African states (e.g., Libya). The principal wild rodent hosts in Africa include gerbils (*Tatera* and *Desmodillus* spp.), swamp rats, various grass mice, multimammate mice (*Mastomys* spp.), and commensal rats (*Rattus* spp.). Gerbil populations are found in open grassland sites, while multimammate mice are more likely to be found in agricultural fields and in commensal association with humans. The principal flea vectors of wild rodent hosts are *Xenopsylla* and *Dinopsyllus* spp., and *X. cheopis* and *X. braziliensis* are the principal vector flea species involving commensal rats and humans.

Asian Plague Foci

The most important Eurasian plague hosts are gerbils (various *Meriones* spp.) in Iran, Kurdistan, Transcaucasia, other areas around the Caspian Sea, and the plains of southeastern Russia; marmots in central Asia, including northeastern China, Mongolia, and Manchuria; and ground squirrels (*Spermophilus* spp.) in Mongolia, north-central China, central Asian plains, and some areas around the Caspian Sea (23, 32). The primary flea vectors are *Xenopsylla* and *Nosopsyllus* spp. on gerbils, various *Oropsylla*, *Rhadinopsylla*, and *Citellophilus* spp. on marmots, and *Citellophilus* and *Neopsylla* spp. on ground squirrels.

In India, the gerbil *T. indica* has been described as the principal wild rodent reservoir host. Although it lives preferentially in open grasslands in its natural state, it may invade agricultural fields and village peripheries. The important commensal rat species are *B. bengalensis*, *Bandicota indica*, *R. rattus*, and *R. norvegicus*. The primary vectors of plague in India are *X. cheopis* and *Xenopsylla astia*.

The principal rodent hosts in Myanmar, Vietnam, and Indonesia are *R. rattus* and the Polynesian rat (*Rattus exulans*). *R. rattus* subsp. *flavipectus* is an important host in southern China. *R. norvegicus* and the bandicoot *B. indicus* have been described as important hosts in Vietnam. *X. cheopis* is the principal vector of plague in southern China, Myanmar, Vietnam, and Indonesia; *X. astia* (a less efficient vector) is also found on rats in Myanmar and Vietnam.

Epidemiology

Distribution of Human Plague

The potential for human plague exists wherever there are zootic foci of infection (Fig. 2.2). Human plague cases are regularly identified in 10 to 15 countries each year (Table 2.1). Plague is a class 1 quarantinable disease (along with cholera and yellow fever) and is subject to the World Health Organization (WHO) International Health Regulations (39). These regulations require prompt reporting of plague cases to WHO. From 1980 through 1994, a total of 18,739 human plague cases (mean of 1,249 per year) and 1,853 deaths (10%) were reported by 24 countries to WHO (Table 2.1) (41). More than half (10,155) of the total number of cases were reported by countries in eastern and southern Africa, approximately a third (5,661) were reported by Asia, and the remaining cases (2,923) were reported by the Americas. Recent epidemic activity has been reported by India, Vietnam, Myanmar, Tanzania, Zaire, Madagascar, Mozambique, and Peru. In 1994, India identified its first cases of plague in nearly 30 years, when 876 bubonic

In India, the gerbil T. indica has been described as the principal wild rodent reservoir host

Table 2.1 Reported cases of plague in humans, by country, 1980–1994[a]

Continent	Country	No. of cases	No. of deaths
Africa	Angola	27	4
	Botswana	173	12
	Kenya	49	10
	Libya	8	0
	Madagascar	1,390	302
	Malawi	9	0
	Mozambique	216	3
	South Africa	19	1
	Tanzania	4,964	419
	Uganda	660	48
	Zaire	2,242	513
	Zambia	1	1
	Zimbabwe	397	31
	Total	10,155	1,344
America	Bolivia	189	27
	Brazil	700	9
	Ecuador	83	3
	Peru	1,722	112
	United States	229	33
	Total	2,923	184
Asia	China	252	76
	India	876	54
	Kazakhystan	10	4
	Mongolia	59	19
	Myanmar	1,160	14
	Vietnam	3,304	158
	Total	5,661	325
World Total		18,739	1,853

[a] From reference 41.

and pneumonic plague cases and 54 deaths were reported from adjoining Maharashtra and Gujurat states in west-central India (40, 41). Vietnam and Myanmar regularly experience both urban and rural plague and reported 1,756 and 727 cases, respectively, in the period from 1990 to 1994. Tanzania reported outbreaks involving 1,293 cases in 1991 and 444 cases in 1994. Zaire reported a total of 1,397 cases in the period from 1991 to 1994. Zimbabwe experienced outbreak activity involving 392 cases in 1994. Madagascar regularly reports cases, averaging 167 cases per year in the period from 1990 to 1994, and in 1995, an outbreak of rat-borne bubonic plague occurred in the port city of Mahajanga.

From 1980 to 1994, the United States reported 229 plague cases (mean of 15 cases per year) and 33 deaths (14%) (40). Although enzootic and epizootic plague occurs in 17 of the states in the contiguous western United States, extending from the Pacific coastal states to the Great Plains states and eastern Texas, 80% of human cases occur in the southwestern states of New Mexico, Arizona, and Colorado, and approximately 10% occur in California (14,24). No plague cases have been reported by Canada or Mexico in recent decades.

Risk Factors for Human Plague

Y. *pestis* readily infects persons of all ages and races, and differences in attack rates are due to differing levels of exposure to infective fleas. Because of their greater likelihood of living and working in close association with rodents, persons with low socioeconomic status have been at greatest risk, especially for urban plague.

In the United States, most plague cases in recent decades have resulted from peridomestic exposures. This trend has been associated with the placement of homes in natural surroundings, with building and landscaping practices that preserve or enhance habitats for plague-susceptible animals (e.g., rock squirrels and wood rats), and with siting of homes near prairie dog colonies (5, 28). Hikers, campers, and hunters in natural areas throughout the western states are at a small but definite risk of exposure to plague, especially during the warmer months of the year. Visitors to public parks and camping sites in mountainous areas of California and Nevada are at special risk of being exposed to epizootic plague in chipmunks and ground squirrels.

Plague can be transmitted to humans as a result of skinning and handling carcasses of wild animals such as rodents, rabbits and hares, prairie dogs, wild cats, and coyotes (11, 31). Such direct inoculation is associated with an increased risk for primary septicemia and high fatality rates. In Mongolia and some areas of northeastern China, the hunting of marmots for fur and food is associated with a relatively high risk for plague. As well, interperson pneumonic spread sometimes occurs in the crowded living spaces of these hunters. Plague, including oropharyngeal plague, can result from the ingestion of undercooked contaminated meat (13) and perhaps from the manual transfer of contaminated fluids to the mouth while handling infected animal tissues.

In the United States, detailed information on exposures for human plague cases is available. From 1950 through 1994, among 364 evaluable patients, 313 (86%) presented as primary lymphadenitic (bubonic) plague, thought to be associated in almost every case with flea bites; 44 (12%) presented with primary septicemic plague, often following handling of infected animal tissues; and 7 (2%) presented with primary pneumonic plague, with evidence suggesting that 6 cases had resulted from inhaling respiratory droplets expelled by infected cats (24).

Tens of thousands of cases of pneumonic plague resulted from two explosive outbreaks in Manchuria in the early part of this century (33). Otherwise, person-to-person spread of plague in modern times has occurred infrequently and in limited outbreaks, usually involving household members and caregivers. The reported outbreak of pneumonic plague in the city of Surat, India, in 1994 (2, 35) most likely involved fewer than 100 cases. Importantly, Y. *pestis* disperses from pneumonic plague patients in respiratory droplets, not as a fine aerosol or as droplet nuclei, and persons who have direct and close (2 m) respiratory exposure are at highest risk of acquiring primary pneumonic plague. Primary plague pneumonia is associated with a copious watery or mucoid sputum that may render these patients more

> Y. *pestis readily infects persons of all ages and races, and differences in attack rates are due to differing levels of exposure to infective fleas*

contagious than those with secondary plague pneumonia, which is usually associated with a thick, tenacious sputum.

Disease

Clinical Illness

Bubonic Plague

Bubonic plague typically has an incubation period of 2 to 6 days, occasionally longer. Early disease manifestations include chills, fever, myalgias, arthralgias, headache, and a feeling of weakness. Within 1 to 2 days of disease onset, the patient notices tenderness and pain in one or more regional lymph nodes proximal to the site of inoculation of the plague bacillus. The femoral and inguinal groups of nodes are most commonly involved, followed (in frequency of occurrence) by axillary and cervical nodes. The enlarging bubo(es) becomes progressively swollen, painful, and tender, sometimes exquisitely so. The surrounding tissue often becomes swollen with edema, and the overlying skin may be reddened, warm, and tense (Fig. 2.3). Inspection of the skin surrounding or distal to the bubo sometimes reveals the site of a flea bite, marked by a small papule, pustule, scab, or ulcer. Larger eschars that are indistinguishable from those caused by tularemia may occur. The bubo of plague is distinguishable from lymphadenitis of most other causes by its rapid onset, extreme tenderness, accompanying signs of toxemia, and absence of cellulitis or obvious ascending lymphangitis. Treated in the uncomplicated state with an appropriate antibiotic, bubonic plague usually responds quickly, with resolution of fever and other systemic manifestations over a 2- to 5-day period. Buboes may take a week or more to resolve.

> *Treated in the uncomplicated state with an appropriate antibiotic, bubonic plague usually responds quickly*

Without specific antimicrobial treatment, bubonic plague patients typically manifest an increasingly toxic state of fever, tachycardia, and lethargy, leading to prostration, agitation, confusion, and, occasionally, convulsions and delirium. Mild forms of bubonic plague, called pestis minor, have been described in South America and elsewhere; in these cases, the patients are ambulatory and only mildly febrile and have subacute buboes.

Septicemic Plague

Septicemic plague is manifest as a rapidly progressive, overwhelming endotoxemia and systemic inflammatory response syndrome (7, 15, 25, 38). Primary septicemia occurs in the absence of an apparent regional lymphadenitis, and the diagnosis of plague is often unsuspected. Patients with septicemic plague frequently present with prominent gastrointestinal symptoms such as nausea, vomiting, diarrhea, and abdominal pain, which makes misdiagnosis likely. Delayed or inappropriate treatment is associated with a high case-fatality rate. In the United States from 1950 to 1994, there were 64 septicemic plague cases with 18 deaths, for a case-fatality rate of 28%. Petechiae, ecchymoses, bleeding, and acral gangrene are usual manifestations of disseminated intravascular coagulation (Fig. 2.4); refractory hypotension, renal shutdown, obtundation, and other signs of shock are preterminal events. Adult respiratory distress syndrome, which can occur at any stage of septicemic plague, may be mistakenly attributed to some other cause, such as hantavirus pulmonary syndrome.

Pneumonic Plague

Pneumonic plague is the most fulminant and fatal form of plague (32, 42). The incubation period for primary pneumonic plague is usually 2 to 4 days, rarely longer. The onset is most often sudden, with chills, fever, headache, body pains, weakness, dizziness, and chest discomfort. Cough, sputum production, increasing chest pain, tachypnea, and dyspnea typically predominate on the second day of illness and may be accompanied by hemoptysis, increasing respiratory distress, cardiopulmonary insufficiency, and circulatory collapse. In primary plague pneumonia, the sputum is typically watery or mucoid, frothy, and blood tinged, but it may become frankly bloody. Chest signs in primary pneumonic plague may indicate localized pulmonary involvement in the early stage, with rapidly developing segmental consolidation before bronchopneumonic spread to other segments and lobes of the same and opposite lung (Fig. 2.5). Liquefactive necrosis and cavitation may develop and can leave significant residual scarring. Secondary plague pneumonia manifests first as a diffuse interstitial pneumonitis, and the sputum is typically scant, inspissated, and tenacious in character. In the United States from 1950 to 1994, a total of 39 cases of secondary pneumonic plague and 7 cases of primary pneumonic plague were recorded without known secondary transmission to contacts. The overall case-fatality rate was 41%. Observers of pneumonic plague patients in the early 20th century remarked on minimal auscultatory findings, the appearance of toxemia, and the frequency of sudden death, compared with patients with other bacterial pneumonias (42).

Pneumonic plague is the most fulminant and fatal form of plague

Meningeal Plague

Meningitis is an unusual manifestation of plague. In the United States, there were 12 (3%) meningitis cases among the 373 plague cases reported in the 45-year period from 1950 to 1994. All cases were complications of bubonic plague and all patients survived. The onset of meningeal plague is often delayed and may be a manifestation of insufficient treatment of the primary illness. The course is not always malignant, and chronic relapsing illness over periods of weeks and even months was described in the preantibiotic era. Patients typically present with fever, headache, meningismus, and pleocytosis.

Pharyngeal Plague

Plague pharyngitis in its early stages may be clinically indistinguishable from more common infectious causes of pharyngitis. The development of characteristic cervical buboes, however, provides an important clue to the true diagnosis.

Pathogenesis of Human Plague

Molecular Basis of Disease

Y. pestis is among the most invasive bacteria known; both chromosome- and plasmid-encoded gene products are most likely involved (see "*Y. pestis* Virulence Factors," above). A lipopolysaccharide endotoxin is thought to be primarily responsible for the pathogenic effects of plague sepsis and associated systemic inflammatory response syndrome, including adult respiratory distress syndrome, cytokine activation, complement cascade and resultant disseminated intravascular coagulation and bleeding, unresponsive shock, and organ failure (7, 15, 25, 38).

Pathology of Human Plague

General

The pathologic lesions of bubonic plague can be organized by following the course of the *Y. pestis* bacilli from the site of inoculation in the skin, through the lymph nodes, where the characteristic buboes arise, to the various lesions that occur following hematogenous spread. Special emphasis must also be focused on the lung, where the lesions of primary pneumonic plague arise. Primary pneumonic plague can be considered a short circuit, bypassing the usual initial bubonic phase and accelerating a final septicemic phase of plague, while causing life-threatening local damage to the lung itself.

Lymph Nodes

In a small minority of cases (6% in a Portuguese series from the turn of the century) (21), there is a primary pustule (or larger plague carbuncle) on the skin at the site of the bite; even more rarely, a primary lymphangitis connects such a skin lesion to the primary bubo. At the beginning of this century, Albrecht and Ghon distinguished between primary buboes "of the first order" (those in the lymph node group draining the area of the infectious bite) from primary buboes "of the second order" (those contiguous to the first group and infected by lymphatic spread). These two types of buboes were distinguished from secondary buboes, those in noncontiguous lymph node groups that were infected by hematogenous spread (1). The primary buboes of the first order show (or, have time to develop) the most complex pattern of histologic reaction in the following ways. (i) The initial change is a thick, proteinaceous exudate that includes bacilli and that distends the subcapsular sinus, expands the interfollicular cords, and clogs the medullary sinus of the node. (ii) In these areas, this exudative pattern eventually gives way to lakes of necrosis, obliterating the lymph node's underlying architecture. (iii) Within the affected lymph node, zones of the contrasting exudative and necrotizing patterns of inflammation are most typically separated by a line of acute hemorrhage. In the exudative phase, the inflammatory infiltrate predominantly includes polymorphonuclear neutrophils (and often less mature myeloid cells, such as metamyelocytes), lymphocytes, and relatively few macrophages (Fig. 2.6). This inflammation involves not only the inter- and perifollicular and medullary lymphoid tissue itself but also the vasculature of the node, promoting a necrotizing vasculitis, which presumably contributes to the rapid development of bacteremia, the lakes of necrosis, and the parenchymal hemorrhage within the node. The same inflammatory infiltrate also invades the connective tissue skeleton of the node, violates its capsule, and extends, primarily along fibrous septa, into the surrounding perinodal fat, where it also involves connective tissue bundles and blood vessels. There is thus both nodal and perinodal, as well as both lymphoid and vascular and both exudative and necrotizing, inflammation in the primary bubo. These pathologic findings correlate with the swollen, tender, painful nodes observed clinically. Plague bacilli are easily seen in all phases of nodal infection. In the initial exudative phase, the bacilli are found both extracellularly and intracellularly in both the inflammatory infiltrate and the areas of exudate without inflammatory response. In the eventual necrotic phase, they contribute a granular texture to the lakes of necrosis. Both tissue Gram stain and Warthin-Starry stain bring out the bipolar intensity of staining at either end of the long axis of the bacillus (Fig. 2.7). However, this appearance is more strikingly demonstrated by use of Giemsa or the more traditional Wayson stain (in which the "safety pin" appearance is seen more clearly).

In secondary buboes, the pathologic changes are usually less complex. In general, the nodal, lymphoid, and exudative components predominate over the extranodal, vascular, and necrotizing elements. As a result, these nodes tend to be smaller, less tender, and not as painful. Sometimes, nodal involvement can be surprisingly subtle; this observation has led to disputes about whether primary septicemic plague is truly without buboes or whether the bubonic phase is just inapparent (16). Such subtle involvement of lymph nodes has also been presented as the histological substrate of pestis minor, a self-limited lymphadenitis caused by Y. *pestis*, an infrequent "peri-plague" syndrome (43).

In secondary buboes these nodes tend to be smaller, less tender, and not as painful

Lung

Because of the clinical and epidemiological implications of pneumonic plague, during the plague outbreaks of the early 20th century, much consideration was given to distinguishing between plague pneumonia with an airway versus a vascular pattern of spread, that is, between a primary versus a secondary (hematogenous) infection with plague bacilli in the lung parenchyma.

The two patterns have several features in common. The lungs, in both primary pneumonic and secondary pneumonic infections, show striking edema and congestion. The edema is thicker with protein than is the edema found with cardiovascular conditions or pneumococcal pneumonia. Lesions, composed of a combination of central exudate and peripheral congestion, produce characteristic yellow and red dots and bands, seen grossly upon the cross-sectioning of lungs from plague victims. The distribution of this pattern tends initially to be lobular, but it can eventually become "lobar by confluence" (3). As with the lymph nodes, all anatomic structures of the lung are affected; bronchi, intralobar septa, and pleural serosa, as well as blood vessels, are involved equally with the lung parenchyma. Thus, exudative and necrotizing bronchitis proximal to foci of parenchymal involvement, pleural exudate overlying these foci, and parenchymal hemorrhage into adjacent lung around the areas of exudate and necrosis are seen. In zones where the thick exudate without inflammatory cells fills alveolar spaces, the exudate has a granular texture under low-power microscopic examination; upon inspection at high power, this texture turns out to be due to fields and drifts of plague bacilli (Fig. 2.8–2.10). In the areas of necrosis, all traces of discernible lung architecture are often lost.

Given these shared features of overwhelming infection, it is sometimes difficult to determine whether the initial inoculum of plague bacilli arrived down the bronchi (as primary pneumonic plague) or through the vasculature (secondary to bubonic or septicemic plague), because hematogenous infection quickly involves the airways, while airway infection quickly involves blood vessels. In both situations, the inflammatory infiltrate is the same: mostly polymorphonuclear neutrophils, interspersed with small round lymphocytes and a few macrophages. Some of the latter are characteristically enlarged and filled with brown pigment.

A variety of different sorts of both pulmonary and extrapulmonary pathologic findings have to be brought into play to separate primary pneumonic from secondary pneumonic *Y. pestis* infection in the lung. The pulmonary features of primary pneumonic (airway) infection are (i) less inflammation and necrosis and more exudation in lobular foci in the lung parenchyma, the latter including "enormous agglomeration of the bacilli in the lungs" (42), rather than the more widely scattered nodules of necrosis typical of secondary hematogenous spread; (ii) tracheal and bronchial mucosal and submucosal hemorrhage, rather than the bronchial ulceration and necrosis typical of septicemic plague lesions on epithelial surfaces; (iii) fibrinous pleuritis and subpleural hemorrhage overlying the zones of exudative pneumonia; (iv) the arrangement of these zones of pneumonia along medium or large bronchi like "flowers of the hydrangea" (37), rather than in a more widespread vascular distribution; (v) more involvement of the hilar lymph nodes, with the characteristic lymph node findings described above, compared with the degree of infection and inflammation found in other, more peripheral lymph node groups; and (vi) more involvement of mediastinal viscera (e.g., the myocardium), with edema and hemorrhage, compared with the degree of similar changes discovered in abdominal viscera. The extrapulmonary features of primary pneumonic plague infection are (i) the absence of buboes, (ii) absence of tonsillar involvement or plague pharyngitis (The latter illustrates a tropism of *Y. pestis* for extranodal, as well as nodal, lymphoid tissue and provides a source for potentially confusing secondary seeding of the lungs via the airway in bubonic plague; the tonsils themselves are usually seeded from the cervical lymph nodes. "Anginose plague" is a designation given to the combination of plague pharyngitis and cervical bubonic plague, another relatively rare presentation of *Y. pestis* infection.), and (iii) evidence of disease in other organs that is much less extensive than that in the lungs.

These criteria reveal that it is especially difficult to separate primary pneumonic plague from bubonic plague with secondary pneumonic involvement when buboes occur in cervical lymph nodes. Fortunately, the cervical bubo is the least frequent presentation of bubonic plague. Otherwise, clinicopathologic correlation can also be helpful in making the critical distinction between bubonic plague with lung involvement versus primary pneumonic plague. Untreated primary pneumonic plague tends to have a shorter fatal course (3 days) than plague pneumonia complicating bubonic plague; in primary pneumonic plague, sputum samples containing the characteristic bacilli or sputum cultures growing Y. *pestis* appear very early in the course of infection (i.e., within 48 h of symptom onset), rather than as evidence of a terminal pneumonia presenting late as a coup de grace.

Other Organ Systems

The anatomic consequences of plague bacteremia are found chiefly in the spleen, liver, and skin; less so in the kidneys, brain, and serosal surfaces of these organs; and least of all in the gastrointestinal tract. (The last is an interesting negative finding because it contrasts with the tropism of other *Yersinia* pathogens of the gut.)

Spleen

The spleen is usually enlarged but relatively firm compared with the consistency of splenic pulp seen in other instances of sepsis. As with other lymphoid organs, there is an initial intense exudate, whose thickness contributes to the relative firmness. The exudate is full of bacilli; subsequent focal necrosis involves all tissue layers and commonly leads to subcapsular hemorrhage and, less frequently, to bands of parenchymal hemorrhage separating and compressing both white pulp and the fibrous trabeculae of the red pulp (Fig. 2.11).

Liver

The liver is also usually enlarged. There is a pattern of hemorrhage around damaged blood vessels that can coalesce peripherally into subcapsular hemorrhage. Scattered foci of necrosis "rich in bacilli" (3) are sometimes superimposed on this underlying hemorrhagic pattern in the hepatic parenchyma.

Skin

Consistent with the findings in the liver (which correlate with the plague bacillus's fibrinolysin [hemorrhage-inducing] virulence factor), secondary skin manifestations of plague are much more frequently due to coagulopathic hemorrhage than to metastatic infection. The coagulopathic lesions are mostly petechiae, which were present in 42% of patients in a large autopsy series (21). The skin lesions of metastatic infection are pustules that may coalesce into the plague "carbuncles," or "blains," which rarely become confluent as "eschars." The latter lesions are vividly described and depicted in historical accounts of plague; however, carbuncles were found in only 9% of autopsies in the series of 110 patients cited above (21).

Secondary skin manifestations of plague are much more frequently due to coagulopathic hemorrhage than to metastatic infection

Kidneys

Hemorrhagic appearances also dominate in renal tissue, particularly just below the capsule and adjacent to the renal calyx. Disseminated intravascular coagulation induced by plague can sometimes also be documented postmortem by the presence of fibrin thrombi in glomerular capillaries. Foci of metastatic infection, either in the interstitium or in the glomeruli, are relatively rare; this is another striking negative finding, given the high volume of renal blood flow.

Brain

Cerebral infection usually seems to seed from the meninges where it arrives by hematogenous spread. Plague meningitis cases in which a "thick, canary yellow, fibrinopurulent exudate" covers the brain have been described.

Serosal Surfaces

Serosal surfaces are frequently involved in coagulopathic hemorrhage caused by plague septicemia

Serosal surfaces are frequently involved in coagulopathic hemorrhage caused by plague septicemia. Examples of this pattern include bleeding into the peri- and epicardium and hemorrhage along the vascular bundles of large vessels in the mediastinum, neck, and retroperitoneum. Exemplifying the other plague pattern of metastatic infection, a transmural vasculitis with intramural bacilli can sometimes also be demonstrated, especially in medium-sized veins.

Gastrointestinal Tract

Again, it is worth remarking that not only the mucosa but also the serosa of the gastrointestinal tract is relatively spared from all the changes just described.

Summary

The morbid anatomist's first task in the study of plague victims is to distinguish the findings of bubonic, septicemic, and pneumonic plague (i) by a careful search for involved lymph nodes to demonstrate the extent and patterns of bubonic inflammation and (ii) by a careful analysis of the lung appearances to distinguish the relatively rare bronchopneumonia of primary pneumonic plague from the relatively common secondary hematogenous pneumonia.

The pathologist can recognize the early exudative and late necrotizing patterns of inflammation in the lymph nodes and the lung, as well as in secondarily involved lymphoid organs (including Waldeyer's ring [tonsils and adenoids] and the spleen); both organs are full of the typical bacilli, which exhibit their "safety pin" pattern of staining.

Elsewhere, the prosector is presented with two patterns of vascular pathology: (i) coagulopathic hemorrhage, striking most often in the liver, and (ii) vasculitic necrotizing infection, present most dramatically, but relatively rarely, in the skin and meninges.

Diagnosis

Except in epidemic situations, a high index of clinical suspicion is required to make a timely diagnosis of plague. A delayed or missed diagnosis is associated with a high case-fatality rate, and infected travelers who seek medical care after they have left areas of endemicity (peripatetic plague cases) are especially at risk (29). Laboratory tests for plague are highly reliable when conducted by persons experienced in working with *Y. pestis*, but such expertise is usually limited to reference laboratories.

Specimen Collection and Processing

When plague is suspected, specimens should be collected promptly for microbiologic studies, chest roentgenograms should be taken to rule out pneumonia, and specific antimicrobial therapy should be started pending confirmation. Diagnostic specimens for smears and culture include blood in all patients, lymph node aspirates in those with suspected buboes, sputum samples or tracheal aspirates in those with suspected pneumonic plague, and cerebrospinal fluid in those with suspected meningitis. A portion of each specimen should be inoculated onto suitable media (see "General Microbiology," above). Smears of each specimen should be stained with a polychromatic stain such as Wayson, Wright, or Giemsa stain and with Gram stain and then examined by using light microscopy. When stained with a polychromatic stain, plague bacilli in clinical specimens demonstrate a characteristic bipolar appearance, often resembling closed safety pins (Fig. 2.12). If possible, the specimens should also be examined by using direct fluorescent-antibody testing (34). An acute-phase serum specimen should be collected for *Y. pestis* antibody testing, and a convalescent-phase specimen should be collected 3 to 4 weeks later. For autopsy cases, tissues, including buboes, samples of solid organs (especially the liver, spleen, and lung), and bone marrow, should be collected for culture and fluorescent-antibody testing. For culture, specimens should be sent to the laboratory either fresh or frozen on dry ice and not in preservatives or fixatives. Cary-Blair or a similar holding medium can be used to transport *Y. pestis*-infected tissues.

Plague patients typically have leukocyte counts of 15,000 to 25,000/mm^3, with a predominance of polymorphonuclear leukocytes and a left shift. Leukemoid reactions with leukocyte counts as high as 100,000/mm^3 can occur.

Laboratory Confirmation

Early laboratory confirmation depends on the isolation of *Y. pestis* from body fluids or tissues. When the patient's condition allows, several blood cultures taken over a 45-min period prior to treatment will usually result in successful isolation of the bacterium. *Y. pestis* strains are distinguishable from other gram-negative bacteria by polychromatic and immunofluorescence staining properties, characteristics of growth on microbiologic media, biochemical profiles, and confirmatory lysis by the *Y. pestis*-specific bacteriophage (34). Laboratory mice and hamsters are susceptible to *Y. pestis* and are used in specialized laboratories to make isolations from contaminated materials and to test for virulence.

In the absence of cultural isolation of *Y. pestis*, plague cases can usually be confirmed by demonstrating a fourfold or greater change in serum antibodies to *Y. pestis* F1 antigen by passive hemagglutination testing. Confirmation is less conclusively made by detecting a serum antibody titer of 128 or greater in a single serum sample from a patient with a compatible illness who has not received plague vaccine. The specificity of a positive passive hemag-

Several blood cultures taken over a 45-min period prior to treatment will usually result in successful isolation of Y. pestis

glutination test is validated by F1 antigen hemagglutination inhibition testing. Some plague patients develop diagnostic levels of antibodies within as few as 5 days after the onset of illness, most seroconvert 1 to 2 weeks after onset, some do not seroconvert until 3 weeks after onset, and <5% fail to seroconvert. Positive serologic titers diminish gradually over months to years. Enzyme-linked immunosorbent assays for detecting immunoglobulin M and immunoglobulin G antibodies to *Y. pestis* are useful in identifying antibodies in early stages of infection and in differentiating between infection and previous immunization.

Treatment and Prognosis

Untreated bubonic plague is fatal in over 50% of patients, and untreated septicemic or pneumonic plague is almost always fatal. The overall case-fatality rate in plague cases in the United States in the past 25 years is approximately 15% (23). Fatalities are almost always due to delays in seeking treatment, misdiagnosis, and delayed or incorrect treatment. Rapid diagnosis and appropriate antimicrobial therapy are essential (Table 2.2).

Streptomycin is the drug of choice for treating plague (9), and gentamicin is an acceptable substitute. Tetracycline and chloramphenicol are effective alternatives to the aminoglycosides. Chloramphenicol is indicated for conditions in which high tissue penetration is important, such as plague meningitis, pleuritis, endopthalmitis, and myocarditis. Chloramphenicol may be used separately or in combination with an aminoglycoside. Penicillins, cephalosporins, macrolides, and fluoroquinolones are relatively ineffective and should not be used. Doxycycline may be as or more effective than other tetracyclines, but controlled trials have not been reported. Trimethoprim-sulfamethoxazole has been used successfully in small series to treat bubonic plague, but it is not considered a first-line choice. In general,

> *Fatalities are almost always due to delays in seeking treatment, misdiagnosis, and delayed or incorrect treatment*

Table 2.2 Plague treatment guidelines[a]

Drug	Dosage	Interval (h)	Route of administration[b]
Streptomycin			
Adults	2 g/day	12	IM
Children	30 mg/kg/day	12	IM
Gentamicin			
Adults	3 mg/kg/day	8	IM or IV
Children	6.0–7.5 mg/kg/day	8	IM or IV
Infants/neonates	7.5 mg/kg/day	8	IM or IV
Tetracycline			
Adult	2 g/day	6	PO
Children ≥9 years	25–50 mg/kg/day	6	PO
Chloramphenicol			
Adults	50 mg/kg/day	6	PO or IV
Children ≥1 year	50 mg/kg/day	6	PO or IV

[a] From reference 17a with permission.
[b] IM, intramuscular; IV, intravenous; PO, oral.

antimicrobial treatment should be continued for 10 days or for at least 3 days after the patient has become afebrile and has made a clinical recovery. Patients begun on intravenous antibiotics may be switched to oral regimens as indicated by clinical response. Improvement is usually evident 2 to 3 days from the start of treatment, even though fever may continue for several more days.

Prevention and Control

General Principles

Surveillance, education, and environmental sanitation are the cornerstones of prevention and control (4, 5, 23). In known plague foci, surveys should be routinely conducted to determine evidence of epizootics. Carnivore serosurveillance can be used as a sensitive indicator of recent rodent plague in an area, as can the finding of Y. pestis infection in animals found dead of apparently natural causes (4, 23, 31). Other means of detecting epizootic plague include identification of infected fleas collected from abandoned burrows and the trapping and testing of live rodents and their fleas for Y. pestis infection. The risks for exposure of humans should be evaluated, and public health advisories, posting of warnings, and flea control measures should be undertaken as warranted.

Surveillance, education, and environmental sanitation are the cornerstones of prevention and control

Personal protective measures include avoiding areas with known epizootic plague; avoiding sick or dead animals; using repellents, insecticides, and protective clothing when potentially exposed to rodent fleas; and using gloves when handling animal carcasses.

To decrease the risk of pneumonic transmission, all suspected plague patients should be managed under respiratory precautions (appropriate to prevent droplet spread) during the first 48 h of antibiotic treatment. After that, standard precautions are adequate. Patients with suspected pneumonic plague should be managed in respiratory isolation until sputum cultures are shown to be negative. Persons caring for sick animals (especially cats) should take precautions to avoid contact with infectious exudates or expelled respiratory secretions. Postexposure treatment with a tetracycline or chloramphenicol for 7 days is recommended for persons who have had a known close exposure to a suspected or known pneumonic plague patient in the prior 6 days. Antibiotic prophylaxis may occasionally be recommended for persons who are unable to avoid visiting or residing in an area where a plague outbreak is in progress or who are caring for plague patients (9).

Sources of food and harborage for rodents should be eliminated in domestic, peridomestic, and working environments, and buildings and food stores should be rodent proofed. Controlling fleas with insecticides is an important public health measure in situations where epizootic plague places humans at risk. This includes dusting and spraying of rodent burrows, rodent runs, and other sites where potentially infected rodents and their fleas are found. In known plague foci, persons should keep their dogs and cats free of fleas and restrained. The decision to control plague by killing rodents should be left to public health authorities and should only be carried out in conjunction with effective flea control. Killing of rodents may promote dispersal of their fleas and can allow colonization of the area by young, more highly plague-susceptible rodent populations.

In the event of a plague epidemic, measures should be taken rapidly to control spread, as described in international regulations and manuals of disease control (4, 39). These measures include delineation of infected areas, enhanced surveillance, laboratory confirmation and reporting of human and animal plague, rapid detection and treatment of cases and exposed contacts, isolation and surveillance of suspected human plague patients and their contacts, and control of fleas and rodents in plague-infected areas, in port facilities, and on ships and other conveyances as indicated. A surveillance system to identify and contain the possible introduction of pneumonic plague into the United States was rapidly established at the time of the reported outbreaks of plague in India in 1994 (22).

Plague Vaccine

A killed, whole-cell plague vaccine is available in the United States (12). Reviews of vaccine use during the Vietnam War provide indirect evidence that the vaccine protects against bubonic plague but does not appear to fully protect against primary pneumonic plague. Primary immunization consists of a series of three injections. Persons with continuing risk may need to monitor their antibody levels and receive booster doses as warranted. The vaccine is moderately reactogenic. With the exception of military personnel, plague vaccine is recommended only for persons at high risk of exposure, such as laboratory personnel who routinely work with *Y. pestis* and persons whose work brings them into regular contact with wild rodents and their fleas in known or suspected plague foci (12). Vaccination is not routinely indicated for persons living in areas where zootic plague occurs, for medical personnel, for travelers to countries that have reported plague cases, or for controlling plague epidemics.

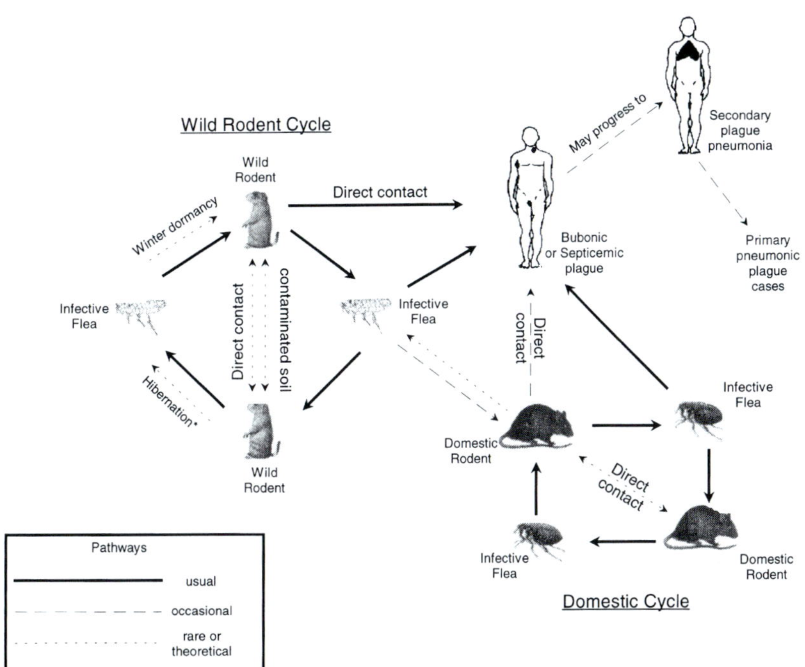

Figure 2.1 Zootic and human plague, demonstrating the interrelationship of the wild rodent and domestic rodent cycles and the routes of incidental infection of humans. The wild rodent cycle is associated with sporadic human plague cases; the domestic rodent cycle is associated with epidemic plague. Adapted from reference 26 with permission.

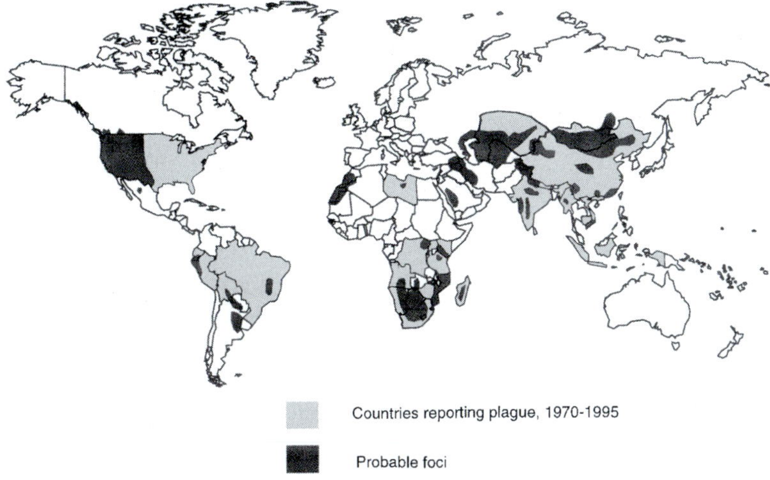

Figure 2.2 Distribution of natural foci of plague. Compiled from the World Health Organization, Centers for Disease Control, and other sources.

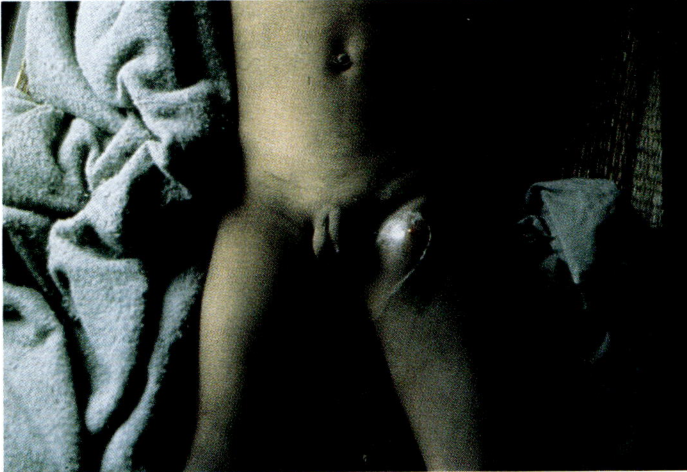

Figure 2.3 Bubonic plague, showing left femoral and inguinal buboes with marked surrounding edema and desquamation.

Figure 2.4   Septicemic plague, with acral gangrene of the digits and ecchymoses of the skin of the hand and arm due to disseminated intravascular coagulation.

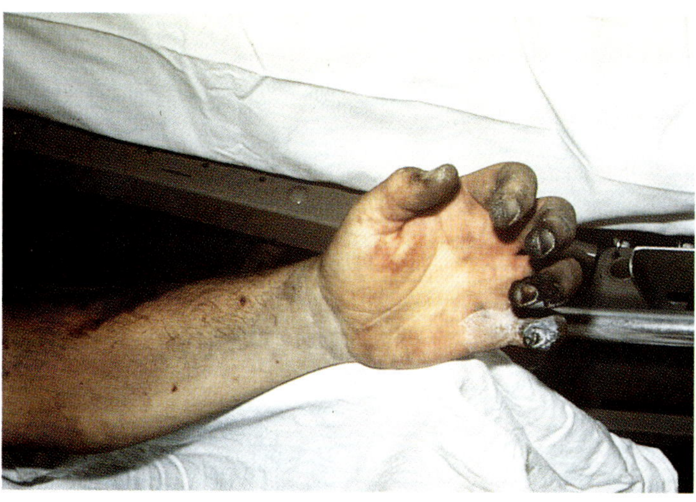

Figure 2.5   Primary plague pneumonia, showing segmental consolidation in the right upper lobe at hospital admission, 3 days after onset of illness.

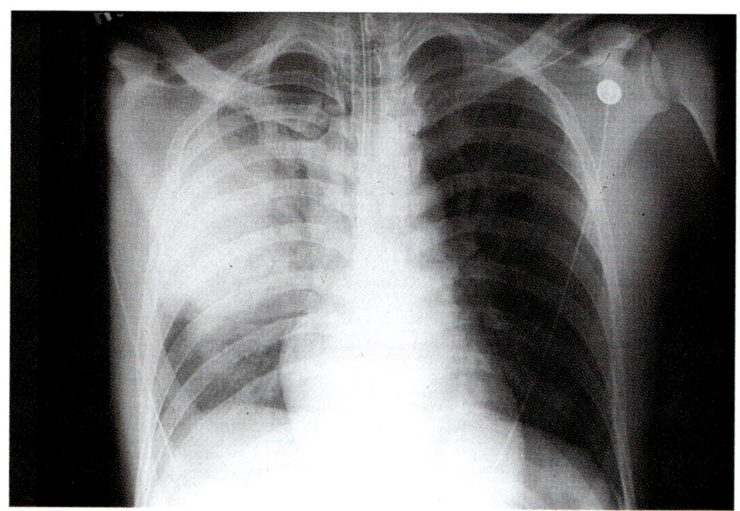

Figure 2.6   Lymph node from monkey experimentally infected with bubonic plague. Dilated blood vessel showing plague bacilli (i) in endothelial cells, (ii) lining apparently the nuclear endothelium, (iii) extending into the vessel lumen, and (iv) contained in circulating (or marginating) polymorphonuclear leukocytes (Brown-Hopps; original magnification, ×250). Armed Forces Institute of Pathology photo no. 1103519.

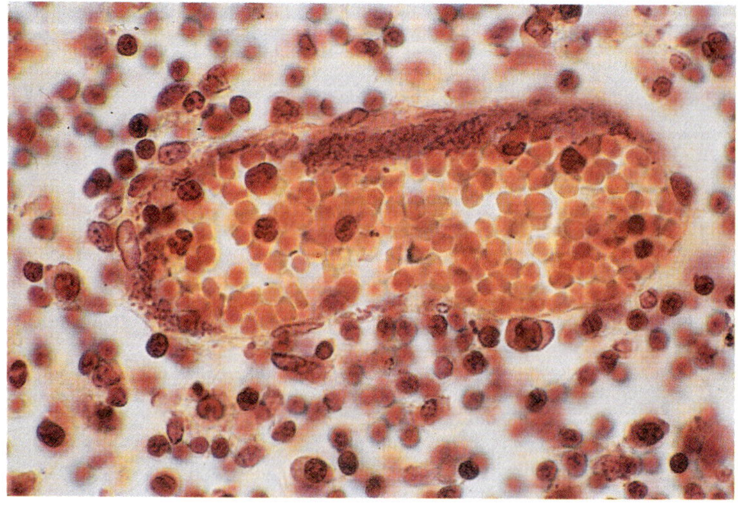

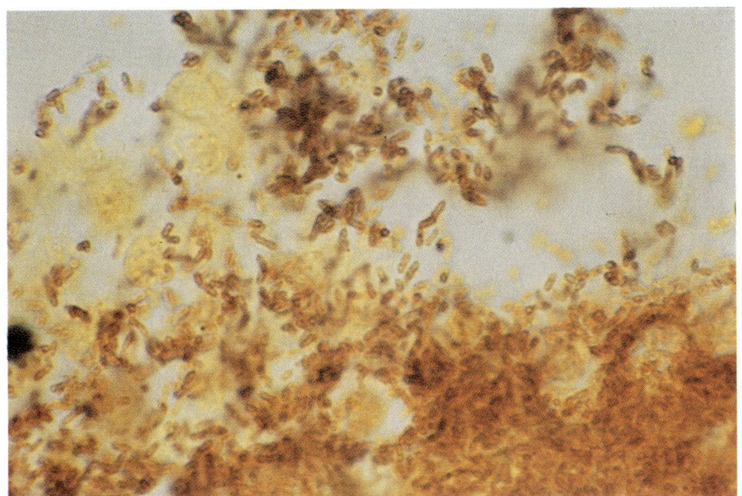

Figure 2.7   Warthin-Starry silver impregnation highlights the polar intensification of silver uptake in plague bacilli, producing a "safety pin" effect. Original magnification, ×400. Photo courtesy of Doug Wear, Armed Forces Institute of Pathology.

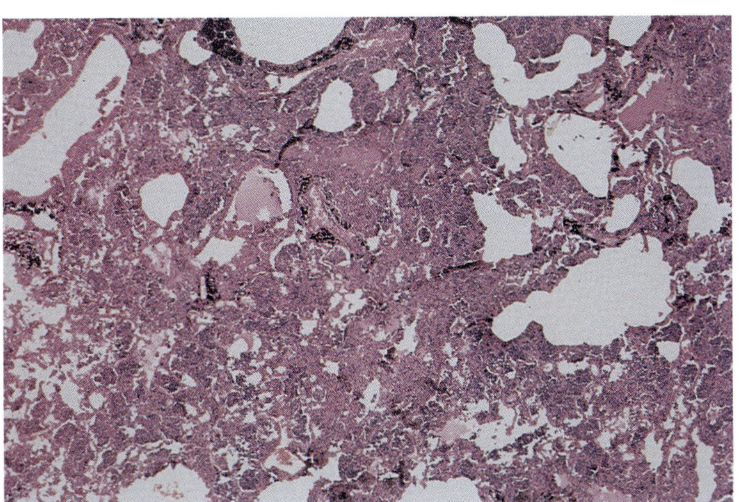

Figure 2.8   Low-power view of lung of patient with pneumonic plague (case from Manchuria epidemic, 1920s). An inflammatory proteinaceous exudate (i) obscures the lung architecture, (ii) invades airways and vasculature as well as the lung parenchyma, and (iii) destroys some interalveolar septa (hematoxylin and eosin stain; original magnification, ×10). Armed Forces Institute of Pathology photo no. 23801, courtesy of Doug Wear.

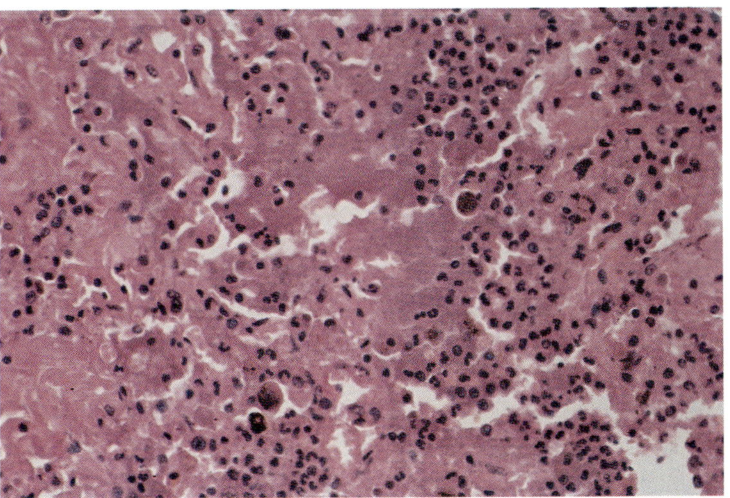

Figure 2.9   Lung from patient with pneumonic plague at higher power than that in Fig. 2.8. Inflammatory exudates are composed mostly of neutrophils (and occasional metamyelocytes) interspersed with lymphocytes and a few macrophages, and they extend along focally necrotic intra-alveolar septae and within alveolar spaces. The inflammatory cells are seen against a background of proteinaceous granular exudate, with fields or "drifts" containing myriad bacteria (hematoxylin and eosin; original magnification, ×100). Armed Forces Institute of Pathology photo no. 23801, courtesy of Doug Wear.

Figure 2.10 Brown-Hopps Gram stain demonstrates a field of plague bacilli in the dense exudate. The organisms fill an alveolar space and drift through the intra-alveolar pores from one alveolus to the next (Brown-Hopps; original magnification, ×250). Armed Forces Institute of Pathology photo no. 23801, courtesy of Doug Wear.

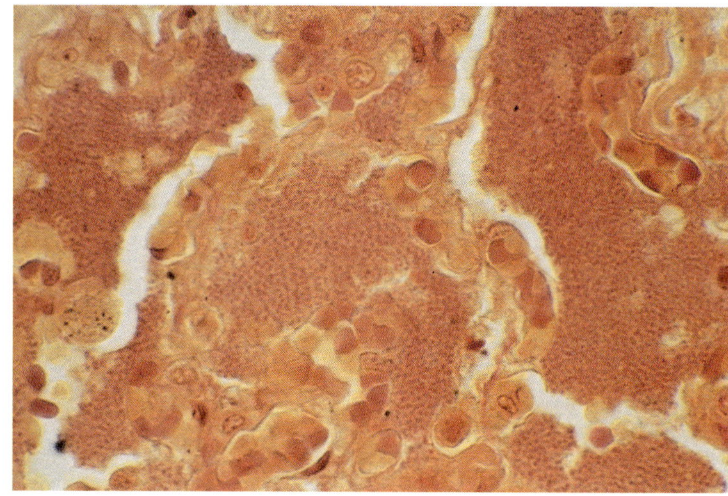

Figure 2.11 High-power view of spleen from patient with septicemic plague. Numerous extracellular bacilli form a column along a fibrous septum extending between blood vessels. Note the presence of two polymorphonuclear leukocytes just above the zone of bacteria in the center of the field (Brown-Hopps; original magnification, ×400). Armed Forces Institute of Pathology photo no. 1993604, courtesy of Doug Wear.

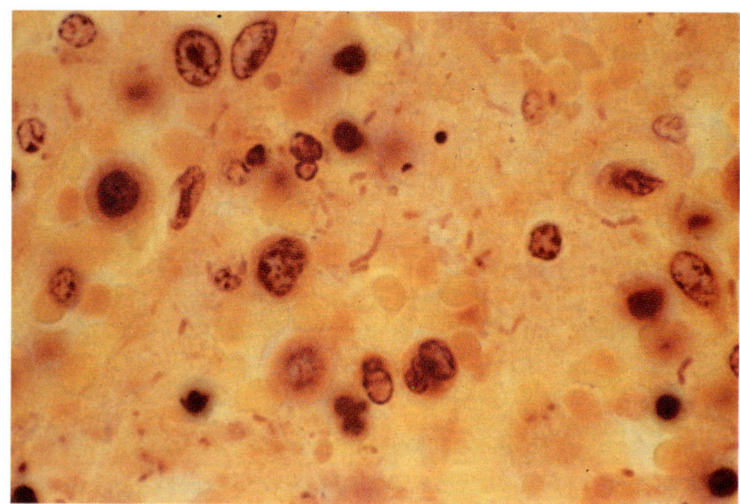

Figure 2.12 Peripheral blood smear from a patient with fatal plague septicemia, demonstrating characteristic bipolar-staining Y. *pestis* bacilli.

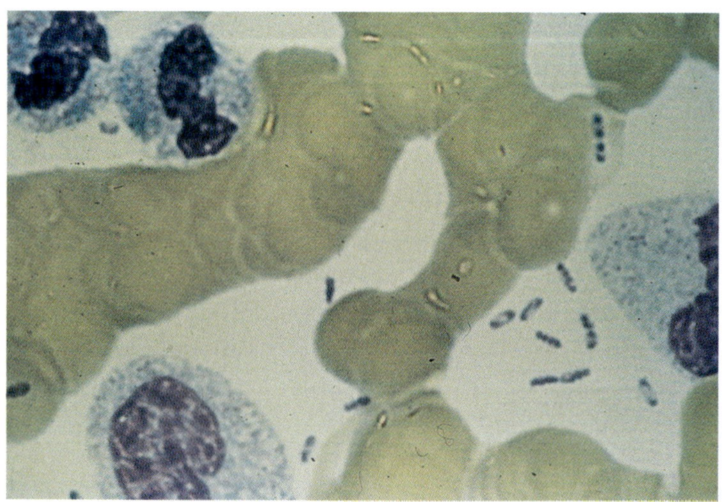

References

1. **Albrecht, H., and A. Ghon.** 1900. *Denkschr. Akad. Wiss. Wien* 1898. Cited in **Pollitzer, R.** 1954. Plague. *WHO Monogr. Ser.* **22:206.**

2. **Anonymous.** 1994. *Plague in India: World Health Organization International Plague Investigative Team Report,* December 9, 1994. World Health Organization, Geneva.

3. **Ash, J. E., and S. Spitz.** 1945. Plague, p. 114–115. *In Atlas of Tropical Diseases.* The W. B. Saunders Co., Philadelphia.

4. **Bahmanyar, M., and D. C. Cavanaugh.** 1976. *Plague Manual.* World Health Organization, Geneva.

5. **Barnes, A. M.** 1982. Surveillance and control of bubonic plague in the United States. *Symp. Zool. Soc. Lond.* **50:**237–270.

6. **Brubaker, R. R.** 1991. Factors promoting acute and chronic diseases caused by yersiniae. *Clin. Microbiol. Rev.* **4:**309–324.

7. **Butler, T.** 1972. A clinical study of bubonic plague: observations of the 1970 Vietnam epidemic with emphasis on coagulation studies, skin histology, and electrocardiograms. *Am. J. Med.* **53:**268–276.

8. **Butler, T.** 1983. *Plague and Other Yersinia Infections.* Plenum Press, New York.

9. **Campbell, G. L., and D. T. Dennis.** Plague and other *Yersinia* infections. *In* K. J. Isselbacher, E. Braunwald, J. D. Wilson, et al. (ed.), *Harrison's Principles of Internal Medicine,* in press. McGraw Hill, New York.

10. **Campbell, G. L., and J. M. Hughes.** 1995. Plague in India: a new warning from an old nemesis. *Ann. Intern. Med.* **122:**151–153.

11. **Centers for Disease Control.** 1984. Winter plague—Colorado, Washington, Texas, 1983–1984. *Morbid. Mortal. Weekly Rep.* **33:**145–148.

12. **Centers for Disease Control and Prevention.** 1996. Prevention of plague. Recommendations of the Advisory Committeee on Immunization Practices (ACIP). *Morbid. Mortal. Weekly Rep.* **45**(RR-14):1–15.

13. **Christie, A. B., T. H. Chen, and S. S. Elberg.** 1980. Plague in camels and goats: their role in human epidemics. *J. Infect. Dis.* **141:**724–727.

14. **Craven, R. B., G. O. Maupin, M. L. Beard, T. J. Quan, and A. M. Barnes.** 1993. Reported cases of human plague infections in the United States, 1970–1991. *J. Med. Entomol.* **30:**758–761.

15. **Crook, L. D., and B. Tempest.** 1992. Plague: a clinical review of 27 cases. *Arch. Intern. Med.* **152:**1253–1256.

16. **Crowell, B. C.** 1915. *Philipp. J. Sci.* **10**(Section B):249. Cited in **Wu, L. -T., J. W. H. Chun, R. Pollitzer, and C. Y. Wu (ed.).** 1936. *Plague: a Manual for Medical and Public Health Workers,* p. 155–156. Weischengshu-National Quarantine Service, Shanghai Station, China.

17. **Dennis, D. T.** 1994. Plague in India. *Br. Med. J.* **309:**893–894.

17a. **Dennis, D. T.** 1996. Plague, p. 124. *In* R. E. Rakel (ed.), *Conn's Current Therapy 1996.* W. B. Saunders, Philadelphia.

18. **Dennis, D. T., and K. Orloski.** 1996. Plague!, p. 160–191. *In 1996 Medical and Health Annual.* Encyclopaedia Brittanica, Inc., Chicago.

19. **Devignat, R.** 1951. Variétés de l'espèce Pasteurella pestis. Nouvelle hypothèse. *Bull. W. H. O.* **4:**247–263.

20. **Eskey, C. R., and V. H. Haas.** 1940. Plague in the western part of the United States. *Public Health Bull.* **254:**1–82.

21. **Franca, C.** 1905. *Zeitsch. Hyg. Infekt.* **52:**129. Cited in **Pollitzer, R.** 1954. Plague. *WHO Monogr. Ser.* **22:**206.

22. **Fritz, C. L., D. T. Dennis, M. A. Tipple, G. L. Campbell, C. R. McCance, and D. J. Gubler.** 1996. Surveillance for pneumonic plague in the United States during an international emergency: a model for control of imported emerging diseases. *Emerg. Infect. Dis.* **2:**30–36.

23. **Gage, K. L.** Plague. *In* L. Collier, A. Balows, H. Sussman, and W. L. Hausler (ed.), *Topley & Wilson's Microbiology and Microbiological Infections,* in press. Arnold, London.

24. **Gage, K. L., S. E. Lance, D. T. Dennis, and J. Montenieri.** 1992. Human plague in the United States: a review of cases from 1988–1992 with comments on the likelihood of increased plague activity. *Border Epidemiol. Bull.* **19:**1–10.

25. **Hull, H. F., J. M. Montes, and J. M. Mann.** 1987. Septicemic plague in New Mexico. *J. Infect. Dis.* **155:**113–118.

26. **Kartman, L., M. I. Goldenberg, and W. T. Hubbert.** 1966. Recent observations on the epidemiology of plague in the United States. *Am. J. Public Health* **56:**1554–1569.

27. **Link, V. B.** 1955. *A History of Plague in the United States of America.* Public Health Monograph no. 26. Government Printing Office, Washington, D. C.

28. **Mann, J. M., W. J. Martone, J. M. Boyce, A. F. Kaufmann, A. M. Barnes, and N. S. Weber.** 1979. Endemic human plague in New Mexico: risk factors associated with infection. *J. Infect. Dis.* **140:**397–401.

29. **Mann, J. M., G. P. Schmid, P. A. Stoesz, M. D. Skinner, and A. F. Kaufmann.** 1982. Peripatetic plague. *JAMA* **247:**47–48.

30. **Perry, R. D., and J. D. Fetherston.** 1997. *Yersinia pestis:* etiologic agent of plague. *Clin. Microbiol. Rev.* **10:**35–66.

31. **Poland, J. D., and A. M. Barnes.** 1979. Plague, p. 523–540. *In* J. H. Steele (ed.), *CRC Handbook Series in Zoonoses. Section A: Bacterial, Rickettsial, and Mycotic Diseases,* vol 2. CRC Press, Boca Raton, Fla.

32. **Pollitzer, R.** 1954. Plague. *WHO Monogr. Ser.* **22:**1.

33. **Pollitzer, R., and K. F. Meyer.** 1961. The ecology of plague, p. 433–501. *In* J. H. May (ed.), *Studies in Disease Ecology.* Hefner, New York.

34. **Quan, T. J., A. M. Barnes, and J. D. Poland.** 1981. Yersinioses, p. 734–735. *In* A. Balows and W. J. Hausler (ed.), *Diagnostic Procedures for Bacterial, Mycotic and Parasitic Infections,* 6th ed. American Public Health Association, Washington, D. C.

35. **Ramalingaswami, V.** 1996. An overview of the work carried out by the Technical Advisory Committee on Plague. *Curr. Sci.* **71:**783–786.

36. **Saxena, V. K., and T. Vergese.** 1996. Ecology of flea-transmitted zoonotic infection in village Mamla, District Beed. *Curr. Sci.* **71:**800–802.

37. **Strong, R. P.** 1912. *Report of the International Plague Conference, Mukden, April, 1911.* Manila Bureau of Printing, Manila, Philippines.

38. **Wenzel, R. P., M. P. Pinsky, R. J. Ulevitch, and L. Young.** 1996. Current understanding of sepsis. *Clin. Infect. Dis.* **22:**407–413.

39. **World Health Organization.** 1983. *International Health Regulations (1969)*. World Health Organization, Geneva.

40. **World Health Organization.** 1994. Plague. *Weekly Epidemiol. Rec.* **69:**295–299.

41. **World Health Organization.** 1996. Human plague in 1994. *Weekly Epidemiol. Rec.* **71:**165–172.

42. **Wu, L.-T.** 1926. A *Treatise on Pneumonic Plague*. League of Nations Health Organization, Geneva.

43. **Wu, L.-T., and H. M. Jettmar.** 1926. North Manchurian Plague Prevention Service reports, vol. 5, p. 1. Cited in **Wu, L.-T., J. W. H. Chun, R. Pollitzer, and C. Y. Wu (ed.).** 1936. *Plague: a Manual for Medical and Public Health Workers*, p. 161. Weischengshu-National Quarantine Service, Shanghai Station, China.

chapter 3

Ehrlichiosis

Jacqueline E. Dawson and Aileen M. Marty

urrently, there are two potentially fatal forms of human ehrlichiosis in the United States. Both of these are caused by tick-borne
pathogens and are characterized by an acute febrile illness similar to Rocky Mountain spotted fever (RMSF) (3, 15). Many
physicians believe that the illness historically diagnosed as "spotless" RMSF
may have been due to one of these ehrlichial species. Indeed, the clinical
presentations of both ehrlichial diseases are extremely similar to that of
RMSF; however, in a minority of ehrlichiosis patients, a rash is also observed. Both of these diseases, human ehrlichiosis due to *Ehrlichia chaffeensis* and human granulocytic ehrlichiosis (HGE), have only recently been
recognized (3, 15).

Ehrlichia sennetsu, the etiologic agent of human sennetsu fever, causes
lymphadenopathy, fever, and lethargy (21). This disease, however, has been
reported only in western Japan, not in North America (20). This led some
investigators to believe that *Ehrlichia canis* was causing infections in human beings (19). It was not until 1990, when *E. chaffeensis* was isolated
and subsequently sequenced, that enough evidence had accumulated to

Jacqueline E. Dawson, Viral and Rickettsial Zoonoses Branch, Division of Viral and Rickettsial Diseases, National Center for Infectious Diseases, Centers for Disease Control and Prevention, 1600 Clifton Road, N.E., Mailstop G-13, Atlanta, GA 30333. **Aileen M. Marty,** Infectious Disease Branch, Armed Forces Institute of Pathology, Washington, DC 20306-6000.

Pathology of Emerging Infections
Edited by C. Robert Horsburgh, Jr., and Ann Marie Nelson
© 1997 American Society for Microbiology, Washington, DC 20005-4171

prove that a new ehrlichial species was infecting human beings in the United States (1, 6). More recently, HGE has been identified in Wisconsin and Minnesota (30). Sequencing of the 16S rRNA gene of the HGE agent revealed a 99.9% similarity with *Ehrlichia phagocytophila* (5), a pathogen of sheep and cattle in Europe, India, and South Africa (29), and a 99.8% similarity with *E. equi*, an equine pathogen in the United States (18).

Because neither form of human ehrlichiosis is reportable, an accurate number of cases is not available. However, prospective studies of human ehrlichiosis due to *E. chaffeensis* have shown rates equal to or in excess of the number of cases of RMSF (16).

Classification

The genus *Ehrlichia* was established in 1945, in honor of the German bacteriologist Paul Ehrlich (14). This genus of obligate intracellular leukocytic parasites was created to distinguish it from other medically significant genera (*Rickettsia*, *Coxiella*, and *Chlamydia*). *Ehrlichia* are members of the family *Rickettsiaceae* and the order *Rickettsiales*, which includes the tribes *Ehrlichieae*, *Rickettsieae*, and *Wolbachieae*. Three species are pathogenic for humans, *E. sennetsu*, *E. chaffeensis*, and the newly recognized HGE agent. The two last agents are the only ones recognized in the United States. *E. chaffeensis* is apparently most closely related to the canine pathogens *E. canis* and *E. ewingii* (1). Similarly, the HGE agent appears to be very closely related, if not identical, to *E. phagocytophila* and *E. equi*, both pathogens in domestic herbivores (5).

Epidemiology of *E. chaffeensis*

Human ehrlichiosis due to *E. chaffeensis* has been diagnosed in more than 400 patients. Ehrlichiosis is particularly common in persons 60 years of age and older, although the median age is 44 years (15). Fatalities have occurred in individuals ranging from 8 to 68 years old. Similar to that seen with other tick-borne diseases, over 70% of patients are men (15).

Cases of ehrlichiosis due to *E. chaffeensis* from 30 states in the United States have been reported since its discovery in 1986. In addition, one case from Portugal (22) and one from Africa (27) have been reported. Most cases occur between May and October, which is suggestive of arthropod transmission. Indeed, Fishbein et al. (16) stated that tick exposure is a common part of the history for human ehrlichiosis patients, and Petersen et al. (24) found that soldiers who tucked their pants into their boots to deter ticks were only half as likely as their cohorts to develop ehrlichiosis. In addition, Everett et al. (13) found a few *Amblyomma americanum* and *Dermacentor variabilis* ticks positive for *E. chaffeensis* by the indirect fluorescent-antibody technique, and Anderson et al. (2) used the polymerase chain reaction (PCR) technique to amplify the *E. chaffeensis* 16S rRNA gene from a pool of *A. americanum*.

Ehrlichiosis is particularly common in persons 60 years of age and older

Epidemiology of HGE

HGE is so recently discovered that little is known about the geographic distribution or reservoir host(s). All 15 cases reported to date (including 2 fatalities) were seen in Minnesota and Wisconsin (3, 5). The patients ranged in age from 29 to 91 years old. Bakken et al. (3) reported that 92% of the patients examined had a history of an arthropod bite within 10 days of onset of illness. Ticks were attached to 67% of the patients and were identified as either *Ixodes scapularis* or *D. variabilis*.

More recently, Reed et al. (25) reported the removal of an adult female *I. scapularis* tick from a clinically ill patient. The tick was analyzed, along with blood from the patient, by PCR. *Ehrlichia* DNA was detected in both samples. While this is not definitive evidence that *I. scapularis* transmits the HGE agent, it does support epidemiologic observations. Reed et al. (25) also reported two additional patients that were seropositive and PCR positive, thus bringing the total number of cases of HGE to 15.

The possibility that *I. scapularis* is the vector of HGE is highly significant, especially considering the role this tick already plays in the transmission of *Borrelia burgdorferi*, the etiologic agent of Lyme disease. Because of the similarity of their initial presentations, discussed below, it is certainly possible that some of the unconfirmed Lyme disease cases actually involve infections with the HGE agent.

The possibility that I. scapularis is the vector of HGE is highly significant, especially considering the role this tick already plays in the transmission of Borrelia burgdorferi, the etiologic agent of Lyme disease

Clinical Syndromes

Ehrlichial diseases are characterized by sudden onset of fever, headache, and malaise. Other commonly encountered symptoms include confusion, myalgia, rigor, sweats, and nausea and/or vomiting (3, 15). Despite the nonspecific signs and symptoms of human ehrlichiosis, laboratory findings are more consistent and frequently include thrombocytopenia, leukopenia, elevated liver enzymes, and occasionally anemia (3, 15). Most patients present between May and October, often with a history of arthropod exposure. Fatalities due to both agents have been reported.

One early case report of human ehrlichiosis ascribed to *E. chaffeensis* documented bone marrow hypoplasia and suggested diminished production of leukocytes, erythrocytes, and platelets (23). Other bone marrow findings have included myeloid hyperplasia, megakaryocytosis, granulomas, marrow histiocytosis, myeloid hypoplasia, pancellular hypoplasia, and normocellular marrow (12). Three postmortem examinations revealed gastrointestinal hemorrhage; mild interstitial pneumonitis; perivascular lymphohistiocytic infiltrates in the lung, liver, kidneys, and heart; and bone marrow hyperplasia. Focal hepatocyte necrosis, hepatocyte dropout, Kupffer cell hyperplasia, and erythrophagocytosis were also observed (10). Immunostaining with biotinylated globulin from a patient convalescing from ehrlichiosis demonstrated the presence of clusters of ehrlichial organisms (morulae) in the splenic cords and sinuses, splenic periarteriolar lymphoid sheaths, hepatic sinusoids, lymph nodes, lung microvasculature, bone marrow, kidney, and epicardium (11).

Less is known about the two fatalities that have been attributed to infection with the HGE agent. Both patients died of multiorgan failure after presenting with cough and pulmonary infiltrates that were obvious upon radiography (3). Diagnosis of the first patient was based upon autopsy findings obtained a week after his death. The second patient's illness was compounded by several factors, including chronic lymphocytic leukemia with Richter's syndrome, high-dose steroid treatment, and previous splenectomy (3).

Diagnosis

Ehrlichia spp. appear as round, dark purple-stained dots or clusters of dots (morulae) in the cytoplasm of leukocytes upon direct microscopic examination of peripheral blood smears or buffy coat preparations stained by Romanowsky-type techniques (e.g., Giemsa, Wright, or Diff-Quik), as shown in Fig. 3.1. Direct examination of such smears is probably useful only during the acute, febrile phase of infection, when organisms are most prevalent. Presence of *E. chaffeensis* in lymphocytes, atypical lymphocytes, band neutrophils, and segmented neutrophils has occasionally been reported, but most organisms are observed in monocytes or macrophages (19, 26).

The search for *E. chaffeensis* via immunohistologic techniques has been made not only with peripheral blood smears but also with formalin-fixed, paraffin-embedded bone marrow biopsy specimens or aspirated marrow. Dumler et al. (12) described use of the biotinylated human anti-*E. chaffeensis*, avidin-alkaline phosphatase or avidin-horseradish peroxidase system. Organisms were detected primarily within histiocytes, but morulae were occasionally present within lymphocytes (12).

The HGE agent has been found only in neutrophils. Direct examination of buffy coats and peripheral blood smears is a lengthy process, as evidenced by the work of Bakken et al. (3), who needed to inspect at least 800 polymorphonuclear granulocytes per smear for evidence of infection with the HGE agent. Immunohistology has also been performed on paraffin-embedded tissue sections from a patient infected with the HGE agent. In order to locate the etiologic agent in the postmortem specimens, equine anti-*E. equi* and bovine anti-*E. phagocytophila* sera were used in a modified immunohistologic method (3). Numerous small (1- to 3-μm-diameter) intracytoplasmic morulae that were not present in control tissues were observed in postmortem spleen and peripheral blood neutrophils (3). The HGE agent has recently been grown in cell culture (17).

The PCR technique has been used to detect both human ehrlichiosis agents known to occur in the United States. PCR primers derived from variable regions of the 16S rRNA gene sequence have been used to amplify DNA from *E. chaffeensis* (1) and the HGE agent (5). In both instances, sensitivity has been increased by using a nested PCR reaction (5, 9). The outside amplification is performed by using either primers derived from a highly conserved region of the 16S rRNA gene sequence or universal primers. The specificity of the assay is dependent upon the inside primers, which bind to the 16S gene of the species in question. Since the HGE agent has only been

> *The search for E. chaffeensis via immunohistologic techniques has been made not only with peripheral blood smears but also with formalin-fixed, paraffin-embedded bone marrow biopsy specimens or aspirated marrow*

amplified from a few patients, the inside primers were designed to amplify a wider group that includes *E. phagocytophila*, *E. equi*, and the HGE agent. As in the case of successful culture, EDTA blood samples for the PCR technique are optimally drawn during the febrile phase of the disease, prior to antibiotic treatment.

Serologic diagnosis of ehrlichial infections is accomplished by using the indirect fluorescent-antibody test (8). Continuously infected macrophage cultures (DH82 cells) are used as the antigen for the *E. chaffeensis* indirect fluorescent antibody test (7). At the Centers for Disease Control and Prevention, human ehrlichiosis due to *E. chaffeensis* is defined by a fourfold change in immunoglobulin G antibody levels. Until 1990, when *E. chaffeensis* was first isolated, *E. canis* was used as the diagnostic antigen. Comparative tests have shown that *E. chaffeensis* antigen is more sensitive for detecting the homologous antibody during the early stages of the disease (4a). Serologically, the HGE agent is detected by testing patients' sera on *E. phagocytophila*-infected neutrophils or *E. equi*-infected leukocytes (5). The majority of patients had a higher antibody titer when *E. equi*-infected cells were used as antigen. However, two patients had a 1:80 titer with *E. phagocytophila* antigen and had a titer of <1:80 with *E. equi* (3).

Pathology and Pathogenesis

Peripheral blood in severely infected patients may display anisocytosis of erythrocytes, decreased platelets with giant platelets, and neutrophils with toxic granulations and Dhole bodies. Differential leukocyte counts show mainly neutrophils, with a large population of neutrophilic bands, few lymphocytes, and increased plasmacytoid lymphocytes. Ehrlichia morulae are in as many as 30% of the mononuclear cells, primarily in monocytes and atypical lymphocytes. Damage to leukocytes and platelets may be direct or indirect. There is experimental evidence for the production of antiplatelet antibodies in canine ehrlichiosis (28).

It is difficult to find ehrlichia morulae in tissues of humans with a normal immune system, but in immunocompromised hosts, morulae can be present in as many as 5 to 10% of perivascular and intravascular mononuclear cells. Morulae of *Ehrlichia* spp. are best demonstrated by using hematoxylin and eosin (H&E) and Brown and Hopps (B&H) stains under oil immersion (Fig. 3.2). B&H staining reveals small, gram-negative, intracellular coccobacilli. There is variable staining with the periodic acid-Schiff technique. Giemsa, Ziehl-Neelsen, Movat, and silver stains are not helpful for demonstrating the organism. In tissues of immunocompetent hosts, *Ehrlichia* spp. are often extremely difficult to find, but they can be quite abundant in those of immunocompromised hosts. Most tissues display accumulations of mononuclear cells, particularly around veins, and vacuolization of parenchymal cells. The predominant perivascular cells are lymphocytes, but plasma cells are also prominent.

Bone marrow may have decreased cellularity, the myeloid/erythroid ratio may be reversed, and there may be erythrophagocytosis and decreased megakaryocytes with ehrlichia morulae in the mononuclear cells. Bone mar-

> *Comparative tests have shown that E. chaffeensis antigen is more sensitive for detecting the homologous antibody during the early stages of the disease*

row biopsy may reveal granulomas (15). The heart may have mild chronic pericarditis and perivascular chronic inflammation with ehrlichia morulae within mononuclear cells of the pericardium and in the perivascular areas. The lung may be congested with extravasation of erythrocytes. Mononuclear cells, edema, and fibrosis may cause a widening of some of the interlobular septi. Focal histiocytic intra-alveolar pneumonia may be present. Perivascular lymphoplasmocytic infiltrations are noted. Morulae are within some intra-alveolar macrophages, atypical perivascular lymphocytes, and type 2 pneumocytes.

The liver retains its lobular architecture, but granulomas may be present (Fig. 3.3). The liver of an ehrlichial patient who became immunocompromised from steroid therapy showed patchy fatty change and hepatocytes with intracytoplasmic vacuoles. Portal areas had chronic inflammatory infiltrates consisting of lymphocytes, atypical lymphocytes, and plasma cells with morulae within atypical lymphocytes. Kidney glomeruli are unremarkable, but the kidney may have chronic interstitial nephritis or tubular casts, as well as morulae within atypical lymphocytes. The spleen may be congested with a heavy mononuclear cell infiltration, and morulae may be visible within mononuclear cells. Brain tissue may also develop a mononuclear meningoencephalitis with congestion and can possibly develop a vasculitis that, if severe, can produce hemorrhage, with ehrlichia morulae within monocytes and lymphocytes (Fig. 3.4). Chronic inflammation is potentially present in virtually every organ.

Immunohistochemistry using monoclonal antibodies against either *E. chaffeensis* or *E. canis* will demonstrate morulae of *E. chaffeensis*, but monoclonal antibodies against *E. sennetsu*, *E. equi*, or *Ehrlichia risticii* are usually negative. Transmission electron microscopy reveals membrane-bound morulae of elementary bodies (Fig. 3.5). The physical appearance of *E. chaffeensis*, as seen by transmission electron microscopy, was indistinguishable from that of *E. canis*, as described in published reports of canine ehrlichiosis. There were, however, rare organisms in some infected cells that had a slightly different appearance. The cause for this difference and how it may relate to the variable staining with the periodic acid-Schiff technique are not known.

The physical appearance of E. chaffeensis, as seen by transmission electron microscopy, was indistinguishable from that of E. canis

Prevention and Treatment

Epidemiologic evidence suggests that both forms of human ehrlichiosis are transmitted by ticks. Therefore, precautions against tick exposure must be taken. A study of military personnel documented that use of permethrin-impregnated clothing is an effective prevention measure (30). However, the availability of this acaricide may be limited in the civilian population. Vaccines are not available for either form of this disease. Recently, Fishbein et al. (15) reported a lower rate of hospitalization, shorter duration of illness, and more rapid defervescence in patients treated with tetracycline than in those treated with other antibiotics. This study also showed that chloramphenicol frequently corrected the pyrexia and other clinical signs within 24 to 48 h. These results contrast with in vitro studies of *E. chaffeensis*, which showed that chloramphenicol was not effective (4).

Conclusion

Because of its nonspecific clinical presentation and varied clinical manifestations, human ehrlichiosis is not commonly recognized by physicians. Since both pathogens are potentially fatal, ehrlichiosis should be considered more frequently in the differential diagnosis of patients with febrile illness after tick exposure, especially if accompanying thrombocytopenia or abnormal liver profiles are present. Patients generally respond to tetracycline therapy within 24 to 48 h after onset of treatment, and complications are rare in promptly treated patients (15).

The PCR technique is a rapid method for confirming the diagnosis of acutely ill, untreated patients. The PCR technique, however, is not widely available; therefore, serologic confirmation is essential. Culture may also be used, but it also is not widely available. To optimize serologic results, acute-phase serum samples should be drawn as early as possible during the acute stage of the disease, and convalescent-phase serum samples should be obtained at least 4 weeks later. Regardless of the currently available testing procedures, the physician must base his or her diagnosis upon clinical and hematologic findings and initiate prompt tetracycline therapy prior to any laboratory confirmation (15). Rapid intervention should help to reduce the morbidity and eliminate the mortality associated with these tick-borne diseases.

Because of its nonspecific clinical presentation and varied clinical manifestations, human ehrlichiosis is not commonly recognized by physicians

Figure 3.1 Peripheral blood smear with three *Ehrlichia* inclusions in mononuclear cell. Wright-Giemsa; original magnification, ×400.

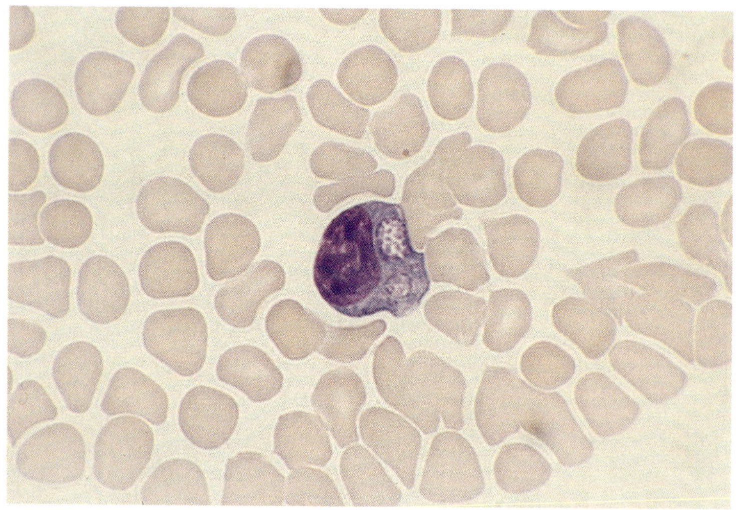

Figure 3.2 Ovary with morula in cytoplasm of lymphocyte (center of figure). H&E; original magnification, ×500.

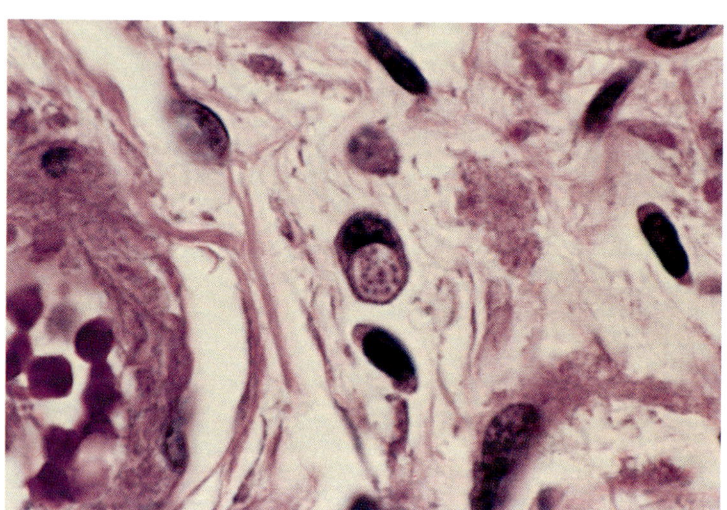

Figure 3.3 Liver with epithelioid cell granulomas, showing the distinctive doughnut shape. H&E; original magnification, ×50.

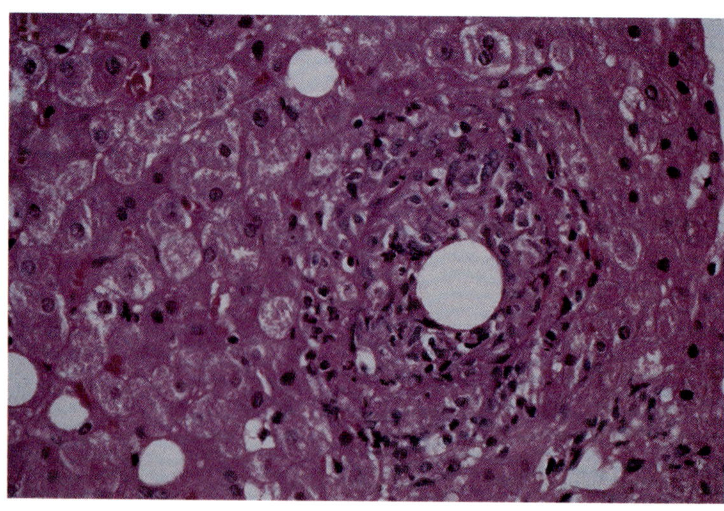

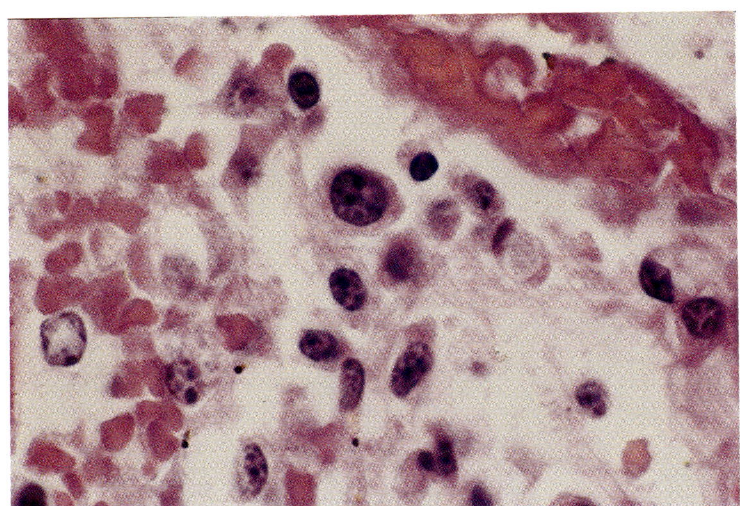

Figure 3.4 Brain with morulae in inflammatory cell in area of hemorrhage. H&E; original magnification, ×400.

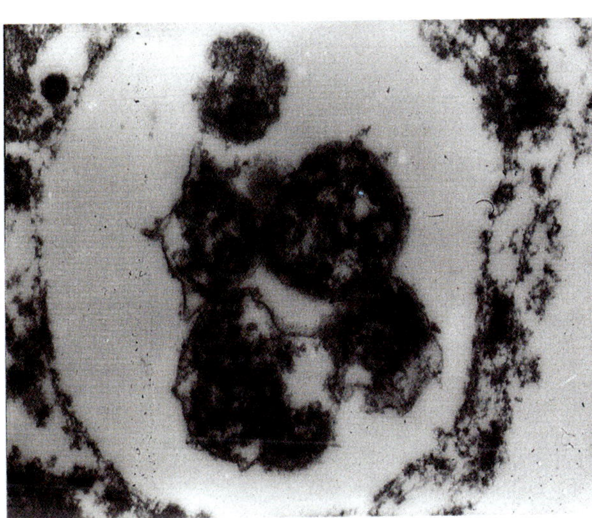

Figure 3.5 Electron micrograph of ehrlichiae in phagosome of a mononuclear cell in the bone marrow. Original magnification, ×21,600.

References

1. **Anderson, B. E., J. E. Dawson, D. C. Jones, and K. H. Wilson.** 1991. *Ehrlichia chaffeensis*, a new species associated with human ehrlichiosis. *J. Clin. Microbiol.* **29:**2838–2842.

2. **Anderson, B. E., K. G. Sims, J. G. Olson, J. E. Childs, J. F. Piesman, C. M. Happ, G. O. Maupin, and B. J. Johnson.** 1993. *Amblyomma americanum*: a potential vector of human ehrlichiosis. *Am. J. Trop. Med. Hyg.* **49:**239–244.

3. **Bakken, J. S., J. S. Dumler, S. M. Chen, M. R. Eckman, L. L. Van Etta, and D. H. Walker.** 1994. Human granulocytic ehrlichiosis in the upper Midwest United States. JAMA **272:**212–218.

4. **Brouqui, P., and D. Raoult.** 1992. In vitro antibiotic susceptibility of the newly recognized agent of ehrlichiosis in humans, *Ehrlichia chaffeensis*. *Antimicrob. Agents Chemother.* **36:**2799–2803.

4a. **Centers for Disease Control and Prevention.** Unpublished data.

5. **Chen, S. -M., J. S. Dumler, J. S. Bakken, and D. H. Walker.** 1994. Identification of a granulocytotropic *Ehrlichia* species as the etiologic agent of human disease. *J. Clin. Microbiol.* **32:**589–595.

6. **Dawson, J., B. E. Anderson, D. B. Fishbein, J. L. Sanchez, C. S. Goldsmith, and K. H. Wilson.** 1991. Isolation and characterization of an *Ehrlichia* sp. from a patient diagnosed with human ehrlichiosis. *J. Clin. Microbiol.* **29:**2741–2745.

7. **Dawson, J. E., and S. A. Ewing.** 1992. Susceptibility of dogs to infection with *Ehrlichia chaffeensis*, causative agent of human ehrlichiosis. *Am. J. Vet. Res.* **53:**1322–1327.

8. **Dawson, J. E., Y. Rikihisa, S. A. Ewing, and D. B. Fishbein.** 1991. Serologic diagnosis of human ehrlichiosis using two *Ehrlichia canis* isolates. *J. Infect. Dis.* **163:**564–567.

9. **Dawson, J. E., D. E. Stallknecht, E. W. Howerth, C. K. Warner, K. L. Biggie, W. R. Davidson, J. M. Lockhart, V. F. Nettles, J. G. Olson, and J. E. Childs.** 1994. Susceptibility of white-tailed deer (*Odocoileus virginianus*) to infection with *Ehrlichia chaffeensis*, the etiologic agent of human ehrlichiosis. *J. Clin. Microbiol.* **32:**2725–2728.

10. **Dumler, J. S.** 1991. Human ehrlichiosis: pathologic findings in three fatal cases, abstr. 510, p. 87A. United States and Canadian Academy of Pathology Annual Meeting, March 17–22, Chicago. United States and Canadian Academy of Pathology, Chicago.

11. **Dumler, J. S., P. Brouqui, and J. Aronson.** 1991. Identification of *Ehrlichia* in human tissue. *N. Engl. J. Med.* **325:**1109–1110.

12. **Dumler, J. S., J. E. Dawson, and D. H. Walker.** 1993. Human ehrlichiosis: hematopathology and immunohistologic detection of *Ehrlichia chaffeensis*. *Hum. Pathol.* **24:**391–396.

13. **Everett, E. D., K. A. Evans, B. Henry, and G. McDonald.** 1994. Human ehrlichiosis after tick exposure. Diagnosis using polymerase chain reaction. *Ann. Intern. Med.* **120:**730–735.

14. **Ewing, S. A.** 1969. Canine ehrlichiosis, p. 331–353. *In* C. A. Brandley and C. E. Cornelius (ed.), *Advances in Veterinary Science and Comparative Medicine.* Academic Press, New York.

15. **Fishbein, D. B., J. E. Dawson, and L. E. Robinson.** 1994. Human ehrlichiosis in the United States, 1985–1990. *Ann. Intern. Med.* **20:**736–743.

16. **Fishbein, D. B., A. Kemp, J. E. Dawson, N. R. Greene, M. A. Redus, and D. H. Fields.** 1989. Human ehrlichiosis: prospective active surveillance in febrile hospitalized patients. *J. Infect. Dis.* **160:**803–809.

17. **Goodman, J. L., C. Nelson, B. Vitale, J. E. Madigan, J. S. Dumler, T. S. Kurtti, and U. G. Munderloh.** 1996. Direct cultivation of the causative agent of human granulocytic ehrlichiosis. *N. Engl. J. Med.* **334:**209–215.

18. **Lewis, G. E.** 1976. Equine ehrlichiosis: a comparison between *E. equi* and other pathogenic species of *Ehrlichia. Vet. Parasitol.* **2:**61–74.

19. **Maeda, K., N. Markowitz, R. C. Hawley, M. Ristic, D. Cox, and J. E. McDade.** 1987. Human infection with *Ehrlichia canis*, a leukocytic rickettsia. *N. Engl. J. Med.* **31:**853–856.

20. **Misao, T., and K. Katsuta.** 1956. Epidemiology of infectious mononucleosis. *Jpn. J. Clin. Exp. Med.* **33:**73–76.

21. **Misao, T., and Y. Kobayashi.** 1954. Studies on infectious mononucleosis. I. Isolation of etiologic agent from blood, bone marrow, and lymph node of a patient with infectious mononucleosis by using mice. *Tokyo Iji Shinshi* **71:**683–686.

22. **Morais, J. D., J. E. Dawson, C. Greene, A. R. Filipe, L. C. Galhardas, and F. Bacellar.** 1991. First European case of ehrlichiosis. *Lancet* **338:**633–634.

23. **Pearce, C. J., M. E. Conrad, P. E. Nolan, D. B. Fishbein, and J. E. Dawson.** 1988. Ehrlichiosis: a cause of bone marrow hypoplasia in humans. *Am. J. Hematol.* **28:**53-55.

24. **Petersen, L. R., L. A. Sawyer, D. B. Fishbein, P. W. Kelley, R. J. Thomas, L. A. Magnarelli, M. A. Redus, and J. E. Dawson.** 1989. An outbreak of ehrlichiosis in members of an Army Reserve Unit exposed to ticks. *J. Infect. Dis.* **159:**562-568.

25. **Reed, K. D., D. H. Persing, and V. Cameron.** 1995. Transmission of human granulocytic ehrlichiosis. *JAMA* **273:**23.

26. **Rynkiewicz, D., and L. X. Liu.** 1994. Human ehrlichiosis in New England. *N. Engl. J. Med.* **330:**292. (Letter.)

27. **Uhaa, I. J., J. D. MacLean, C. R. Greene, and D. B. Fishbein.** 1992. A case of human ehrlichiosis acquired in Mali: clinical and laboratory findings. *Am. J. Trop. Med. Hyg.* **46:**161-164.

28. **Waner, T., S. Harris, D. J. Weiss, H. Bark, and A. Keysary.** 1995. Demonstration of serum antiplatelet antibodies in experimental acute canine ehrlichiosis. *Vet. Immunol. Immunopathol.* **48:**17-82.

29. **Woldehiwet, Z.** 1983. Tick-borne fever. *Vet. Res. Commun.* **6:**163-175.

30. **Yevich, S. J., J. L. Sanchez, R. F. DeFraites, C. Rives, J. E. Dawson, I. J. Uhaa, B. J. Johnson, and D. B. Fishbein.** 1997. Seroepidemiology of infections due to spotted fever group rickettsiae and *Ehrlichia* species in military personnel exposed in areas of the United States where such infections are endemic. *J. Infect. Dis.* **171:**1266–1273.

chapter 4

Microsporidia

David A. Schwartz and Ralph T. Bryan

The term "microsporidia" is used to refer to obligate intracellular protozoan parasites which belong to the order *Microsporida* of the phylum *Microspora*. Microsporidia are ubiquitous in the environment, and they infect a broad range of invertebrates and vertebrates. The taxonomic nomenclature of the microsporidia is complex and rapidly changing, and to date, more than 100 genera and more than 1,000 species have been described. Microsporidia are characterized by the production of spores that contain a unique coiled polar filament through which infective sporoplasm is injected into the host cell (6, 10, 70, 89). Microsporidia are considered true eukaryotes because they have a nucleus with a nuclear membrane, an intracytoplasmic membrane system, and chromosome separation on mitotic spindles. However, they also share some features with prokaryotes, including the lack of mitochondria, Golgi membranes, peroxisomes, and prokaryotic-type ribosomes. These features suggest that the microsporidia are very ancient organisms (6, 70, 89).

David A. Schwartz, Departments of Pathology and Medicine (Infectious Diseases), Emory University School of Medicine, Atlanta, GA 30303, and Centers for Disease Control and Prevention, Atlanta, GA 30333. **Ralph T. Bryan,** National Center for Infectious Diseases, Centers for Disease Control and Prevention, Atlanta, GA 30333.

Pathology of Emerging Infections
Edited by C. Robert Horsburgh, Jr., and Ann Marie Nelson
© 1997 American Society for Microbiology, Washington, DC 20005-4171

In humans, infections with members of the phylum *Microspora* constitute a group of rapidly emerging parasitic diseases which occur predominantly, but not exclusively, in severely immunosuppressed persons with AIDS (6, 10, 70, 89). Six genera of microsporidia from humans have been described; four of these—*Enterocytozoon, Encephalitozoon, Pleistophora,* and *Trachipleistophora*—are reported to infect patients with AIDS (6, 39, 53, 75). *Vittaforma corneum* (formerly *Nosema corneum*), *Nosema connori,* and *Nosema ocularum* have also been identified as human pathogens, but they have not yet been reported to occur in human immunodeficiency virus (HIV)-infected persons (89). The initial descriptions of microsporidial infections in AIDS patients occurred in 1985. Subsequently, the number of reported cases and the clinical spectrum of disease have increased remarkably. For example, although *Enterocytozoon bieneusi* was not described prior to 1985, it has now become one of the most frequently identified pathogens in the intestinal tract of patients infected with HIV (42, 52, 89).

In many hospitals throughout the world, however, microsporidial infection is often either not suspected or incorrectly diagnosed. The diagnosis of microsporidiosis may be difficult for several reasons: the organisms are minute (the smallest species infecting humans are 1 to 2.5 µm) and not easily seen in biopsy, cytology, or stool specimens when routine stains are used; ultrastructural examination is not practical for use as a screening method and is frequently unavailable; serological testing is not currently useful as an indicator of active infection; and the specialized methods of diagnosis, including tissue culture, antibody staining, and molecular pathology techniques, are currently available in only a few specialized laboratories (67).

Microsporidial infections are a significant cause of morbidity and, occasionally, mortality in patients with AIDS. In addition, they are being identified in patients with posttransplant immunosuppression and in immunocompetent persons with traveler's diarrhea (11, 61, 64, 65, 79, 86). It is increasingly important for physicians and laboratorians to be knowledgeable regarding the clinical presentation, methods for diagnosis, and therapy of these agents.

Microsporidia Infecting Humans

Enterocytozoon bieneusi

E. bieneusi was initially described by Desportes and colleagues as a new species of microsporidian occurring in the intestines and stool of AIDS patients with chronic diarrhea (24). It shares the family *Enterocytozoonidae* with one other organism, *Enterocytozoon salmonis,* an intranuclear parasite of salmonid fish (89).

E. bieneusi is one of the most prevalent intestinal pathogens identified in patients with AIDS, and the organisms can spread into the hepatobiliary tree to infect biliary and pancreatic duct epithelial cells. The most common anatomic location of *E. bieneusi* is within the cytoplasm of superficial lining epithelial cells of the small intestine. *Enterocytozoon* infection is associated with chronic diarrhea and wasting syndrome. In patients with hepatobiliary infection, it can cause papillary stenosis, sclerosing cholangitis of both intra-

Although Enterocytozoon bieneusi was not described prior to 1985, it has now become one of the most frequently identified pathogens in the intestinal tract of patients infected with HIV

and extrahepatic bile ducts, and acalculous cholecystitis (51, 56, 58, 89). Unlike other microsporidial species causing infections in HIV-infected patients, *E. bieneusi* rarely produces systemic infections (88–90).

E. bieneusi is the smallest microsporidian reported to infect humans. All developmental stages are formed in direct contact with the host cell cytoplasm, and no sporophorous vesicles or pansporoblastic membranes are present. It produces elongated nuclei early in development which are unique to this genus. The proliferative and sporogonial stages are rounded, multinucleated plasmodia measuring up to 6 μm in diameter. Also unique to this genus is the presence of electron-dense discs which are precursors to the polar tubule and anchoring discs. The mature spores are oval, measure approximately 1 to 1.6 μm in length and 0.7 to 1 μm in width, and contain five to seven turns of the coiled polar tubule which appear in two rows by electron microscopy (Fig. 4.1 and 4.2) (89).

Encephalitozoon (Septata) intestinalis

E. intestinalis was first identified from AIDS patients with diarrhea by Cali and colleagues in 1993 (12). The agent was initially named *Septata intestinalis* because of the ultrastructural observation of unique septations occurring between spores in the cytoplasm of infected cells. It is the second most prevalent microsporidial infection in AIDS patients reported. In a study from the United States, the ratio of intestinal infection with *E. intestinalis* to that with *E. bieneusi* was 1:10 (42). A recent German investigation of 20 HIV-positive patients with intestinal microsporidiosis, including persons both with and without diarrhea, also found that *E. intestinalis* infection occurs at approximately 10% of the frequency of *Enterocytozoon* infection (80). *E. intestinalis* is present throughout the small intestine, where developing stages and spores are found in the cytoplasm of enterocytes and in fibroblasts, macrophages, and endothelial cells of the lamina propria (12, 54, 55, 70, 80). It can also infect the colon and hepatobiliary tree. Similar to that seen with *E. bieneusi*, the most common clinical presentation of *E. intestinalis* infection is severe chronic diarrhea which often progresses to malabsorption and wasting syndrome. Unlike *E. bieneusi*, however, *E. intestinalis* frequently disseminates to involve other organs, including the bronchi, renal tubules, nasal epithelium, and the eye (36, 50, 89).

E. intestinalis has developmental stages which are somewhat similar to those of the other two species of *Encephalitozoon* which infect humans (*E. cuniculi* and *E. hellem*). Meronts of *Encephalitozoon* spp. proliferate by cellular elongation and development of cytoplasmic invaginations between nuclei. Sporonts also divide by fission. Similar to that of *E. hellem* and *E. cuniculi*, sporogony of *E. intestinalis* occurs in the cytoplasm within a parasitophorous vacuole of host origin. The proliferative cells of *E. intestinalis* are uni-, bi-, or tetranucleated. Sporogony is tetrasporous. The most obvious diagnostic ultrastructural feature that characterizes *E. intestinalis* is the formation of a parasite-secreted fibrillar matrix surrounding the developing organisms. This gives the parasitophorous vacuole a septated, or honeycombed, appearance (Fig. 4.3). Another unique finding is the presence of tubular appendages, up to 1.2 μm in length and 50 nm in diameter, which

The most common clinical presentation of E. intestinalis infection is severe chronic diarrhea which often progresses to malabsorption and wasting syndrome

originate from the sporont surface and end in a bulbular structure. The mature spores of *E. intestinalis* measure 2.0 by 1.2 µm and contain a single row of polar tubule coils with four to seven turns (89).

Recommendations were made to change the taxonomic status of this agent from *S. intestinalis* to *E. intestinalis* on the basis of the results of genetic and immunological analyses (37); most authors now designate this agent *E. intestinalis* in the medical literature.

Encephalitozoon cuniculi

E. cuniculi, the first microsporidian to be recognized as a parasite of mammals, was initially described as an infection in rabbits in 1922. It has a broad host range, infecting birds, carnivores, rodents, and other mammals, including primates (6, 70, 89). In nonhuman hosts, *E. cuniculi* has a predilection for the brain and kidneys, but it also infects macrophages, the vascular endothelium, and epithelial cells in a variety of organs.

Encephalitozoon infections of humans were rarely reported prior to the AIDS pandemic (4, 9, 48). Prior to the identification of *E. hellem* as a separate species in 1991, all *Encephalitozoon* infections in patients with AIDS were believed to be due to *E. cuniculi*. Most of these patients had microsporidial keratoconjunctivitis, but extraocular infections due to *E. cuniculi* in one patient with hepatitis and another with peritonitis were described (13, 14, 82, 89, 95). Since 1991, most human infections with *Encephalitozoon* spp. have been found to be due to *E. hellem* (25, 71). A patient with widely disseminated *E. cuniculi* infection, including involvement of the central nervous system, heart, kidneys, spleen, lymph nodes, adrenal glands, and trachea, has recently been reported (49). In the few cases of human infection by *E. cuniculi* which have been confirmed by molecular or antigenic analysis, there have been no confirmed instances of transmission of microsporidial infections from animals to humans (21, 35).

E. cuniculi develops in an intracytoplasmic parasitophorous vacuole bounded by a membrane presumably of host cell origin. The nuclei of all stages of both *E. cuniculi* and *E. hellem* are unpaired. Meronts divide by binary fission, are round to ovoid structures measuring 2 to 6 by 1 to 3 µm, and lie in close proximity to the vacuolar membrane. Sporonts lie free in the center of the vacuole and divide into two sporoblasts which then mature into spores. The spores of both *E. hellem* and *E. cuniculi* measure 2 to 2.5 by 1 to 1.5 µm and have five to seven turns of the coiled polar tubule in a single row (6, 89).

Encephalitozoon hellem

E. hellem is a newly described microsporidian which is morphologically indistinguishable by light and electron microscopy from *E. cuniculi* (70). Before 1991, it was assumed that all human isolates of *Encephalitozoon* spp. causing infection were *E. cuniculi*. However, in that year, Didier and colleagues utilized biochemical and antigenic methods to describe a new species of *Encephalitozoon*, named *E. hellem*, from the eyes of three patients with AIDS and keratoconjunctivitis (25). Shortly thereafter, the first patient with disseminated infection and renal failure due to *E. hellem* was

> *Prior to the identification of E. hellem as a separate species in 1991, all Encephalitozoon infections in patients with AIDS were believed to be due to E. cuniculi*

described (67), and following this, a second patient with systemic *E. hellem* infection and bronchiolitis was reported (72). The potential of *E. hellem* to cause disseminated disease in patients with AIDS has now been clearly demonstrated (6, 67, 68, 70, 72, 89). Infections of the trachea, bronchus, lungs, kidneys, ureters, bladder, prostate, nose and paranasal sinuses, cornea, conjunctiva, liver, and peritoneum have been described (70, 89). Unlike *E. cuniculi*, *E. hellem* has never been isolated from a nonhuman host, and little is known of the epidemiology or source of infection with this agent. However, an autopsy of one untreated patient with disseminated *E. hellem* infection demonstrated numerous organisms within the lining epithelium of almost the entire length of the tracheobronchial tree, suggesting a respiratory tract portal of entry and dissemination (67).

The developmental stages and ultrastructural features of *E. hellem* are similar to those of *E. cuniculi* (Fig. 4.4).

Pleistophora sp.

Pleistophora sp. is a microsporidial parasite of insects and fish, including neon tetras, a common aquarium fish. *Pleistophora* sp. has been isolated from the skeletal muscles of two patients (16, 45), one of whom had confirmed AIDS.

Pleistophora sp. develops within the cytoplasm of host skeletal muscle cells. The parasite secretes a thick, amorphous vesicle, surrounding and isolating itself from the host cell cytoplasm. This is termed a sporophorous vesicle. The nuclei of all developmental stages are unpaired, and merogonic proliferation results in multinucleated plasmodia. Sporogony is multisporous and produces large numbers of spores within the sporophorous vesicle. Mature spores measure 2.8 by 3.2 to 3.4 μm and have 9 to 12 coils of the polar tubule (70, 89).

Trachipleistophora hominis

A newly identified microsporidian species, *T. hominis*, has been described as an agent of myositis and disseminated disease in patients with AIDS, adding to the growing list of microsporidial pathogens of humans (32, 39, 94). The initial recognition of this new genus and species of microsporidian occurred in 1996, when it was isolated from the skeletal muscle of a patient with AIDS and myositis (39). Since then, it has also been identified as causing ring-enhancing lesions of the cerebrum and hippocampus, associated with seizures and other symptoms referable to the central nervous system (32, 94). Auopsy of these patients has revealed disseminated disease also involving the heart, thyroid, pancreas, parathyroids, liver, spleen, bone marrow, and lymph nodes. In culture, meronts of this microsporidian have two to four nuclei and divide by binary fission. A sporophorous vesicle, in which sporoblasts are formed by repeated binary fission, is present. The number of sporoblasts, and later spores, within the sporophorous vesicle varies from 2 to greater than 32. Mature spores measure 4.0 by 2.4 μm and have a prominent posterior vacuole. This parasite differs from *Pleistophora* sp. in that it does not form multinucleated sporogonial plasmodia and the sporophorous vesicle enlarges during sporogony and its wall is not multilayered.

The initial recognition of T. hominis occurred in 1996, when it was isolated from the skeletal muscle of a patient with AIDS and myositis

Vittaforma (Nosema) corneae

Nosema spp. are well-described parasites of a variety of invertebrates. Human ocular disease caused by *Nosema corneum*, which has recently been reassigned to the genus *Vittaforma*, has been reported (77). Rare human infections caused by other *Nosema* spp. have also been described (see below).

> *The ultrastructural features of V. corneae are sufficient to distinguish this parasite from the other microsporidian pathogens of humans*

The ultrastructural features of *V. corneae* are sufficient to distinguish this parasite from the other microsporidian pathogens of humans. Development of the parasite takes place in direct contact with the host cell cytoplasm. Nuclei are diplokaryotic, sporogony is polysporoblastic, and sporonts are ribbon shaped, constricting to give rise to linear arrays of sporoblasts. Each parasite is enveloped by a complete cisterna of host endoplasmic reticulum. The spores of *V. corneae* measure 3.8 by 1 μm and have five to seven turns of the coiled polar tubule (77, 89).

Nosema spp.

N. connori infection was first described in 1973, associated with disseminated infection in an athymic child which involved almost all of the tissues examined at autopsy. Not all stages of the parasite were seen, and only sporoblasts with immature and mature spores could be identified in these tissues. The mature spores of *N. connori* are diplokaryotic, measure 4 to 4.5 by 2 to 2.5 μm, and have approximately 11 turns of the coiled polar tubule. This microsporidian develops in direct contact with the host cell cytoplasm. Another *Nosema* species, *N. ocularum*, was identified from biopsy samples from a person with a corneal ulcer. The spores measured 3 by 5 μm and contained polar tubules with 11 to 12 turns (89).

Uncharacterized Microsporidia

Microsporidian pathogens of humans which are not sufficiently characterized to be confidently assigned to a known genus are designated with the collective term *Microsporidium*. These include *Microsporidium africanum*, a parasite found in the stroma of a perforated corneal ulcer from a woman from Botswana, and *Microsporidium ceylonensis*, isolated from a corneal ulcer in a young boy from Sri Lanka (6, 10, 89).

Epidemiology

Human microsporidial infections are globally dispersed and have been documented in persons from all continents except Antarctica. Recently, increasing numbers of patients with microsporidial infections from tropical and developing nations have been reported (10, 83). It has become clear that although microsporidiosis appears to occur most frequently in severely immunocompromised persons infected with HIV, it is emerging as an important infection in other immunosuppressed patients (e.g., organ transplant recipients), as well as in immunocompetent individuals. Unfortunately, very little is currently known about risks for infection or modes of transmission.

The documentation of microsporidial spores in urine and respiratory secretions, in addition to the presence of spores in stool and duodenal aspirates, suggests a potential role for person-to-person transmission (67, 72, 84, 88, 91). Fecal-oral contamination may play a role in the transmission of intestinal microsporidiosis; reports of "asymptomatic" *E. bieneusi* intestinal infections (enteric carriage) support this idea (60). Thus, it is likely that *E. bieneusi* is acquired by ingestion, similar to acquisition of other enteric protozoa, such as *Giardia, Isospora, Entamoeba,* and *Cryptosporidium* spp. Also, the extensive genitourinary tract involvement seen with *E. hellem* and *E. intestinalis* infections raises the possibility of person-to-person transmission by sexual means (17, 74).

The occurrence of pulmonary infections suggests that microsporidial infections can be acquired by inhalation or transmitted via aerosolized respiratory secretions, and histopathologic evidence for respiratory acquisition has been reported (67, 90, 91). The presence of *Encephalitozoon* spores in urine and respiratory secretions has also led to the suggestion that ocular infections with this agent may be acquired by external autoinoculation, perhaps by contaminated fingers (63, 71).

Ingestion or inhalation of spore-laden urine contaminating animal cages is an established means of *E. cuniculi* transmission in rabbits and other laboratory animals, suggesting that comparable forms of environmental exposure could lead to human infections. The presence of spores in surface water samples also suggests the possibility of environmentally acquired infection, but no human-infecting microsporidia have yet been identified from such sources (3). It has been suggested that microsporidia are likely to be waterborne pathogens, but there are currently no epidemiologic or environmental data to support this claim.

Transmission of *E. cuniculi* in many mammalian hosts, including blue foxes, dogs, and squirrel monkeys, occurs by transplacental infection. Although transplacental transmission of *E. cuniculi* occurs in rabbits and rodents, most infections in these mammals probably occur by another mechanism following birth. No confirmed or suspected cases of congenital microsporidiosis in humans have been reported.

Transmission of E. cuniculi in many mammalian hosts occurs by transplacental infection

Human microsporidiosis may be a zoonotic disease, but definitive proof is still lacking. Animal reservoirs for *E. cuniculi* are well known, but *E. hellem* and *E. intestinalis* have been confirmed only in human hosts. *E. cuniculi* was the first microsporidian to be reported as a parasite of mammals, and human infections confirmed by immunological or nucleic acid methods have been reported (21, 35). Initial reports of *Encephalitozoon* sp.-associated keratoconjunctivitis mentioned that cat or bird ownership was common among case patients, but a causal association has never been confirmed (15, 67). Despite this lack of proof, seemingly identical strains of *E. cuniculi* have recently been isolated from three HIV-infected patients and nine rabbits, strongly suggesting that at least *E. cuniculi* is a zoonotic parasite (22). *E. bieneusi* has recently been identified in the hepatobiliary tract and intestines of simian immunodeficiency virus-infected rhesus monkeys, but the epidemiologic significance of this remains unclear (1b, 46a).

E. hellem from a nonhuman host has never been reported. However, this agent is morphologically similar to *E. cuniculi*. Thus, it is possible that infections which were diagnosed prior to the initial description of *E. hellem* in 1991 and which were thought to be due to *E. cuniculi* were, in fact, due to the latter microsporidian. Patients with *E. hellem* infections usually present with ocular, sinonasal, and tracheobronchial infections, suggestive of an upper respiratory mechanism of acquiring the infection. Because these patients often have disseminated infection and shed infective spores in the urine, there is a possibility of autoinoculation or human-to-human infection via contaminated fingers. *E. hellem* and *E. bieneusi* infections in cohabitating patients with AIDS have been observed (personal observation).

Clinical Findings

HIV/AIDS Patients

E. bieneusi

E. bieneusi has frequently been associated with chronic diarrhea and/or biliary illness in severely immunodeficient HIV-infected patients, particularly in those with CD4+ cell counts below 50 to 100/mm^3 and otherwise unexplained chronic diarrhea (10, 30, 52, 53, 58). *E. bieneusi*-associated diarrhea is, however, being seen and reported more frequently even in patients with relatively preserved CD4+ cell counts (59, 81).

Chronic diarrhea, anorexia, and weight loss are the most commonly reported clinical manifestations of *E. bieneusi* infections in persons with AIDS. Patients typically report from 3 to 10 bowel movements per day, but daily stool frequency may range from 1 to over 20. Stools are loose to watery and, unless the patient is coinfected with invasive intestinal pathogens, nonbloody and without fecal leukocytes (2, 6, 8, 31, 51–53, 89, 93). Diarrhea may be worsened by foods and may be more frequent in the morning (2). Diarrhea tends to develop gradually in most patients and may be less voluminous than that seen in patients with cryptosporidiosis. The increased stool frequency (with incontinence in severe cases), malabsorption, and weight loss associated with *E. bieneusi* infections often result in a protracted debilitating illness that impacts severely on the infected person's quality of life (2, 92). Prolonged diarrhea for up to 48 months has been reported, and others have documented persistent *E. bieneusi* infections of 21 to 24 months (92). Laboratory evidence for intestinal malabsorption is common, including one report of zinc deficiency (75). CD4+ lymphocyte counts are usually low (<100 cells/mm^3).

Other signs and symptoms reported in association with *E. bieneusi* intestinal infections include abdominal pain, nausea, vomiting, and fever. These findings are often seen in patients with concomitant biliary infection, which typically produces clinical manifestations consistent with cholangitis or cholecystitis. *E. bieneusi* is now recognized as at least one cause of AIDS-related sclerosing cholangitis (57, 58) and has been implicated in at least two cases of chronic acalculous cholecystitis (6, 8, 41, 89). In most patients with recognized biliary *E. bieneusi* infection, chronic diarrhea is also present and right upper quadrant abdominal pain is common. Clinical jaundice is rarely evident. Imaging procedures (abdominal ultrasonography and computerized tomography, endoscopic ultrasonography, and ERCP) often reveal dilatation of both intrahepatic and common bile ducts, irregularities of the bile duct wall, and gall bladder abnormalities such as wall thickening, distension, or the presence of sludge. Papillary stenosis may also be present. Laboratory values for serum alkaline phosphatase, gamma glutamyltrans-

> *E. bieneusi has frequently been associated with chronic diarrhea and/or biliary illness in severely immunodeficient HIV-infected patients*

ferase, and aspartate and alanine aminotransferases are usually elevated (2 to 3 times the upper limit of normal), but bilirubin is usually normal (58).

In the only reported case of pulmonary involvement with *E. bieneusi*, Weber and colleagues described a patient with chronic diarrhea who developed a persistent cough (with scant, nonpurulent sputum), dyspnea, and wheezing. A chest roentgenogram revealed minimal interstitial infiltrates and a small pleural effusion. Spores of *E. bieneusi* were detected in bronchoalveolar lavage fluid, transbronchial biopsy specimens, stool, and ileal biopsy specimens. Death of the patient was attributed to severe wasting syndrome (90).

Although reports of deaths directly attributable to *E. bieneusi* are rare, reported mortality rates in patients with intestinal *E. bieneusi* are as high as 56% (30, 51); death rates in persons with biliary infections may be even higher (58).

E. intestinalis

Diarrheal and biliary illness associated with enteric *E. intestinalis* infection is similar to that seen with *E. bieneusi*, with the exception that acute colitis in a case of *E. intestinalis* infection has been described in at least instance (29). *E. intestinalis* has also been shown to disseminate, particularly to the kidneys (12, 54, 55, 80). Leukocyturia is relatively common and sometimes is associated with dysuria or frequency (36, 50). Recent reports suggest, however, that the complete clinical spectrum of *E. intestinalis* infections is still being described and will likely parallel that of the other human-infecting *Encephalitozoon* species (see "*E. hellem* and *E. cuniculi*," below) and will likely include sinusitis, bronchitis, and keratoconjunctivitis (36, 50, 78). Prostatitis and purulent urethritis have also been reported (17, 50).

> *E. intestinalis has been shown to disseminate, particularly to the kidneys*

E. hellem and E. cuniculi

In persons infected with *E. hellem* or *E. cuniculi*, keratoconjunctivitis has often been the first and most commonly recognized clinical manifestation. Symptoms include dry eyes, foreign body sensation, ocular pain, excessive tearing, blurred vision, and photophobia, all of which may range from mild to severe (6, 13–15, 71, 89, 91). Purulent discharge is absent unless the microsporidial infection is accompanied by bacterial superinfection. Ophthalmologic slit lamp examination often reveals a characteristic diffuse, superficial, punctate keratopathy. Infection is frequently bilateral, but not all patients exhibit keratopathy, as cases with only mild conjunctivitis have been reported (71, 91). Corneal ulceration rarely, if ever, occurs. Coexisting cytomegalovirus retinitis may be present (in three of seven patients in one report [71]), but retinal involvement with *Encephalitozoon* spp. has not been reported.

Although most known cases of HIV-associated *E. hellem* or *E. cuniculi* infection were initially diagnosed because of symptomatic keratoconjunctivitis, it now appears that ocular disease rarely, if ever, occurs in the absence of systemic microsporidial infection (21, 43, 67, 72, 82, 91, 95). As with *Enterocytozoon* infection, CD4+ lymphocyte counts in AIDS patients with these infections are generally low. Severity may range from essentially asymptomatic infection to chronic rhinosinusitis to lethal respiratory or renal failure. Currently, the spectrum of recognized *E. hellem-* and *E. cuniculi*-associated disease in AIDS patients includes bronchiolitis (46, 72), sinusitis (21, 43), nephritis (21, 67), cystitis/ureteritis (67), urethritis and prostatitis (74), hepatitis (82), and peritonitis (95). Cerebritis associated with seizures has recently been associated with *E. cuniculi* infection (23, 49). Asymptomatic *E. cuniculi* infection of the gastrointestinal tract (35) and *E. cuniculi*-associated interstitial pneumonitis (22) have also been reported.

Pleistophora sp.

A single case of myositis due to *Pleistophora* sp. has been reported in a 33-year-old Haitian man with AIDS and a history of *Pneumocystis* pneumonia. He developed diffuse myalgias and muscular weakness that began in his calves and spread to the posterior thighs and upper extremities. Physical examination revealed cachexia, proximal muscular tenderness, apparently normal strength and tone in all muscles, and a normal neurological examination. Laboratory tests were notable for elevated serum levels of creatinine phosphokinase (2,914 U/liter), aldolase (21.1 U/liter), lactate dehydrogenase (527 U/liter), and myoglobin (958 g/liter). Motor and sensory nerve conduction studies were consistent with mild lower extremity axonal neuropathy; electromyography suggested a diffuse, active myopathic process with denervation characteristic of inflammatory myopathy. Muscle biopsies revealed focal areas of atrophic muscle fibers containing clusters of microsporidia and scant inflammatory infiltrates. All developmental stages of *Pleistophora* sp. were present (16).

T. hominis

The few reported patients with *T. hominis* infection have presented either with diffuse myalgia and muscular weakness as a result of microsporidial myositis or with symptoms referable to the central nervous system (seizures, declining mental status) as a result of brain involvement (32, 39, 94)

Non-HIV-Infected Immunosuppressed Hosts

Human microsporidial infections remain relatively rare outside of HIV-infected populations, even in persons with other forms of immunosuppression. To date, four patients with systemic microsporidial infection and documented or presumed cellular immunodeficiency other than AIDS have been described: a 3-year-old child with systemic *Encephalitozoon* infection and cellular immune deficiency of unknown etiology (4); a 4-month-old boy with thymic aplasia and systemic *Nosema* infection (47); a 9-year-old boy who presented with symptoms of recurrent fever, loss of consciousness, headache, and convulsions and had an *Encephalitozoon* sp. isolated from his cerebrospinal fluid and urinary sediments (48); and a 20-year-old male with muscular infection due to *Pleistophora* sp. (45).

In addition to these four cases, a few patients with presumably localized microsporidial infections and non-HIV-associated immunosuppression have been recently reported. All infections were associated with diarrheal syndromes without obvious evidence for systemic dissemination. One case oc-

> *H*uman microsporidial infections remain relatively rare outside of HIV-infected populations, even in persons with other forms of immunosuppression

curred in a liver transplant recipient; *E. bieneusi* was implicated (65). In 1996, *E. bieneusi* was diagnosed in an HIV-negative heart-lung transplant recipient who developed diarrhea and massive weight loss (61). No other etiologic agent was identified, and the infection persisted despite treatment with albendazole. *E. cuniculi* infection of a transplanted kidney was recently diagnosed by polymerase chain reaction and light and electron microscopy in a female patient approximately 7 months after receiving a kidney/pancreatic transplant. In addition to renal failure, she also had encephalitis and cardiomyopathy of uncertain etiology (69a).

Immunocompetent Hosts

A few isolated case reports have confirmed that microsporidium-associated diarrheal illness does occur in HIV-negative, otherwise healthy, immunocompetent persons. The first case reported was that of a 26-year-old German medical student who had traveled through Egypt and Jordan in 1992. He sought medical attention 2 days after returning with complaints of a 7-day history of nonbloody diarrhea. Stool parasite examinations revealed microsporidial spores. Stool electron microscopy confirmed the presence of *E. bieneusi*. Further electron microscopy detected no enteropathogenic viruses, and routine bacterial cultures were negative. His diarrhea was self-limited and resolved without treatment after 2 weeks. A comprehensive laboratory evaluation revealed no evidence of immunosuppression (64).

Another report from Germany describes the case of a 3-year-old Turkish girl who had accompanied her family on a return trip to rural Turkey in 1994. While in Turkey, she developed profuse watery diarrhea, nausea, and vomiting. Upon her return to Germany, she was hospitalized for weight loss and dehydration. Stool parasite examination revealed both *Cryptosporidium parvum* and *E. bieneusi* (the latter was confirmed by electron microscopy). A search for other parasitic, bacterial, or viral enteropathogens was negative. The girl was HIV negative, and lymphocyte subset analysis and immunoglobulin levels were normal. Her diarrhea resolved within 6 weeks without specific antiparasitic therapy; repeat stool examinations at that time revealed neither parasite (79).

A third case occurred in a 26-year-old nurse from Switzerland who developed watery diarrhea, nausea, abdominal pain, and fever. Comprehensive stool examinations revealed only *E. bieneusi*. Serologic assays for hepatitis A, B, C, and E, cytomegalovirus, Epstein Barr virus, and HIV were negative; CD4+ lymphocyte counts were normal. Her illness resolved spontaneously after 14 days (33).

Pathology

The Eye and Ocular Adnexa

E. hellem and *E. cuniculi* are the microsporidia most frequently isolated from the eye in patients with AIDS (6, 70, 71, 89). In these patients, characteristic microsporidian spores are present in the corneal and conjunctival epithelium of ocular biopsies (Fig. 4.5). Unlike *V. (Nosema) corneae* ocular infections which occur in immunocompetent persons, *Encephalitozoon* infections do not extend beyond the level of the corneal or conjunctival epithelium (70). Because *E. hellem* and *E. cuniculi* cannot be distinguished by morphological features alone, immunofluorescent-antibody or molecular pathological methods should be performed on biopsies or cytological specimens from the eye if a species-level diagnosis is desired (70, 71, 75).

E. intestinalis from the conjunctiva of one patient with AIDS has recently been identified; this organism can be easily confused with other *Encephalitozoon* species in biopsy or cytological specimens unless fluorescent-antibody staining or electron microscopy is performed.

V. corneae can produce ocular infections that are characterized by deep, stromal infections of the cornea in otherwise healthy, non-HIV-infected patients. Of four patients with severe keratitis reported, corneal ulcers occurred in two. Histologic findings in patients with corneal infection have varied from intact stromal lamellae with scant inflammation to necrotizing keratitis. The organisms have been found both free in the corneal stroma and within the cytoplasm of histiocytes, but never within epithelial cells, as is seen with *Encephalitozoon* spp. (89).

N. ocularum has been reported to be associated with a corneal ulcer and keratitis in an immunocompetent person following removal of an ocular foreign body (13). The infection was identified following corneal biopsy.

Respiratory Tract

Respiratory tract infection due to microsporidia is associated almost exclusively with disseminated disease produced by members of the genus *Encephalitozoon* (46, 70). Three microsporidian species, *E. hellem*, *E. cuniculi*, and *E. intestinalis*, have been reported to infect the respiratory tract. However, our understanding of the spectrum of pathologic changes in the lungs of persons with microsporidiosis has been limited, because the identification of these agents as pulmonary pathogens has occurred only recently and because only a limited number of cases have been examined by biopsy or autopsy.

Several patients with microsporidian infection of the upper respiratory tract, including sinus and nasal infections, have been documented (Fig. 4.6 and 4.7). The pathologic features of sinonasal microsporidiosis are nonspecific and include rhinitis, sinusitis, and nasal polyposis (43, 69, 70).

Microsporidial infection of the lower respiratory tract, either with or without symptoms, appears to be a common component of disseminated microsporidiosis (Fig. 4.8 and 4.9) (6, 46, 70–73, 91). A recent study of patients presenting with keratoconjunctivitis due to *E. hellem* showed a significant number of persons had microsporidian spores present in sputum, even though they had no pulmonary symptoms (71). A patient with AIDS, disseminated *E. hellem* infection, microsporidian spores present in sputum, and no respiratory symptoms has also been described (91).

In addition to asymptomatic respiratory tract colonization, several AIDS patients with symptomatic *Encephalitozoon* sp.-associated pulmonary disease have been described (46). Autopsy of the initial patient with disseminated *E. hellem* infection revealed massive numbers of microsporidian spores that were present diffusely throughout the entire length of the tracheobronchial

V. corneae can produce ocular infections that are characterized by deep, stromal infections of the cornea in otherwise healthy, non-HIV-infected patients

tree, extending into terminal bronchioles and associated in some areas with an erosive tracheitis, bronchitis, and bronchiolitis (67). This confluent pattern of microsporidial colonization of the superficial tracheobronchial mucosa, extending into terminal bronchioles, was suggestive of a respiratory mechanism of acquisition (Fig. 4.9). The pulmonary findings from this case have been confirmed by subsequent biopsies of patients having pulmonary *E. hellem* infections, which demonstrated bronchiolitis with or without pneumonia (46, 72). In addition to *E. hellem*, *E. cuniculi* pulmonary infection has been reported in an AIDS patient with bronchiolitis and pneumonia, which was confirmed by fluorescent-antibody and nucleic acid analysis (21). Microsporidian spores were present in the bronchial lining and alveolar spaces of an open lung biopsy, in the soft tissues of the maxillary sinus, and beneath a chronic tongue ulcer.

E. cuniculi pulmonary infection has been reported in an AIDS patient with bronchiolitis and pneumonia

E. intestinalis can also infect the respiratory tract, where it is associated with a clinical presentation similar to those of *E. hellem* and *E. cuniculi* (50, 54). There are scant data available on the pulmonary pathologic findings of *E. intestinalis* infection; however, spores in bronchial epithelial cells and from bronchoalveolar lavage fluid have been described (54).

E. bieneusi has been identified in a bronchial biopsy and bronchoalveolar lavage specimen from one AIDS patient with pulmonary symptoms (90). However, the occurrence of lung involvement in patients infected with *Enterocytozoon* spp. is probably very rare.

Genitourinary Tract

Urinary tract microsporidiosis appears to be common in patients with *Encephalitozoon* infections (6, 36, 50, 70, 89). In patients with AIDS and *Encephalitozoon* infections, there is frequently simultaneous infection of the eyes, urinary tract, and bronchial tree, although many persons will not have symptoms referable to the kidneys or bladder (6, 70, 75, 89). The autopsy of a patient with disseminated *E. hellem* infection revealed that the urinary tract was the most severely affected system (Fig. 4.10 and 4.11) (67). The kidneys showed a geographic pattern of chronic and granulomatous interstitial nephritis, composed mostly of plasma cells and lymphocytes, with lesser numbers of histiocytes and neutrophils. Extensive tubular necrosis was present, and the lumina of many necrotic tubules was filled with amorphous, granular material. Coalescence of inflammatory cells around some necrotic tubules resulted in microabscesses and poorly formed granulomas. Tissue Gram stain revealed that microsporidian spores were concentrated in necrotic renal tubules and, to a lesser extent, in the interstitium. The glomeruli were spared (67, 70).

Because of the propensity for *Encephalitozoon* spp. to infect the renal tubular epithelium, spores can be transported in urine from the kidneys to the lower urinary tract, resulting in necrotizing ureteritis, cystitis, and urethritis. Microsporidian spores can be identified in macrophages, urothelial cells, and extracellularly in the bladder and ureteral mucosa. The majority of persons with urinary tract involvement will be diagnosed by urine cytology (Fig. 4.12); however, bladder and renal biopsy techniques can also be used to establish the diagnosis (70, 75).

Genital tract infection by microsporidia, consisting of a large, central prostatic abscess, in one patient with severe urinary tract involvement due to *E. hellem* has been described (74). This abscess probably resulted from extension of an infection of the prostatic urethral mucosa. Spores were present within necrotic abscess material and adjacent granulation tissue and in inflamed prostatic glands. The frequency of prostatic involvement in persons with disseminated microsporidiosis is not known.

Gastrointestinal and Hepatobiliary Tracts

Intestinal infection is the most prevalent type of human microsporidial infection (6, 10, 52, 89). In some studies, microsporidiosis is responsible for up to 50% of cases of idiopathic diarrhea occurring in AIDS patients (6, 89). Three microsporidian agents from the intestinal tract, *E. bieneusi*, *E. intestinalis*, and, in one patient, *E. cuniculi*, have been described (6, 12, 24, 35, 36, 42, 50, 51, 53–56, 70, 80, 88, 89).

The vast majority of microsporidial intestinal infections are caused by *E. bieneusi*. In infected individuals, *E. bieneusi* is present throughout the length of the small intestine and is found in the superficial lining enterocytes (Fig. 4.13) (56). Similar to other tissues, the spores cannot be well visualized using standard hematoxylin and eosin staining (70). Because *E. bieneusi* does not produce active enteritis, ulceration, or other histologic abnormalities specific for intestinal infection, its presence is often not suspected unless tissue Gram staining, modified chromotrope, or other stains for microsporidia are performed (70, 88). *Enterocytozoon* infection is usually focal, and spores may be very scarce (70). In rare instances, spores are present beneath the epithelium in the lamina propria, but this has not been shown to represent a risk factor for disseminated infection (66).

The intestines are frequently, if not always, involved in cases of *E. intestinalis* infection (Fig. 4.14) (36, 50). Similar to *E. bieneusi*, *E. intestinalis* does not produce any specific endoscopic or tissue abnormality. Unlike *E. bieneusi*, however, *E. intestinalis* can be seen in biopsies to infect not only enterocytes but also cells in the lamina propria, including endothelial cells, fibroblasts, and macrophages (Fig. 4.15). *E. intestinalis* can also infect the large bowel (29). In well-prepared paraffin-embedded sections and in plastic-embedded semi-thin sections, the parasitophorous vacuole can often be seen surrounding the developing spores and separating them from the host cell cytoplasm. The observation of a parasitophorous vacuole can permit a tentative diagnosis of *E. intestinalis* infection in intestinal tissue (70, 75).

One patient with disseminated *E. cuniculi* infection which involved the small intestine has been described. Microsporidian spores were present in the superficial enterocytes, but there were no gastrointestinal symptoms (35).

Simultaneous infection of the gastrointestinal tract by *E. bieneusi* and *E. intestinalis* has been described, although this is rare. A coexistent infection with microsporidia and *Cryptosporidium* spp. is more commonly seen (42, 89). Coinfection with *E. bieneusi* and *Giardia lamblia* in a patient with AIDS and chronic diarrhea has been diagnosed from a small intestinal biopsy by histological methods (38).

> *Intestinal infection is the most prevalent type of human microsporidial infection*

Microsporidia, usually *E. bieneusi* but also *E. intestinalis*, can infect the biliary tract (6, 8, 58, 89). Infections of nonparenchymal liver cells and the epithelium of bile ducts and (rarely) the gall bladder have been reported. Infections of the biliary tract may result in sclerosing cholangitis, bile duct dilatation, papillary stenosis, and acalculous cholecystitis. In addition to these microsporidian agents, there has been a report of granulomatous hepatitis due to *E. cuniculi* in a patient with AIDS (82).

Central Nervous System

Two immunocompetent children with central nervous system disease due to *E. cuniculi* have been reported (4, 48). No tissue was available for examination, but a microsporidian species identified as *E. cuniculi* was identified from centrifuged urine in one patient (4).

Four autopsied patients with AIDS and seizures with microsporidial infection of the brain were recently described. Lesions of the gray matter of the cortical ribbon and deep cerebral nuclei had central areas of necrosis. Microsporidian spores were abundant in astrocytes and within macrophages in the necrotic foci. In two patients, *E. cuniculi* was identified in cerebral lesions (23, 49), and the other cases were due to *T. hominis* (32, 94).

Other Tissues

Microsporidial infection of the peritoneum due to *E. cuniculi* has been described (95). At autopsy, a 20-cm lobulated inflammatory mass of the omentum, which contained focal necrosis, nongranulomatous inflammation, and microsporidian spores, was found. The species identity of this microsporidian was not confirmed by antigenic or nucleic acid methods.

Rare microsporidian spores were identified in the soft tissues beneath a tongue ulcer in an AIDS patient with disseminated, confirmed *E. cuniculi* infection (35); it is not known whether a microsporidium was the etiologic agent of ulceration.

Two male patients with AIDS and microsporidian infections of the bone have been identified (34). Painful, radiographically lytic lesions of the left mandible and temporal bone were present. Rare organisms were identified in necrotic tissue, but the species of microsporidian could not be determined.

Inflammatory myositis due to *Pleistophora* sp. has occurred in two patients with AIDS (16, 45) and in one patient with *T. hominis* infection (39). Biopsies taken from deltoid and quadriceps muscles revealed atrophic and degenerating skeletal muscle fibers which were focally infiltrated by clusters of microsporidia measuring up to 3.4 μm in length. There was an associated mild inflammatory infiltrate composed of plasma cells, lymphocytes, eosinophils, and histiocytes.

Disseminated *N. connori* infection associated with *Pneumocystis carinii* pneumonia was diagnosed at the time of autopsy of a 4-month-old athymic male infant (47). Microsporidia were found in the alveolar septa of the lungs; in the smooth muscle; in the interstitium of the muscularis of the stomach, appendix, and small and large intestines; and in the arterial walls in the urinary bladder, kidney, liver, adrenal glands, diaphragm, and myocardium.

Laboratory Diagnosis

Microsporidian spores can be difficult or impossible to identify in biopsy or autopsy tissues and cytological specimens using routine stains

Microsporidian spores can be difficult or impossible to identify in biopsy or autopsy tissues and cytological specimens using routine stains such as hematoxylin and eosin or the Papanicolaou stain. Thus, special procedures to exclude the presence of microsporidiosis must be performed (70, 75). Gram stains of cytological and tissue specimens are usually adequate to demonstrate microsporidian spores. The spores usually stain strongly gram positive but may occasionally stain weakly gram positive or gram negative. Weber's chromotrope stain (88) and its modifications are also useful for staining microsporidian spores in stool, cytological specimens, and, to a lesser extent, biopsy specimens. Using either Gram or Weber's stain, microsporidian spores will often show a belt-like stripe extending around the equatorial diameter of the spore. In addition, microsporidian spores have a polar granule visible at the anterior end of the spore when stained by the periodic acid-Schiff method. Other staining methods, including the Steiner silver, modified trichrome blue, and Giemsa stains, have been successfully used by investigators to demonstrate microsporidian spores (36, 68). Some authors prefer using chemofluorescent optical brightening agents (e.g., Uvitex 2B, Calcofluor white) for identification of microsporidia (26). With any of the staining techniques, it is important that microsporidian spores not be confused with yeasts or bacteria. Microsporidian spores have a uniform oval shape and a regular size and are nonbudding.

The use of exfoliative and aspiration cytologic methods to detect human microsporidiosis is assuming increasing importance as the clinical spectrum of infection widens. Although there are some important exceptions (for example, myositis caused by *Pleistophora* and *Trachipleistophora* spp.), microsporidial infections in humans generally affect mucosal and epithelium-lined tissues and are thus often amenable to diagnosis by relatively safe, noninvasive cytologic techniques. Tissues which are often infected with microsporidia and which can be diagnosed by cytologic methods include the intestinal and biliary epithelium, the epithelium of the cornea and conjunctiva, the epithelium of the sinonasal and tracheobronchial region, the renal tubular epithelium and urothelium, and the prostate. Cytology is especially suited for screening patients who are at high risk for microsporidial infection and for evaluating the efficacy of novel treatments of microsporidiosis. The specific technique (e.g., lavage, scrape, smear, swab, fluid concentrate) used for obtaining cytologic material for diagnosis is dependent on the site of infection.

In ocular infections, cytological preparations, including scrape, smear, and swab specimens of the conjunctiva or cornea, are ideal for demonstrating microsporidian spores (70, 71, 75). Cytology has proven useful not only in the primary diagnosis of microsporidial keratoconjunctivitis, but also as an objective follow-up technique to assess the efficacy of experimental treatment for microsporidial keratoconjunctivitis.

Cytologic examination of small intestinal lavage fluid obtained during endoscopy appears to be a sensitive method for diagnosis of *E. bieneusi* infection. Examination of small intestinal endoscopic brush specimens of the mucosa has also been demonstrated to be a sensitive nonbiopsy method for diagnosis of intestinal microsporidiosis.

Sputum cytology is a valuable screening technique for respiratory tract microsporidiosis. Bronchoalveolar lavage may be useful in patients with suspected lower respiratory tract microsporidiosis, in patients with evidence of focal radiographic disease, and in persons with negative repeat sputum examinations in whom there is a strong suspicion of microsporidial bronchiolitis. As with formalin-fixed biopsies, slides of sputum and lavage fluid can be stained with specific fluorescent-antibody stains to establish the species of the microsporidian. In endoscopically obtained transbronchial biopsies, microsporidian spores are best identified in the bronchial or bronchiolar epithelium. In well-oriented sections of the tracheobronchial epithelium, spores are concentrated in the supranuclear, or subapical, region of infected host cells. Microsporidia can also be found within the alveolar spaces (46, 62, 67, 68, 72, 75).

Diagnosis of hepatobiliary tract microsporidiosis is usually made by biopsy, cholecystectomy, or cytology. Biliary aspiration performed through the ampulla of Vater at the time of endoscopy has been successfully used as a noninvasive method for cytologic diagnosis of biliary tract infection with *E. bieneusi* (75).

Stool Examination

Stool examination for microsporidial spores using special stains is the safest and least expensive method for screening patients for intestinal infection due to *Enterocytozoon* or *E. intestinalis*. The two most commonly used methods for detection of microsporidian spores in stool are the chromotrope (trichrome) stain and its modifications (88) and fluorochrome stains. The differences in the sizes of the two major intestinal microsporidia, *E. bieneusi* and *E. intestinalis*, often permit a tentative diagnosis of the genus from light microscopic examination of stool. The microsporidian should be identified to the level of genus, because *E. intestinalis* has a propensity for dissemination and a drug sensitivity pattern different from that of *E. bieneusi*. Electron microscopic examination has been successfully used for confirmation of microsporidian spores in feces, but it can be time-consuming to use this method to perform a genus- or species-level identification (6, 70, 75, 89).

Stool examination for microsporidial spores using special stains is the safest and least expensive method for screening patients for intestinal infection due to Enterocytozoon or E. intestinalis

Tissue Culture

The in vitro cultivation of several microsporidian agents which infect humans has been of enormous benefit, both in the understanding of the biologic aspects of the host cell-parasite relationship (Fig. 4.12, 4.16, and 4.17) and in developing immunologic reagents for use in clinical diagnosis. Unfortunately, microsporidial tissue culture is available in only a few specialized laboratories, and it is not practical to use this method for routine clinical diagnosis. Microsporidia that have been successfully cultivated from patients with AIDS include *E. hellem*, *E. cuniculi*, *E. intestinalis*, and *T. hominis* (24, 25, 39, 72, 84). *E. bieneusi* has been propagated only in short-term cultures (85).

Immunofluorescence

Although fluorescent-antibody diagnostic reagents are not currently available to most laboratories, they constitute an important method for the species-level identification of *E. cuniculi*, *E. hellem*, *E. intestinalis*, and some other microsporidial species (Fig. 4.8 and 4.11) (35, 67, 68, 70, 72, 75, 84). These studies can be performed on cytologic and biopsy specimens, including fresh tissues and specimens fixed in formalin, ethanol, or methanol. Unfortunately, antiserum to *E. bieneusi* has not yet been developed.

Nucleic Acid-Based Methods

There has been rapid progress in the development of nucleic acid-based diagnostic methods for microsporidial infections. The polymerase chain reaction has been successfully used for the diagnosis of *E. cuniculi*, *E. hellem*, *and E. intestinalis* in a variety of clinical specimens, including biopsy tissues, bronchoalveolar lavage fluid, and urine (20, 21, 84).

A set of primers, termed EBIEF1 and EBIER1, have recently been made that are based upon the small ribosomal subunit of *E. bieneusi* (18, 19). Amplification of *E. bieneusi* templates with this primer pair results in a 607-bp diagnostic DNA fragment. These primers are highly sensitive and specific, and diagnosis of *E. bieneusi* in specimens of infected fresh stool as well as stool which has been maintained for short periods of time in formalin has been successfully made. When these techniques become more widely available, the true extent of microsporidial infections in AIDS patients, in recipients of organ transplants and other immunocompromised patients, and in immunocompetent persons will undoubtedly become evident.

Therapy

Experience in the therapy of human microsporidiosis is limited, and blinded, placebo-controlled comparative treatment trials have not been published

Experience in the therapy of human microsporidiosis is limited, and blinded, placebo-controlled comparative treatment trials have not been published. Virtually all published studies to date have involved severely immunosuppressed, HIV-infected patients. Early attempts at treating intestinal *E. bieneusi* infection met with limited success. Preliminary reports of a good clinical response among patients treated with metronidazole (30) could not be confirmed. Some reports have suggested that treatment with albendazole may lead to improvement of diarrhea and weight gain in some patients, even though parasites were still present in biopsy specimens of the small intestine and microsporidial spores were still detected in stool specimens obtained after treatment (5, 27).

The clinical outcome in general, however, has not been favorable. More recently, one brief report suggested that the antiprotozoal agent furazolidone may be useful for treating patients with *E. bieneusi*-associated diarrhea, while another found the antiemetic thalidomide to be effective. Three patients treated with furazolidone (100 mg orally four times a day for 20 days) experienced cessation of diarrheal stools after 12 days of therapy, and microsporidial spores were no longer detectable in stool specimens. One patient, however, relapsed (28). On the basis of evidence that thalidomide reduces tumor necrosis factor levels, investigators in the United Kingdom treated 12 patients with thalidomide (100 mg nightly for 3 weeks). All patients improved, as evidenced by decreased bowel frequency, transition from liquid to semisolid stools, and decreased weight loss. One patient relapsed (76).

Yet another recent study suggests that atovaquone may be useful in treating patients with *E. bieneusi*-associated diarrhea. Investigators in Atlanta, Ga., monitored eight patients who had received atovaquone (750 mg orally three times a day for at least 4 weeks). All experienced resolution of diarrhea and significant weight gain, despite the fact that spores were still detectable in follow-up stool specimens and in some cases also in intestinal biopsies. Control of diarrhea and other gastrointestinal symptoms appeared to be dependent upon continuation of the medication (1).

Preliminary observations of possibly curative treatment of infections caused by *E. intestinalis* and other *Encephalitozoon* spp. with albendazole have led to an increasing number of reports confirming the efficacy of this drug for these infections (17, 27, 29, 36, 44, 50, 78, 87). Several isolated case reports have described clinical and parasitologic cures using albendazole (400 mg orally twice or three times a day for 2 weeks to 3 months) for disseminated *E. intestinalis* infections with clinical manifestations that included sinusitis, keratoconjunctivitis, enteritis, and urethritis (17, 40, 78, 87). Similarly, case series with two to seven patients each have described successful results using albendazole (400 mg twice a day) for periods ranging from 2 to 4 weeks in patients with disseminated *E. intestinalis* infections. In most cases, reductions in parasite burden or parasitologic cures accompanied clinical improvement. In others, however, cessation of therapy resulted in clinical relapse that required reinstitution of therapy, albeit at lower, suppressive doses. Outright treatment failures were rare (29, 36, 50).

Experience in treating *E. hellem* and *E. cuniculi* infections has been similar to that reported for *E. intestinalis*. One report describes the resolution of renal failure, sinusitis, bronchiolitis, and keratoconjunctivitis in a patient infected with *E. cuniculi* who was treated with albendazole (200 mg twice a day) for 16 months (21). *E. cuniculi*-associated interstitial pneumonitis was also treated successfully with albendazole in another recently reported case (22).

Although initial reports of successful topical therapy for *E. hellem*-associated keratoconjunctivitis were quite promising (63), subsequent experience with systemic albendazole therapy indicates that this will likely become the treatment of choice for *Encephalitozoon* infections in general. The choice of albendazole over topical therapy makes particular sense when one considers that such infections are almost always systemic in nature and rarely, if ever, limited to superficial ocular structures.

Prevention of Infection

Data to support effective preventive strategies are limited, and there is currently no vaccination available or under clinical trial. Nevertheless, the presence of infective spores in various bodily fluids suggests that body substance precautions in health care settings and general attention to hand

Although initial reports of successful topical therapy for E. hellem-associated keratoconjunctivitis were quite promising, subsequent experience with systemic albendazole therapy indicates that this will likely become the treatment of choice for Encephalitozoon infections in general

washing and other personal hygiene measures may be helpful in preventing primary infections. Hand washing may be particularly important in the prevention of ocular infections, which may occur as a result of inoculation of conjunctival surfaces by fingers contaminated with respiratory fluids or urine. Whether respiratory precautions for persons documented to have spores in sputum or other respiratory secretions might be effective is unknown. Similarly, precautions pertinent to environmental or zoonotic exposure to microsporidia are as yet undefined (7).

Prevention of recurrent disease due to microsporidia also requires further study. The data reviewed above suggest that albendazole may be curative in many patients infected with *Encephalitozoon* spp. and that maintenance therapy may be useful in suppressing the clinical manifestations of intestinal *E. bieneusi* infections.

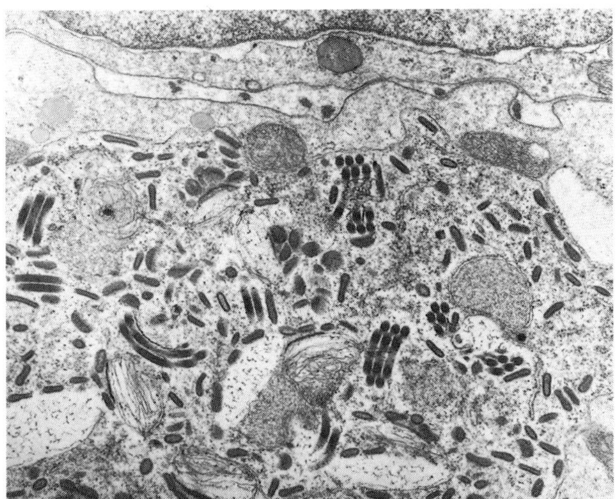

Figure 4.1 Enterocyte containing developmental stages of *E. bieneusi*, including electron-dense discs, nuclei, and electron-lucent inclusions. Magnification, ×38,000.

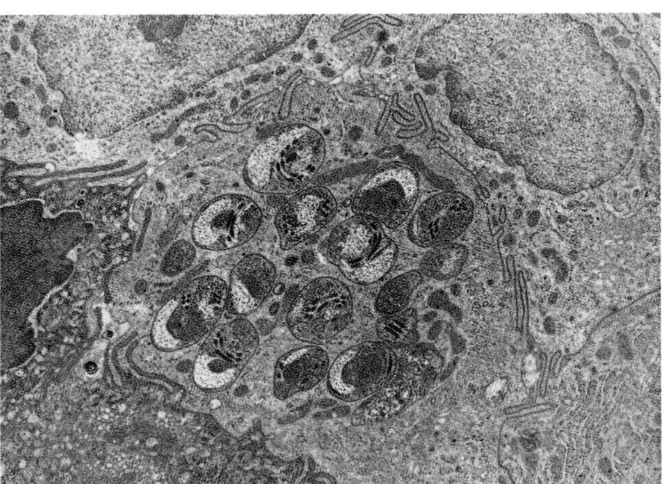

Figure 4.2 Sporoblasts (immature spores) of *E. bieneusi* showing the characteristic double layer of coiled polar tubules. All stages develop in direct contact with the host cell cytoplasm. Magnification, ×25,000.

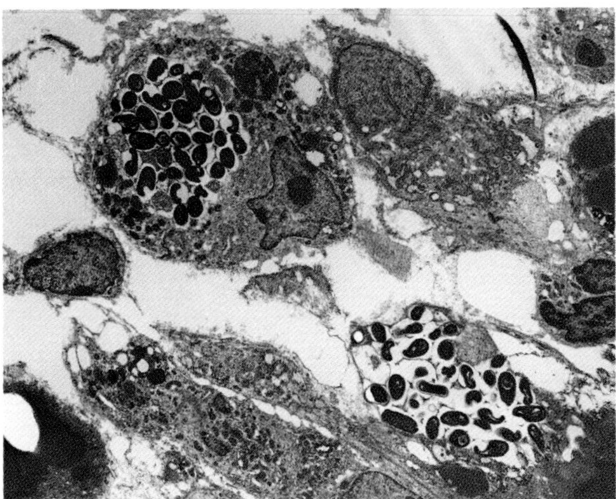

Figure 4.3 Small intestinal lamina propria macrophages containing parasitophorous vacuoles of *E.intestinalis*. The fibrillar matrix between spores gives the vacuole a honeycombed, or septated, appearance. Magnification, ×7,400 (from reference 72 with permission).

Figure 4.4 Immature and mature spores of *E. hellem* in a parasitophorous vacuole from an infected renal tubular epithelial cell. Note the high concentration of spores in this vacuole. Magnification, ×25,000.

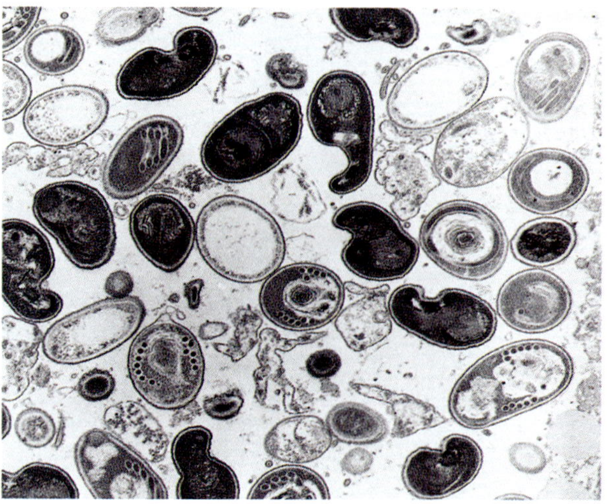

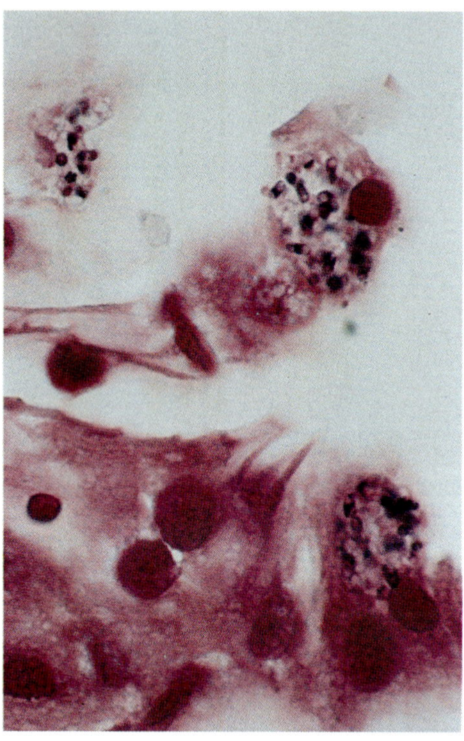

Figure 4.5 Conjunctival biopsy showing gram-positive spores of *E. hellem* in epithelial cells (tissue Gram stain; magnification, ×1,000) (from reference 1a).

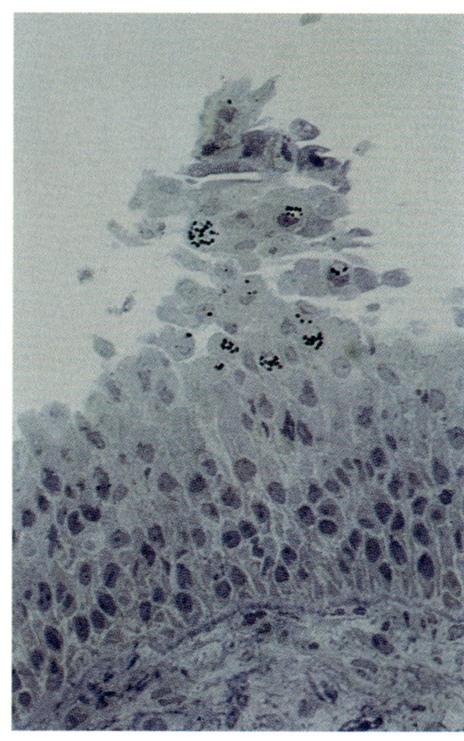

Figure 4.6 *E. hellem* spores are present in the cytoplasm of superficial epithelial cells in the nasal mucosa from a patient with microsporidial rhinitis (semi-thin plastic-embedded section; toluidine blue; magnification, ×40).

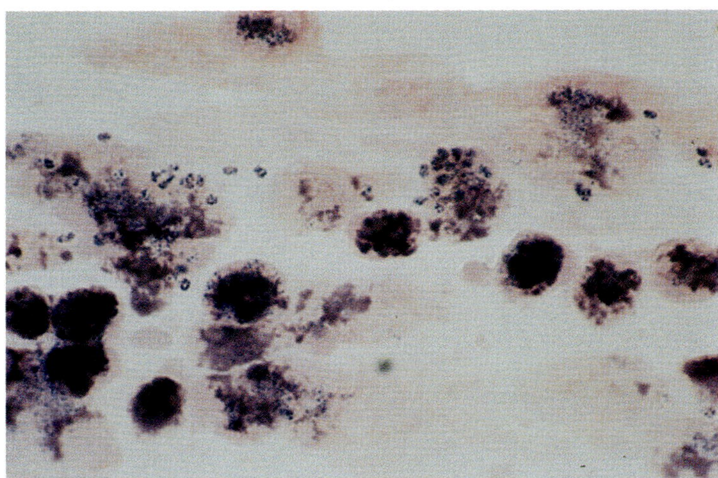

Figure 4.7 Smear of nasal discharge demonstrating numerous gram-positive spores of *E. hellem* (Gram stain; magnification, ×1,000).

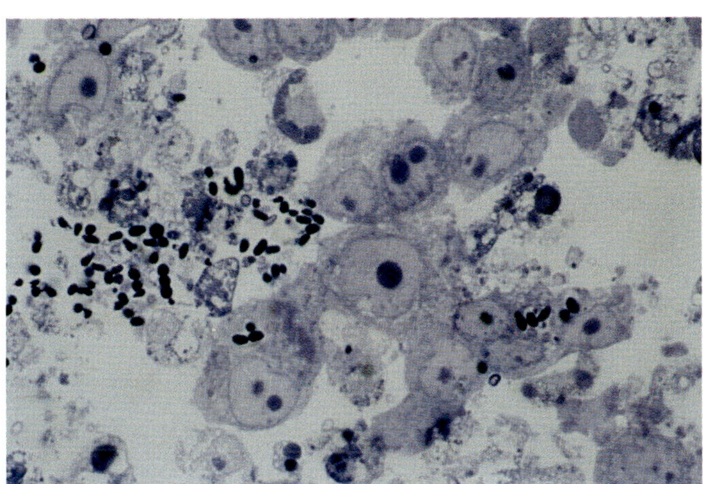

Figure 4.8 Fluorescent-antibody staining of sputum using rabbit antibody to *E. hellem*, showing strong reactivity with spores. Slender polar tubules are seen extruding from the apices of two spores (antibody to *E. hellem*; magnification, ×1,000) (from reference 72 with permission).

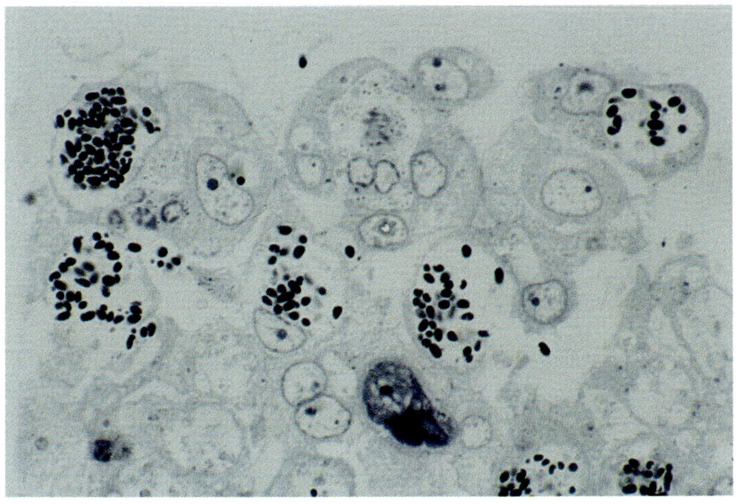

Figure 4.9 Plastic-embedded semi-thin section of tracheal mucosa with *E. hellem* infection. The parasitophorous vacuole is seen as a clear zone in the cytoplasm, surrounding the spores (toluidine blue; magnification, ×400).

Figure 4.10 Spores of *E. hellem* within a necrotic renal tubule from an AIDS patient with disseminated infection (Steiner silver stain; magnification, ×1,200).

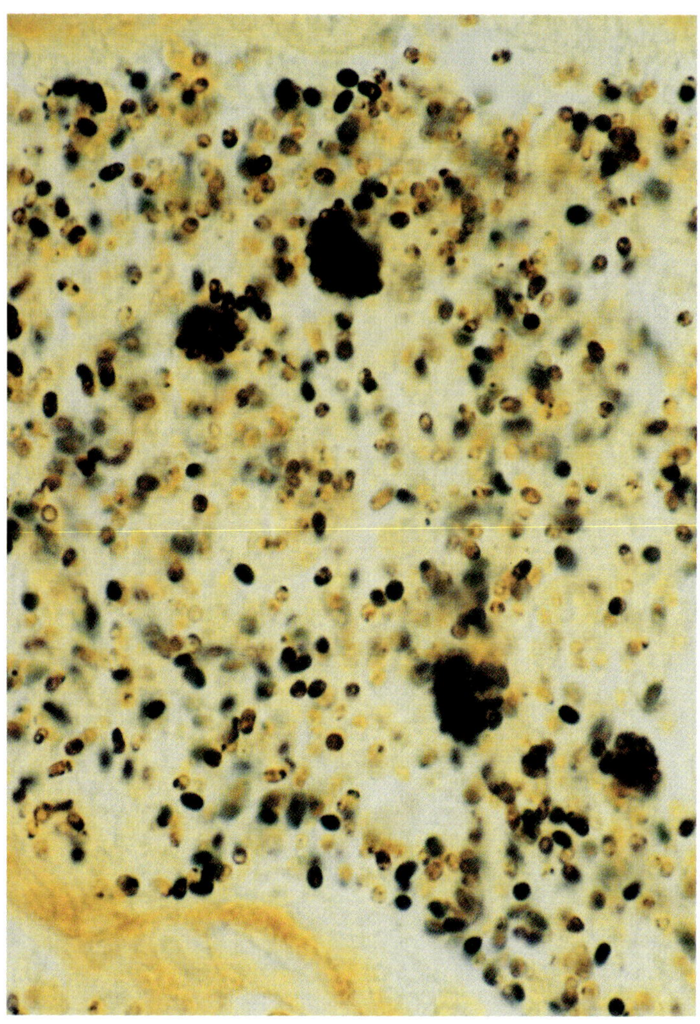

Figure 4.11 Renal tubular epithelium from a patient with disseminated *E. hellem* infection, showing brightly staining clusters of intraepithelial spores (rabbit antibody to *E. hellem*; magnification, ×1,000).

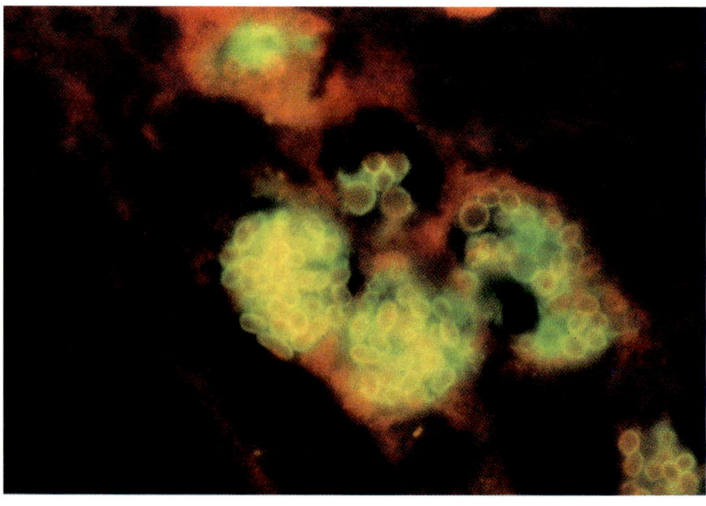

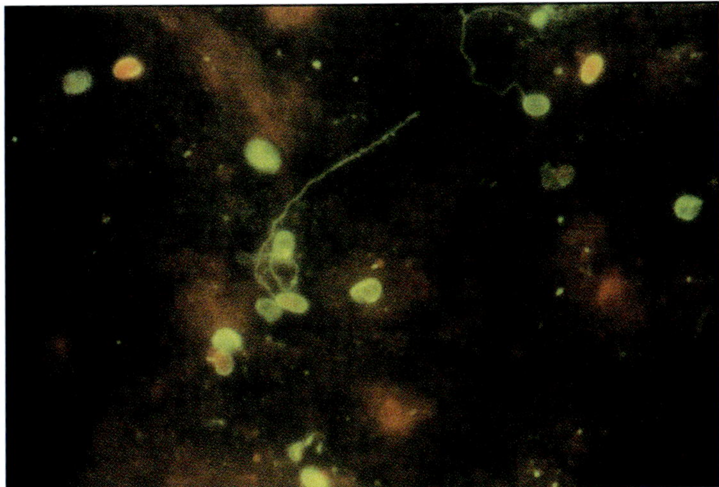

Figure 4.12 *E. hellem* isolated from the urine of an AIDS patient with disseminated infection and grown in a tissue culture system using monkey kidney cells. The ovoid spores are seen within cells and free in the culture media. Tissue culture of microsporidia has been valuable in the understanding the biology of these organisms and the production of diagnostic reagents (semi-thin plastic-embedded section; toluidine blue; magnification, ×1,000).

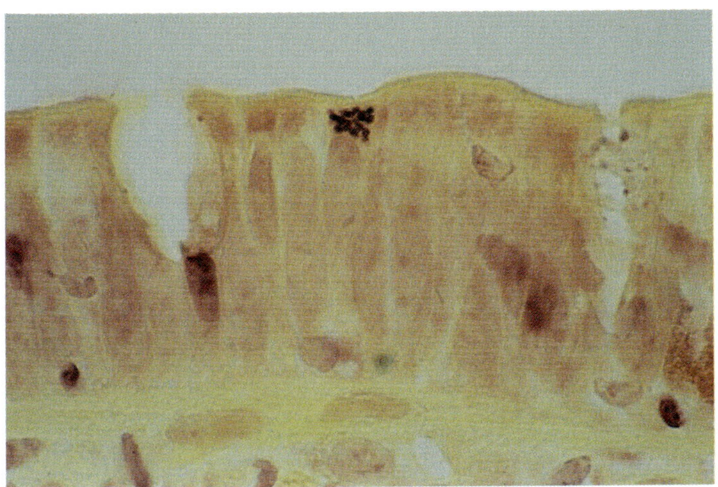

Figure 4.13 Typical appearance of *E. bieneusi* in an infected epithelial cell from a small intestinal mucosal biopsy specimen using tissue Gram staining. The spores are almost always present in the supranuclear region of lining enterocytes (tissue Gram stain; magnification, ×600).

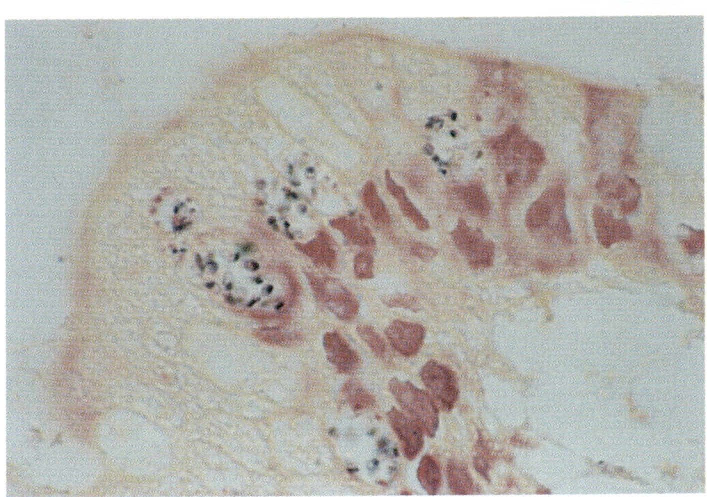

Figure 4.14 Small intestinal mucosal biopsy showing numerous enterocytes infected with *E. intestinalis*. The spores of this microsporidian are larger than those of *Enterocytozoon* spp., and the parasitophorous vacuole of *E. intestinalis* is visible as a clear zone surrounding the spores (tissue Gram stain; magnification, ×400).

Figure 4.15 Duodenal biopsy of *E. intestinalis* infection. Spores are clearly seen in parasitophorous vacuoles within lining enterocytes and also within a macrophage in the lamina propria (semi-thin plastic-embedded section; toluidine blue; magnification, ×400).

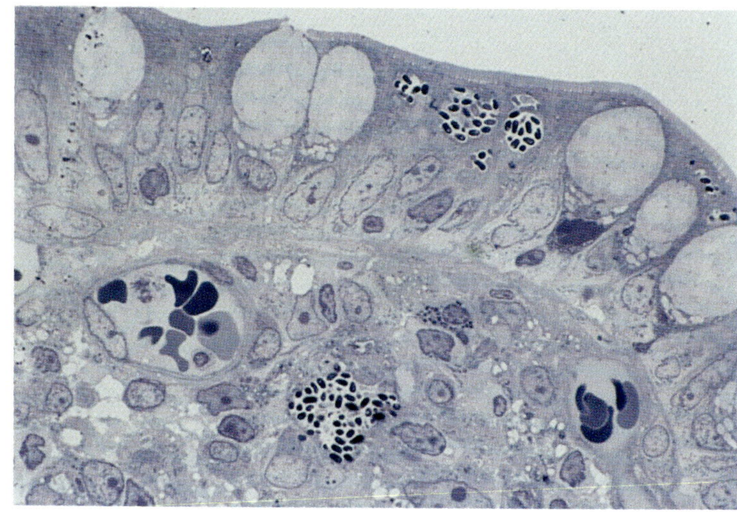

Figure 4.16 Monolayer of human lung fibroblasts showing two cells which are distended by spores and developing stages of *E. hellem* (phase contrast microscopy; magnification, ×600) (from reference 70 with permission).

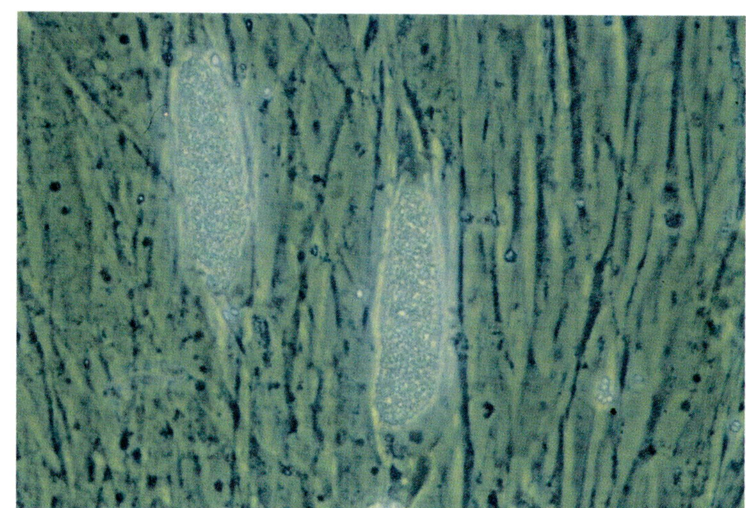

Figure 4.17 Scanning electron micrograph of parasitophorous vacuole of *E. hellem* containing numerous spores. The specimen was isolated from bronchoalveolar lavage fluid of an infected patient and inoculated into monkey kidney cell culture. Bar = 10 µm. (From reference 72 with permission. Photograph courtesy of Dr. Gordon Leitch.)

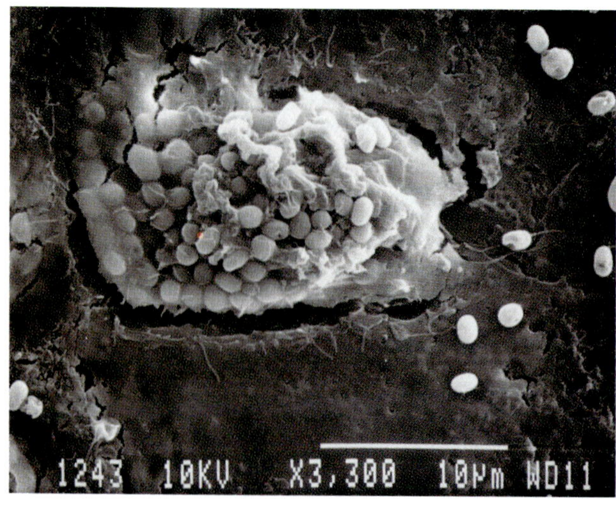

References

1a. **Albrecht, H., I. Sobottka, and D. A. Schwartz.** 1995. Microsporidiose, p. 1–33. *In* H. Jager (ed.), *AIDS und HIV-Infektionen.* Ecomed, Landsberg, Germany.

1b. **Anderson, D. C., S. A. Klumpp, A. J. DaSilva, N. J. Pieniazek, H. M. McClure, and D. A. Schwartz.** Naturally-acquired *Enterocytozoon bieneusi* (Microsporida) hepatobiliary infection in rhesus monkeys with simian immunodeficiency virus (SIV): a possible animal model of disease. Submitted for publication.

1. **Anwar-Bruni, D. M., S. E. Hogan, D. A. Schwartz, C. M. Wilcox, R. T. Bryan, and J. L. Lennox.** 1996. Atovaquone is effective treatment for the symptoms of gastrointestinal microsporidiosis in HIV-1 infected patients. *AIDS* **10**:619–625.

2. **Asmuth, D. M., P. C. DeGirolami, M. Federman, C. R. Ezratty, D. K. Pleskow, G. Desai, and C. A. Wanke.** 1994. Clinical features of microsporidiosis in patients with the acquired immunodeficiency syndrome. *Clin. Infect. Dis.* **18**:819–825.

3. **Avery, S. W., and A. H. Undeen.** 1987. The isolation of microsporidia and other pathogens from concentrated ditch water. *J. Am. Mosq. Control Assoc.* **3**:54–58.

4. **Bergquist, N. R., G. Stintzing, L. Smedman, and T. Waller.** 1984. Diagnosis of encephalitozoonosis in man by serological tests. *Br. Med. J.* **288**:902.

5. **Blanshard, C., D. S. Ellis, D. G. Tovey, S. Dowell, and B. G. Gazzard.** 1992. Treatment of intestinal microsporidiosis with albendazole in patients with AIDS. *AIDS* **6**:311–313.

6. **Bryan, R. T.** 1995. Microsporidia, p. 2513–2524. *In* G. L. Mandell, J. E. Bennett, and R. Dolin (ed.), *Principles and Practice of Infectious Diseases.* Churchill Livingstone, New York.

7. **Bryan, R. T.** 1995. Microsporidiosis as an AIDS-related opportunistic infection. *Clin. Infect. Dis.* **21**:S62–S65.

8. **Bryan, R. T., D. A. Schwartz, D. Rimland, L. Gorelkin, A. Johnson, J. M. Lyons, and T. Grimland for the Enteric Opportunistic Infections Working Group.** 1993. Endoscopic, surgical, and postmortem evaluation of the natural history and anatomic distribution of *Enterocytozoon bieneusi* infection in a patient with AIDS, abstr. no. PO-B10-1445, p. 376. *In* 9th International Conference on AIDS, Berlin.

9. **Bryan, R. T., and R. Weber.** 1993. Microsporidia. Emerging pathogens in immunodeficient patients. *Arch. Pathol. Lab. Med.* **117**:1243–1245.

10. **Bryan, R. T., R. Weber, and D. A. Schwartz.** Microsporidia. *In* R. L. Guerrant, D. J. Krongstad, J. H. Maguire, D. H. Walker, and P. F. Weller (ed.), *Tropical Infectious Diseases: Principles, Pathogens, and Practice,* in press. Churchill Livingstone, New York.

11. **Bryan, R. T., R. Weber, and D. A. Schwartz.** 1997. Microsporidiosis in patients who are not infected with human immunodeficiency virus. *Clin. Infect. Dis.* **24**:534–535.

12. **Cali, A., D. P. Kotler, and J. M. Orenstein.** 1993. *Septata intestinalis* N. G., N. Sp., an intestinal microsporidian associated with chronic diarrhea and dissemination in AIDS patients. *J. Eukaryot. Microbiol.* **40**:101–112.

13. **Cali, A., D. M. Meisler, C. Y. Lowder, R. Lembach, L. Ayers, P. M. Takvorian, I. Rutherford, D. L. Longworth, J. T. McMahon, and R. T. Bryan.** 1991. Corneal microsporidioses: characterization and identification. *J. Protozool.* **38:**215S.

14. **Cali, A., D. M. Meisler, I. Rutherford, C. Y. Lowder, J. T. McMahon, D. L. Longworth, and R. T. Bryan.** 1991. Corneal microsporidiosis in a patient with AIDS. *Am. J. Trop. Med. Hyg.* **44:**463–468.

15. **Centers for Disease Control.** 1990. Microsporidian keratoconjunctivitis in patients with AIDS. *Morbid. Mortal. Weekly Rep.* **30:**188–189.

16. **Chupp, G. L., J. Alroy, L. S. Adelman, J. C. Breen, and P. R. Skolnik.** 1993. Myositis due to *Pleistophora* (microsporidia) in a patient with AIDS. *Clin. Infect. Dis.* **16:**188–189.

17. **Corcoran, G. D., J. R. Isaacson, C. Daniels, and P. L. Chiodini.** 1996. Urethritis associated with disseminated microsporidiosis: clinical response to albendazole. *Clin. Infect. Dis.* **22:**592–593.

18. **da Silva, A. J., F. J. Bornay-Llinares, C. del Aguila de la Puente, G. S. Visvesvara, D. A. Schwartz, S. B. Slemenda, and N. J. Pieniazek.** Sensitive diagnosis of *E. bieneusi* (microsporidia) infections by PCR in unfixed and fixed stool samples using primers based on the region coding for small subunit ribosomal RNA. *Arch. Pathol. Lab. Med.* **121,** in press.

19. **daSilva, A. J., D. A. Schwartz, G. S. Visvesvara, H. de Moura, S. B. Slemenda, and N. J. Pieniazek.** 1996. Sensitive PCR diagnosis of infections by *Enterocytozoon bieneusi* (microsporidia) using primers based on the region coding for small subunit rRNA. *J. Clin. Microbiol.* **34:**986–987.

20. **da Silva, A. J., S. B. Slemenda, G. S. Visvesvara, D. A. Schwartz, C. M. Wilcox, S. Wallace, and N. J. Pieniazek.** 1997. Detection of *Septata intestinalis* (Microsporida) Cali et al. 1993 using polymerase chain reaction primers targeting the small subunit ribosomal RNA coding region. *Mol. Diagnosis* **2:**47–52.

21. **De Groote, M. A., G. S. Visvesvara, M. L. Wilson, N. J. Pieniazek, S. B. Slemenda, A. J. daSilva, G. J. Leitch, R. T. Bryan, R. T. Visvesvara, and R. Reves.** 1995. Polymerase chain reaction and culture confirmation of disseminated *Encephalitozoon cuniculi* in a patient with AIDS: successful therapy with albendazole. *J. Infect. Dis.* **171:**1375–1378.

22. **Deplazes, P., A. Mathis, R. Baumgartner, I. Tanner, and R. Weber.** 1996. Immunologic and molecular characteristics of *Encephalitozoon*-like microsporidia isolated from humans and rabbits indicate that *Encephalitozoon cuniculi* is a zoonotic parasite. *Clin. Infect. Dis.* **22:**557–559.

23. **Deplazes, P., A. Mathis, C. Müller, and R. Weber.** 1996. Molecular epidemiology of *Encephalitozoon cuniculi*, a zoonotic microsporidian infecting HIV-seropositive persons. *Joint Meeting Am. Soc. Parasitol. and Soc. Protozool.,* Tucson, Ariz.

24. **Desportes, I., Y. Le Charpentier, A. Galian, F. Bernard, B. Cochand-Priollet, A. Lavergne, P. Ravisse, and R. Modigliani.** 1985. Occurrence of a new microsporidian: *Enterocytozoon bieneusi* ng, nsp, in the enterocytes of a human patient with AIDS. *J. Protozool.* **32:**250–254.

25. **Didier, E. S., P. J. Didier, D. N. Friedberg, S. M. Stenson, J. M. Orenstein, R. W. Yee, F. W. Tio, R. M. Davis, C. Vossbrinck, N. Millichamp, and J. A. Shadduck.** 1991. Isolation and characterization of a new human microsporidian, *Encephalitozoon hellem* (n. sp.), from three AIDS patients with keratoconjunctivitis. *J. Infect. Dis.* **163:**617–621.

26. Didier, E. S., J. M. Orenstein, A. Aldras, D. Bertucci, L. B. Rogers, and F. A. Janney. 1995. Comparison of three staining methods for detecting microsporidia in fluids. *J. Clin. Microbiol.* **33:**3138–3145.

27. Dieterich, D. T., E. A. Lew, D. P. Kotler, M. A. Poles, and J. M. Orenstein. 1994. Treatment with albendazole for intestinal disease due to *Enterocytozoon bieneusi* in patients with AIDS. *J. Infect. Dis.* **169:**178–183.

28. Dionisio, D., G. Sterrantino, M. Meli, M. Trotta, D. Milo, and F. Leoncini. 1995. Use of furazolidone for the treatment of microsporidiosis due to *Enterocytozoon bieneusi* in patients with AIDS. *Recenti Prog. Med.* **86:**394–397.

29. Dore, G. J., D. J. Marriott, M. C. Hing, J. L. Harkness, and A. S. Field. 1995. Disseminated microsporidiosis due to *Septata intestinalis* in nine patients infected with the human immunodeficiency virus: response to therapy with albendazole. *Clin. Infect. Dis.* **21:**70–76.

30. Eeftinck Schattenkerk, J. K. M., T. Van Gool, R. J. Van Ketel, J. F. W. M. Bartelsman, C. L. Kuiken, W. J. Terpstra, and P. Reiss. 1991. Clinical significance of small-intestinal microsporidiosis in HIV-1-infected individuals. *Lancet* **337:**895–898.

31. Field, A. S., M. C. Hing, S. T. Milliken, and D. J. Marriott. 1993. Microsporidia in the small intestine of HIV-infected patients. *Med. J. Aust.* **158:**390–394.

32. Field, A. S., D. J. Marriott, S. T. Milliken, B. J. Brew, E. U. Canning, J. G. Kench, P. Darveniza, and J. L. Harkness. 1996. Myositis associated with a newly described microsporidian, *Trachipleistophora hominis*, in a patient with AIDS. *Clin. Microbiol.* **34:**2803–2811.

33. Flepp, M., B. Sauer, R. Luthy, and R. Weber. 1995. Human microsporidiosis in HIV-seronegative, immunocompetent patients, abstract LM25, p. 49. *In Program and Abstracts of the 35th Interscience Conference on Antimicrobial Agents and Chemotherapy.* American Society for Microbiology, Washington, D. C.

34. Frankel, S. S., B. M. Wenig, R. Neafie, B. M. Shmookler, and A. M. Nelson. 1996. Microsporidiosis of the skull and mandible in patients with acquired immunodeficiency syndrome, abstr. 751, p. 129A. *In Abstracts of United States and Canadian Academy of Pathology Annual Meeting,* Washington, D. C.

35. Franzen, C., D. A. Schwartz, G. S. Visvesvara, A. Müller, A. Schwenk, B. Salzberger, G. Fätkenheuser, G. Mahrle, V. Diehl, and M. Schrappe. 1995. Immunologically confirmed disseminated asymptomatic *Encephalitozoon cuniculi* infection of the gastrointestinal tract in a patient with AIDS. *Clin. Infect. Dis.* **2:**1480–1484.

36. Gunnarsson, G., D. Hurlbut, P. C. DeGirolami, M. Federman, and C. Wanke. 1995. Multiorgan microsporidiosis: report of five cases and review. *Clin. Infect. Dis.* **21:**37–44.

37. Hartskeerl, R. A., T. Van Gool, A. R. J. Schuitema, E. S. Didier, and W. J. Terpstra. 1995. Genetic and immunological characterization of the microsporidian *Septata intestinalis* Cali, Kotler and Orenstein, 1993: reclassification to *Encephalitozoon intestinalis*. *Parasitology* **110:**277–285.

38. Hewan-Lowe, K., B. Furlong, M. Sims, and D. A. Schwartz. 1997. Coinfection with *Giardia lamblia* and *Enterocytozoon bieneusi* in a patient with AIDS and chronic diarrhea. *Arch. Pathol. Lab. Med.* **121:**417–422.

39. Hollister, W. S., E. U. Canning, E. Weidner, A. S. Field, J. Kench, and D. J. Marriott. 1996. Development and ultrastructure of *Trachipleistophora hominis*, n. g., n. sp., after *in vitro* isolation from an AIDS patient and inoculation into athymic mice. *Parasitology* **112:**143–154.

40. Joste, N. E., J. D. Rich, K. J. Busam, and D. A. Schwartz. 1996. Autopsy verification of *Encephalitozoon intestinalis* (microsporidiosis) eradication following albendazole therapy. *Arch. Pathol. Lab. Med.* **120:**199–203.

41. Knapp, P. E., J. R. Saltzman, and P. Fairchild. 1996. Acalculous cholecystitis associated with microsporidial infection in a patient with AIDS. *Clin. Infect. Dis.* **22:**195–196.

42. Kotler, D. P., and J. M. Orenstein. 1994. Prevalence of intestinal microsporidiosis in HIV-infected individuals referred for gastroenterological evaluation. *Am. J. Gastroenterol.* **89:**1998–2001.

43. Lacey, C. J. N., A. Clark, P. Frazer, T. Metcalfe, G. Bonsor, and A. Curry. 1992. Chronic microsporidian infection in the nasal mucosae, sinuses, and conjunctivae in HIV disease. *Genitourin. Med.* **68:**179–181.

44. Lecuit, M., E. Oksenhendler, and C. Sarfati. 1994. Use of albendazole for disseminated microsporidian infection in patient with AIDS. *Clin. Infect. Dis.* **19:**332–333.

45. Ledford, D. K., M. D. Overman, A. Gonzalvo, A. Cali, S. W. Mester, and R. F. Lockey. 1985. Microsporidiosis myositis in a patient with acquired immunodeficiency syndrome. *Ann. Intern. Med.* **102:**628–630.

46. Lucas, S. B., D. A. Schwartz, and P. S. Hasleton. 1996. Pulmonary parasitic diseases, p. 316–319. *In* P. S. Hasleton (ed.), *Spencer's Pathology of the Lung*, 5th ed. McGraw-Hill, Inc., New York.

46a. Mansfield, K. G., A. Carville, D. Shvetz, J. MacKey, S. Tzipori, and A. A. Lackner. 1997. Identification of an *Enterocytozoon bieneusi*-like microsporidian parasite in simian-immunodeficiency-virus-inoculated macaques with hepatobiliary disease. *Am. J. Pathol.* **150:**1395–1405.

47. Margileth, A. M., A. J. Strano, R. Chandra, R. Neafie, M. Blum, and R. M. McCully. 1973. Disseminated nosematosis in an immunologically compromised infant. *Arch. Pathol.* **95:**145–150.

48. Matsubayashi, H., T. Koike, T. Mikata, and S. Hagiwara. 1959. A case of *Encephalitozoon*-like body infection in man. *Arch. Pathol.* **67:**181–187.

49. Mertens, R. B., E. S. Didier, M. C. Fishbein, D. C. Bertucci, L. B. Rogers, and J. M. Orenstein. 1997. Disseminated *Encephalitozoon cuniculi* microsporidiosis: infection of the brain, heart, kidneys, trachea, adrenal glands, urinary bladder, spleen, and lymph nodes in a patient with AIDS. *Mod. Pathol.* **10:**68–77.

50. Molina, J.-M., E. Oksenhendler, B. Beauvais, C. Sarfati, A. Jaccard, F. Derouin, and J. Modaï. 1995. Disseminated microsporidiosis due to *Septata intestinalis* in patients with AIDS: clinical features and response to albendazole therapy. *J. Infect. Dis.* **171:**245–249.

51. Molina, J.-M., C. Sarfati, B. Beauvais, M. Lémann, A. Lesourd, F. Ferchal, I. Casin, P. Lagrange, R. Modigliani, F. Berouin, and J. Modaï. 1993. Intestinal microsporidiosis in human immunodeficiency virus-infected patients with chronic unexplained diarrhea: prevalence and clinical and biologic features. *J. Infect. Dis.* **167:**217–221.

52. Navin, T. R., R. Weber, D. Rimland, J. M. Roberts, D. G. Addiss, S. P. Wahlquist, S. E. Hogan, D. J. Vugia, D. D. Juranek, D. A. Schwartz, C. M. Wilcox, J. M. Stewart, S. E. Thompson, and R. T. Bryan for the Enteric Opportunistic Infections Working Group. Declining CD4 T lymphocyte counts are associated with increasing likelihood of enteric parasitosis and chronic diarrhea: results of a 3-year longitudinal study. Submitted for publication.

53. **Orenstein, J. M., J. Chiang, W. Steinberg, P. D. Smith, H. Rotterdam, and D. P. Kotler.** 1990. Intestinal microsporidiosis as a cause of diarrhea in human immunodeficiency virus-infected patients. A report of 20 cases. *Hum. Pathol.* **21**:475–481.

54. **Orenstein, J. M., D. T. Dieterich, and D. P. Kotler.** 1992. Systemic dissemination by a newly recognized intestinal microsporidia species in AIDS. *AIDS* **6**:1143–1150.

55. **Orenstein, J. M., M. Tenner, A. Cali, and D. P. Kotler.** 1992. A microsporidian previously undescribed in humans, infecting enterocytes and macrophages, and associated with diarrhea in an acquired immunodeficiency syndrome patient. *Hum. Pathol.* **23**:722–728.

56. **Orenstein, J. M., M. Tenner, and D. P. Kotler.** 1992. Localization of infection by the microsporidian *Enterocytozoon bieneusi* in the gastrointestinal tract of AIDS patients with diarrhea. *AIDS* **6**:195–197.

57. **Pol, S., C. Romana, S. Richard, F. Carnot, J.-L. Dumont, H. Bouche, G. Pialoux, M. Stern, J. -F. Pays, and P. Berthelot.** 1992. *Enterocytozoon bieneusi* infection in acquired immunodeficiency syndrome-related sclerosing cholangitis. *Gastroenterology* **102**:1778–1781.

58. **Pol, S., C. A. Romana, S. R. Richard, P. Amouyal, I. Desportes-Livage, F. Carnot, J.-F. Pays, and P. Berthelot.** 1993. Microsporidia infection in patients with the human immunodeficiency virus and unexplained cholangitis. *N. Engl. J. Med.* **328**:95–99.

59. **Rabeneck, L., G. M. Genta, F. Gyorkey, J. E. Clarridge, P. Gyorkey, and L. W. Foote.** 1995. Observations on the pathological spectrum and clinical course of microsporidiosis in men infected with human immunodeficiency virus: a follow-up study. *Clin. Infect. Dis.* **20**:1229–1235.

60. **Rabeneck, L., F. Gyorkey, R. M. Genta, P. Gyorkey, L. W. Foote, and J. M. H. Risser.** 1993. The role of microsporidia in the pathogenesis of HIV-related chronic diarrhea. *Ann. Intern. Med.* **119**:895–899.

61. **Rabodonirina, M., M. Bertocchi, I. Desportes-Livage, L. Cotte, H. Levrey, M. A. Piens, G. Monneret, M. Celard, J. F. Mornex, and M. Mojon.** 1996. *Enterocytozoon bieneusi* as a cause of chronic diarrhea in a heart-lung transplant recipient who was seronegative for human immunodeficiency virus. *Clin. Infect. Dis.* **23**:114–117.

62. **Remadi, S., J. Dumais, K. Wafa, and W. MacGee.** 1995. Pulmonary microsporidiosis in a patient with the acquired immunodeficiency syndrome. A case report. *Acta Cytol.* **39**:1112–1116.

63. **Rosberger, D. F., O. N. Serdarevic, R. A. Erlandson, D. A. Schwartz, G. S. Visvesvara, and R. T. Bryan.** 1993. Successful treatment of microsporidial keratoconjunctivitis with topical fumagillin in a patient with AIDS. *Cornea* **12**:261–265.

64. **Sandfort, J., A. Hannemann, H. Gelderblom, K. Stark, R. L. Owen, and B. Ruf.** 1994. *Enterocytozoon bieneusi* infection in an immunocompetent patient who had acute diarrhea and who was not infected with the human immunodeficiency virus. *Clin. Infect. Dis.* **19**:514–516.

65. **Sax, P. E., J. D. Rich, W. S. Pieciak, and Y. M. Trnka.** 1995. Intestinal microsporidiosis occurring in a liver transplant recipient. *Transplantation* **60**:617–618.

66. **Schwartz, D. A., A. Abou-Elella, C. M. Wilcox, L. Gorelkin, G. S. Visvesvara, S. E. Thompson, R. Weber, and R. T. Bryan for the Enteric Opportunistic Infections Working Group.** 1995. The presence of *Enterocytozoon bieneusi* spores in the lamina propria of small bowel biopsies with no evidence of disseminated microsporidiosis. *Arch. Pathol. Lab. Med.* **119:**424–428.

67. **Schwartz, D. A., R. T. Bryan, K. O. Hewan-Lowe, G. S. Visvesvara, R. Weber, A. Cali, and P. Angritt.** 1992. Disseminated microsporidiosis (*Encephalitozoon hellem*) and acquired immunodeficiency syndrome: autopsy evidence for respiratory acquisition. *Arch. Pathol. Lab. Med.* **116:**660–668.

68. **Schwartz, D. A., R. T. Bryan, and G. S. Visvesvara.** 1994. Diagnostic approaches for *Encephalitozoon* infections in patients with AIDS. *J. Eukaryot. Microbiol.* **41:**59S–60S.

69. **Schwartz, D. A., A. Cali, D. P. Rosberger, G. S. Visvesvara, and R. T. Bryan.** 1993. A nasal microsporidian with unusual morphologic features from a patient with AIDS, p. 384, abstr. no. PO-B10-1495. *In Proceedings of the 9th International Conference on AIDS*, Berlin.

69a. **Schwartz, D. A., H. S. Goodman, R. T. Bryan, et al.** Unpublished data.

70. **Schwartz, D. A., I. Sobottka, G. J. Leitch, A. Cali, and G. S. Visvesvara.** 1996. Pathology of microsporidiosis. Emerging parasitic infections in patients with the acquired immunodeficiency syndrome. *Arch. Pathol. Lab. Med.* **120:**173–188.

71. **Schwartz, D. A., G. S. Visvesvara, M. C. Diesenhouse, R. Weber, R. L. Font, L. A. Wilson, G. Corrent, D. F. Rosberger, P. C. Keenen, H. E. Grossniklaus, K. Hewan-Lowe, and R. T. Bryan.** 1993. Ocular pathology of microsporidiosis: role of immunofluorescent antibody for diagnosis of *Encephalitozoon hellem* in biopsies, smears, and intact globes from seven AIDS patients. *Am. J. Ophthalmol.* **115:**285–292.

72. **Schwartz, D. A., G. S. Visvesvara, G. J. Leitch, L. Tashjian, M. Pollack, J. Holden, and R. T. Bryan.** 1993. Pathology of symptomatic microsporidial (*Encephalitozoon hellem*) bronchiolitis in the acquired immunodeficiency syndrome: a new respiratory pathogen diagnosed from lung biopsy, bronchoalveolar lavage, sputum, and tissue culture. *Hum. Pathol.* **24:**937–943.

73. **Schwartz, D. A., G. S. Visvesvara, R. Weber, and R. T. Bryan.** 1993. Pulmonary microsporidiosis—an emerging opportunistic infection in AIDS, abstract no. WS-B14-6, p. 96. *In Proceedings of the 9th International Conference on AIDS*, Berlin.

74. **Schwartz, D. A., G. Visvesvara, R. Weber, and R. T. Bryan.** 1994. Male genital tract microsporidiosis and AIDS: prostatic infection with *Encephalitozoon hellem. J. Eukaryot. Microbiol.* **41:**61S.

75. **Schwartz, D. A., G. S. Visvesvara, R. Weber, C. M. Wilcox, and R. T. Bryan.** 1994. Microsporidiosis in HIV positive patients: current methods for diagnosis using biopsy, cytologic, ultrastructural, immunological and tissue culture techniques. *Folia Parasitol.* **41:**91–99.

76. **Sharpstone, D., A. Rowbottom, M. Nelson, and B. Gazzard.** 1995. The treatment of microsporidial diarrhea with thalidomide. *AIDS* **9:**658–659.

77. **Silveira, H., and E. U. Canning.** 1995. *Vittaforma corneae* N. Comb. for the human microsporidium *Nosema corneum* Shadduck, Meccoli, Davis & Font, 1990, based on its ultrastructure in the liver of experimentally infected athymic mice. *J. Eukaryot. Microbiol.* **42:**158–165.

78. **Sobottka, I., H. Albrecht, H. Schafer, J. Schottelius, G. S. Visvesvara, R. Laufs, and D. A. Schwartz.** 1995. Disseminated *Encephalitozoon (Septata) intestinalis* infection in a patient with AIDS: novel diagnostic approaches and autopsy-confirmed parasitological cure following treatment with albendazole. *J. Clin. Microbiol.* **33:**2948–2952.

79. **Sobottka, I., H. Albrecht, J. Schottelius, M. Bentfeld, R. Laufs, and D. A. Schwartz.** 1995. Self-limited traveller's diarrhea due to a dual infection with *Enterocytozoon bieneusi* and *Cryptosporidium parvum* in an immunocompetent HIV-negative child. *Eur. J. Clin. Microbiol. Infect. Dis.* **14:**919–920.

80. **Sobottka, I., D. A. Schwartz, J. Schottelius, G. S. Visvesvara, N. J. Pieniazek, C. Schmetz, N. P. Kock, R. Laufs, and A. Albrecht.** Prevalence and clinical significance of intestinal microsporidiosis in German HIV-infected patients. Submitted for publication.

81. **Sowerby, T. M., C. N. Conteas, O. G. W. Berlin, and J. Donovan.** 1995. Microsporidiosis in patients with relatively preserved CD4 counts. *AIDS* **9:**975.

82. **Terada, S., R. Reddy, L. J. Jeffers, A. Cali, and E. R. Schiff.** 1987. Microsporidian hepatitis in the acquired immunodeficiency syndrome. *Ann. Intern. Med.* **107:**61–62.

83. **Vangool, T., E. Luderhoff, K. J. Nathoo, C. F. Kiire, J. Damkert, and P. R. Mason.** 1995. High prevalence of *Enterocytozoon bieneusi* infections among HIV-positive individuals with persistent diarrhea in Harare, Zimbabwe. *Trans. R. Soc. Trop. Med. Hyg.* **89:**478–480.

84. **Visvesvara, G. S., G. J. Leitch, A. J. da Silva, G. P. Croppo, H. Moura, S. Wallace, S. B. Slemenda, D. A. Schwartz, D. Moss, R. T. Bryan, and N. J. Pieniazek.** 1994. Polyclonal and monoclonal antibody and PCR-amplified small-subunit rRNA identification of a microsporidian, *Encephalitozoon hellem*, isolated from an AIDS patient with disseminated infection. *J. Clin. Microbiol.* **32:**2760–2768.

85. **Visvesvara, G. S., G. J. Leitch, N. J. Pieniazek, A. J. da Silva, S. Wallace, S. B. Slemenda, R. Weber, D. A. Schwartz, L. Gorelkin, C. M. Wilcox, and R. T. Bryan for the Enteric Opportunistic Infections Working Group.** 1995. Short term *in vitro* culture and molecular analysis of the microsporidian, *Enterocytozoon bieneusi*. *J. Eukaryot. Microbiol.* **42:**506–510.

86. **Wanke, C. A., P. DeGirolami, and M. Federman.** 1996. *Enterocytozoon bieneusi* infection and diarrheal disease in patients who were not infected with human immunodeficiency virus—case report and review. *Clin. Infect. Dis.* **23:**816–818.

87. **Wanke, C. A., and A. R. Mattia.** 1993. A 36-year-old man with AIDS, increase in chronic diarrhea, and intermittent fever and chills. Case records of the Massachusetts General Hospital (Case 51-1993). *N. Engl. J. Med.* **329:**1946–1954.

88. **Weber, R., R. T. Bryan, R. L. Owen, C. M. Wilcox, L. Gorelkin, and G. S. Visvesvara.** 1992. Improved light-microscopical detection of microsporidia spores in stool and duodenal aspirates. *N. Engl. J. Med.* **326:**161–166.

89. **Weber, R., R. T. Bryan, D. A. Schwartz, and R. Owen.** 1994. Human microsporidian infections. *Clin. Microbiol. Rev.* **7:**426–461.

90. **Weber, R., H. Kuster, R. Keller, T. Bächi, M. A. Spycher, J. Briner, E. Russi, and R. Lüthy.** 1992. Pulmonary and intestinal microsporidiosis in a patient with the acquired immunodeficiency syndrome. *Am. Rev. Respir. Dis.* **146:**1603–1605.

91. **Weber, R., H. Kuster, G. S. Visvesvara, R. T. Bryan, D. A. Schwartz, and R. Lüthi.** 1993. Disseminated microsporidiosis due to *Encephalitozoon hellem*: pulmonary colonization, microhematuria, and mild conjunctivitis in a patient with AIDS. *Clin. Infect. Dis.* **17:**415–419.

92. **Weber, R., A. Muller, M. A. Spycher, M. Opravil, R. Ammann, and J. Briner.** 1992. Intestinal *Enterocytozoon bieneusi* microsporidiosis in an HIV-infected patient: diagnosis by ileo-colonoscopic biopsies and long-term follow up. *Clin. Invest.* **70:**1019–1023.

93. **Weber, R., B. Sauer, R. Luthy, and D. Nadal.** 1993. Intestinal coinfection with *Enterocytozoon bieneusi* and *Cryptosporidium* in a human immunodeficiency virus-infected child with chronic diarrhea. *Clin. Infect. Dis.* **17:**480–483.

94. **Yachnis, A. T., J. Berg, A. Martinez-Salazar, B. S. Bender, L. Diaz, A. M. Rojian, T. A. Eskin, and J. M. Orenstein.** 1996. Disseminated microsporidiosis especially infecting the brain, heart and kidneys. Report of a newly recognized pansporoblastic species in two symptomatic AIDS patients. *Am. J. Clin. Pathol.* **106:**535–543.

95. **Zender, H. O., E. Arrigoni, J. Eckert, and Y. Kapanci.** 1989. A case of *Encephalitozoon cuniculi* peritonitis in a patient with AIDS. *Am. J. Clin. Pathol.* **92:**352–356.

chapter 5

Hantavirus Pulmonary Syndrome

Clarence J. Peters and Sherif R. Zaki

n May 1993, the deaths of several previously healthy individuals from a rapidly progressive illness were reported by health care workers in the southwestern United States (3). The patients developed an influenza-like illness, which was followed by a rapidly progressive pulmonary edema, respiratory insufficiency, and shock. By using immunoassays, investigators at the Centers for Disease Control and Prevention (2) detected antibodies cross-reactive to known hantavirus antigens in the serum of the patients, suggesting a previously unrecognized hantavirus as the cause of the disease (2). This observation was quickly confirmed by the demonstration of hantavirus antigens and nucleic acid sequences in autopsy tissues by using immunohistochemical and polymerase chain reaction techniques (1, 4, 15, 18, 27, 28). The causative agent was isolated at the Centers for Disease Control and Prevention from a deer mouse, *Peromyscus maniculatus*, the natural reservoir and vector of this zoonotic virus, and has been subsequently named Sin Nombre virus (SNV) (8, 11). The disease is now known as hantavirus pulmonary syndrome (HPS), and as of January 1996, 124 cases in 24

Clarence J. Peters, Special Pathogens Branch, Centers for Disease Control and Prevention, 1600 Clifton Road, N.E., Mailstop A-26, Atlanta, GA 30333. **Sherif R. Zaki,** Infectious Disease Pathology Activity, National Center for Infectious Diseases, Centers for Disease Control and Prevention, 1600 Clifton Road, N.E., Mailstop G-32, Atlanta, GA 30333.

Pathology of Emerging Infections
Edited by C. Robert Horsburgh, Jr., and Ann Marie Nelson
© 1997 American Society for Microbiology, Washington, DC 20005-4171

states have been confirmed, with a case-fatality rate of 50%. Hantavirus infections are caused by a group of closely related, trisegmented, negative-sense RNA viruses of the family *Bunyaviridae* (21–23). Several known serotypes of these viruses are distributed throughout the world, and each is associated with a different primary rodent reservoir (Table 5.1) (9, 23).

Epidemiology

The reservoir for SNV is the widely distributed deer mouse

The reservoir for SNV is the widely distributed rodent *P. maniculatus* (deer mouse), and SNV infection is endemic in the area of distribution of the deer mouse. Related but distinct hantaviruses (e.g., Bayou virus and Black Creek Canal virus) have been associated with human cases outside the range of *P. maniculatus* in Louisiana, Florida, and Rhode Island (Fig. 5.1). These include Black Creek Canal virus from *Sigmodon hispidus* (Florida), Bayou virus from *Oryzomys palustrus* (Louisiana), and a virus referred to as NY-1 from *Peromyscus leucopus* that may be a distinct virus or a subtype of SNV. In addition, medical investigators working in South America have found three foci of HPS in Argentina, one in Brazil, and one in Paraguay (Fig. 5.2). The order *Rodentia*, family *Muridae*, has three main subfamilies: *Murinae*, *Arvicolinae*, and *Sigmodontinae*. The proliferation of "new" hantaviruses promises to continue and there is even a possibility that each species of sigmodontine rodent has a hantavirus of its own. To date, all HPS cases have been determined to be caused by viruses known or suspected to have sigmodontine rodents as their reservoir, which suggests that there may be some association between the rodent subfamily and the clinical manifestations.

Hantavirus infection in humans may be caused by inhalation of aerosols of rodent saliva or excreta, by inoculation into broken skin, or, less commonly, by rodent bites. There have been no documented cases of transmission through human-to-human contact, nor has occupational transmission by health care workers been documented. Laboratory workers practicing universal precautions while processing routine clinical materials are not considered to be at increased risk for hantavirus infection. However, laboratory-acquired infections among persons who handled infected wild or laboratory rodents have occurred. Therefore, laboratory work that may result in cell culture propagation of hantaviruses should be conducted in a biosafety level 3 facility, and animal work requires additional safeguards.

Table 5.1 Characteristics of the major known hantaviruses

Virus	Geographic region	Reservoir	Human pathology	Mortality (%)
Hantaan	Asia	Field mouse	Renal	5–15
Seoul	Worldwide	Norway rat	Renal	1
Puumala	Northern Europe	Bank vole	Renal	1
Prospect Hill	United States	Meadow vole	No known disease	
Sin Nombre	North America	Deer mouse	Pulmonary	50

Clinical

All hantavirus-associated illnesses reported prior to the outbreak of HPS were characterized by various degrees of fever and renal involvement, with or without hemorrhagic manifestations, and are referred to collectively as hemorrhagic fever with renal syndrome (HFRS) (16, 17). Hantaan virus causes the most severe and often fatal form of HFRS, formerly known as Korean hemorrhagic fever in Korea and epidemic hemorrhagic fever in Japan and China. Seoul virus, which is distributed worldwide, causes a less severe form of the disease and has been diagnosed most frequently in Asia. Puumala virus is the agent responsible for the mildest form of HFRS, referred to as nephropathia epidemica, in Scandinavia and Western Europe. Prospect Hill virus is indigenous to the United States, but it has not been associated with human disease. Infection with the newly recognized SNV, the causative agent of HPS, follows a much more aggressive course (Fig. 5.3) (10, 27). Death occurs early as a result of noncardiogenic pulmonary edema and adult respiratory distress syndrome. The onset is abrupt, with fever, cough, headache, and myalgia followed by rapidly developing respiratory failure (Table 5.2). Table 5.3 compares the clinical features of HFRS with those of HPS.

Infection with the newly recognized SNV, the causative agent of HPS, follows a much more aggressive course. Death occurs early as a result of noncardiogenic pulmonary edema and adult respiratory distress syndrome

Pathophysiology

The histopathologic findings in the lungs are characteristic of the illness; however, the degree of involvement has varied among patients (19, 25, 27). Microscopic examination of the lung reveals a mild to moderate interstitial pneumonitis with variable degrees of congestion, edema, and mononuclear cell infiltration (Fig. 5.4). The cellular infiltrate is composed of a mixture of small and enlarged mononuclear cells with the appearance of immunoblasts.

Table 5.2   Frequency of reported prodromal symptoms for 42 fatal HPS cases (7)

Symptom	Frequency	
	No. of occurrences/total no. of cases	%
Fever	41/42	98
Myalgias	24/42	57
Vomiting	18/42	43
Weakness/fatigue	14/42	33
Cough	13/42	31
Diarrhea	12/42	29
Nausea	12/42	29
Shortness of breath	11/42	26
Headache	10/42	24
Dizziness	5/42	12
Rhinorrhea	4/42	10
Abdominal pain	3/42	7
Chest pain	3/42	7
Numbness (digits, extremities)	2/42	5

Table 5.3 Comparison of HFRS and HPS

Parameter	HFRS	HPS
Major target organ	Kidney	Lung
Secondary target organs	Lung, right atrium, anterior pituitary, liver	Kidney, ?
First-phase clinical illness	Febrile	Febrile = "prodrome"
Second-phase clinical illness	Shock	Shock, pulmonary edema
Evolution of clinical illness	Oliguria, polyuria, convalescence	Recovery
Mortality (%)	1–15	52

Focal hyaline membranes as well as extensive intra-alveolar edema, fibrin, and variable numbers of inflammatory cells can be observed. Another observation in HPS cases is the presence of variable numbers of immunoblasts within the red pulp and periarteriolar sheaths of the spleen and paracortex and within sinuses of lymph nodes and peripheral blood (Fig. 5.5). Although no single pathognomonic lesion that would permit certain histopathologic diagnosis of SNV infection is found, the overall pattern of histopathologic lesions and hematologic findings associated with HPS appears to be distinct from that of other diseases (19, 24, 27). However, the differential diagnosis may be difficult, especially in the context of a histopathologic spectrum of HPS that is wider than initially suspected, and the presence of some overlapping histologic and hematologic features in various infectious and noninfectious disease processes. Hantavirus antigens can be detected by immunohistochemistry of formalin-fixed tissues using specific monoclonal and polyclonal antibodies. Antigens are primarily localized within the endothelium of capillaries throughout various tissues, with marked accumulations within the lung (Fig. 5.6) (27, 28). High densities of hantavirus antigens in follicular dendritic cells within lymphoid follicles of spleen and lymph nodes can also be detected (Fig. 5.7) (27).

Electron microscopy studies confirm the infection of endothelial cells and macrophages in the lungs of HPS patients (12, 27). The virus or virus-like particles observed in HPS tissues are infrequent and are extremely difficult to identify because of the considerable degree of pleomorphism and because of the postmortem deterioration of tissues (Fig. 5.8). Typical hantaviral inclusions, on the other hand, are seen more frequently, and their identity can be confirmed by immunolabeling. Similar inclusions in epithelial cells of patients with HFRS have been observed and are considered to be ultrastructural markers of hantavirus-infected cells (Fig. 5.9).

Diagnosis

Although the hematologic features of thrombocytopenia, hemoconcentration, left-shifted neutrophilic leukocytosis, and presence of atypical lymphocytes in peripheral smears may suggest a diagnosis of HPS, there are no definite symptoms and signs that can reliably distinguish HPS from other forms of noncardiogenic pulmonary edema or adult respiratory distress syndrome at the time of presentation. Efforts to identify clinical and laboratory features that distinguish HPS from other infections with similar manifestations and to develop improved diagnostic methods for rapid early diagnosis are ongoing. Currently, virus-specific diagnosis and confirmation are accomplished through a combination of serology (presence of hantavirus-specific immunoglobulin M or rising titers of immunoglobulin G), polymerase chain reaction for hantavirus RNA, and immunohistochemistry for hantavirus antigens (15, 25, 27).

Treatment

Supportive treatments, such as dialysis and circulatory and respiratory support, are the basis of therapy. Severe hypoxia and overhydration should be avoided or prevented. Controlled studies suggest that ribavirin is effective in the treatment of Hantaan virus infection if administered early. Intravenous ribavirin has been made available under an open label protocol for suspected cases of HPS. Comparison of treated and untreated patients showed no significant difference in survival, but the groups were not matched or randomized. The National Institute of Allergy and Infectious Diseases is sponsoring a double-blind, randomized trial of intravenous ribavirin at selected centers to definitively determine whether the drug has any utility in treatment of HPS.

The clinical condition of HPS patients can deteriorate within a matter of hours, and monitoring of recognized cases during the first 48 h of illness should be intensive. Hypoxia during HPS may be managed by nonrebreathing masks, but often it will require intubation. Another important element of HPS therapy is avoidance of overhydration while treating the hypotension and possible shock. Studies of Hantaan virus infection during the Korean War as well as initial observations of HPS show a pattern unlike that of septic shock. Cardiac output is depressed, and systemic vascular resistance is increased. Administration of large quantities of crystalloid may well lead to exacerbation of the pulmonary edema. Early use of invasive monitoring and pressors may be indicated. Colloid and corticosteroids were used in the 1950s in treatment of HFRS, but their efficacy in HPS is unknown.

Supportive treatments, such as dialysis and circulatory and respiratory support, are the basis of therapy

Conclusion

HPS is an emerging infectious disease that continues to be recognized in the United States and elsewhere. Although the initial cases of HPS were recognized in the southwestern United States, additional cases have been identified in other regions of the United States and Canada (Fig. 5.1) (5, 6, 7). Evidence for different hantavirus genetic strains and the spectrum of associated illnesses in North America continue to evolve. Several species of rodents have been identified as reservoirs for hantaviruses in the United States (1, 13, 14, 20). Retrospective fatal cases of HPS have been identified as early as 1978, suggesting that recent environmental and ecologic changes are primarily responsible for the recent recognition of this new hantavirus and for the occurrence of the HPS outbreak in the Southwest (26, 29).

Figure 5.1 Location of HPS cases in North America as of March 1996, showing the distribution of *P. maniculatus*, the deer mouse, in green and brown. Note that several cases have been identified outside the range of the deer mouse. Rodent distributions were obtained from reference 1a.

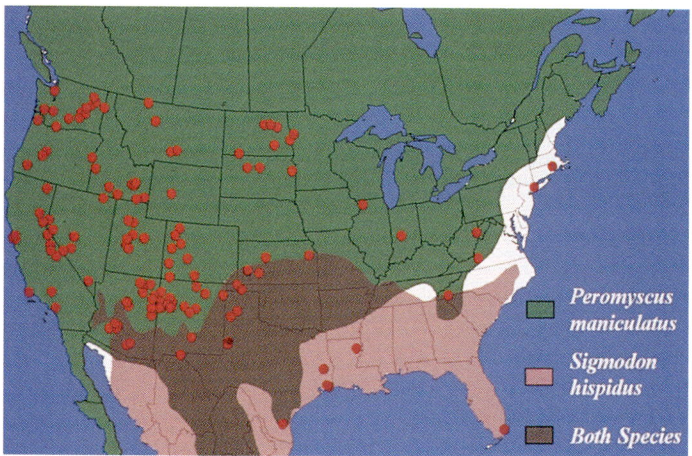

Figure 5.2 Location of three hantaviruses identified in rodents of Central and South America. Sites of recognized HPS cases are also indicated.

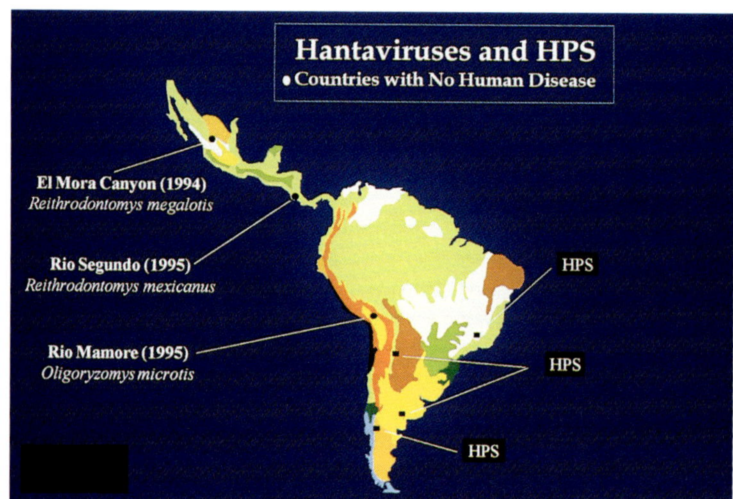

Figure 5.3 Epidemic curve of human HPS cases in the United States, May 1993 through March 1996. Thirty-two additional cases (19 deceased) with onset before 1993 are not shown.

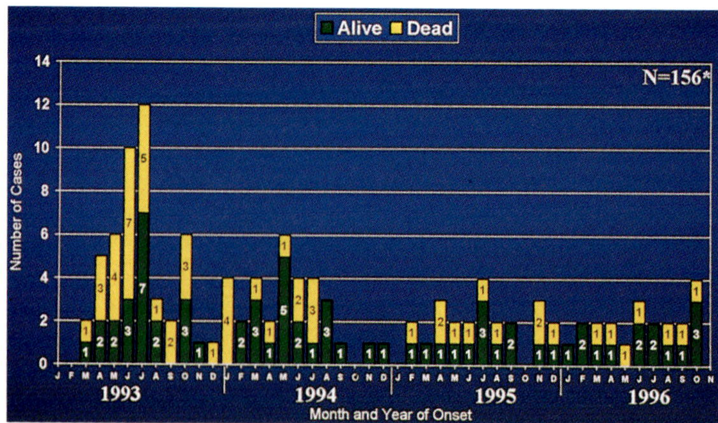

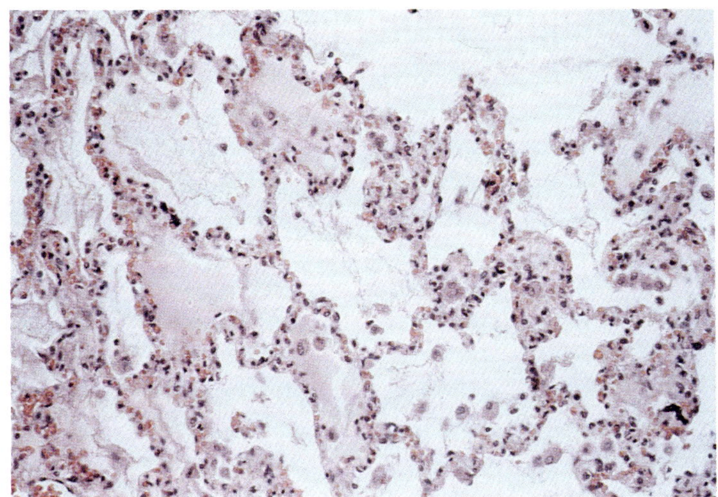

Figure 5.4A Low-power micrograph showing interstitial pneumonitis and intra-alveolar edema (hematoxylin and eosin stain; original magnification, ×50).

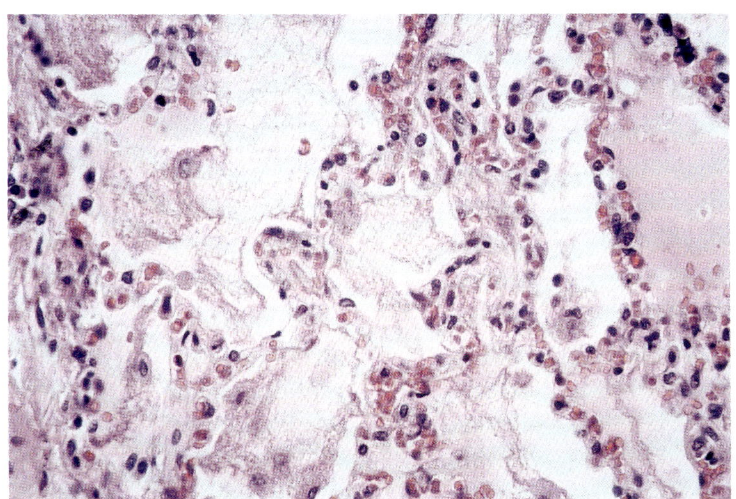

Figure 5.4B Higher magnification showing intra-alveolar fibrin deposits and mononuclear cellular infiltrate (hematoxylin and eosin stain; original magnification, ×100).

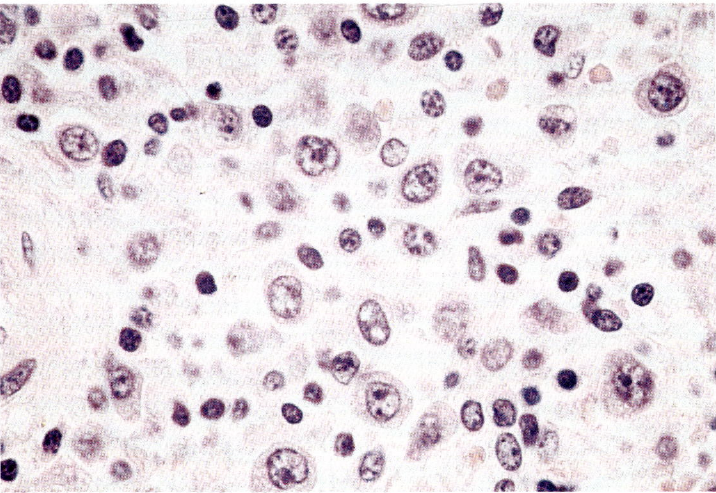

Figure 5.5A Immunoblasts in the periarteriolar sheath of the spleen. Note prominent nucleoli and high nucleus-to-cytoplasm ratio (hematoxylin and eosin stain; original magnification, ×100).

Figure 5.5B Peripheral blood immunoblasts with deeply basophilic cytoplasm, high nucleus-to-cytoplasm ratio, and prominent nucleoli.

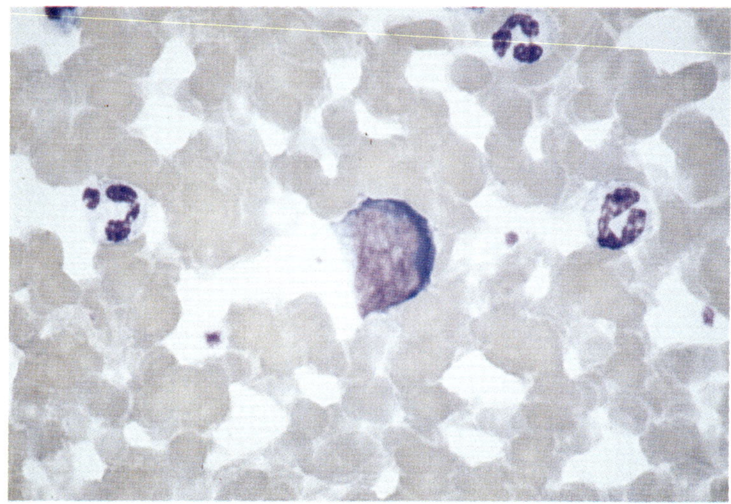

Figure 5.6A Lung showing predominantly endothelial staining in pulmonary microvasculature (rabbit anti-SNV serum; original magnification, ×250).

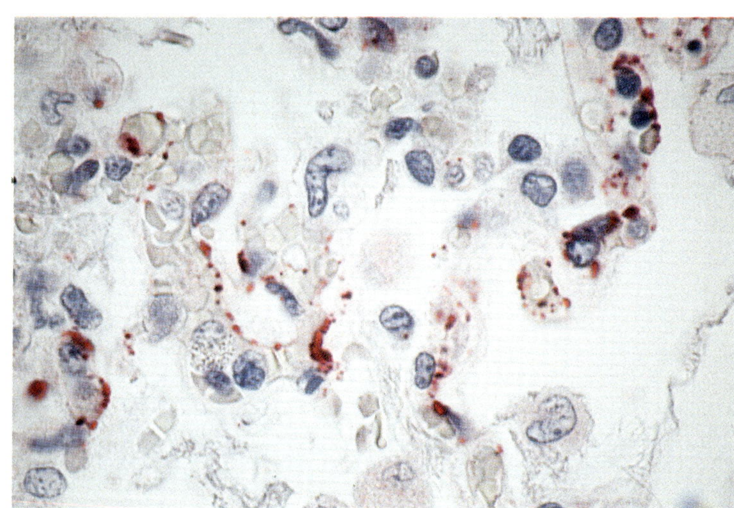

Figure 5.6B Prominent endothelial staining in interstitial capillaries of the renal medulla (rabbit anti-SNV serum; original magnification, ×100).

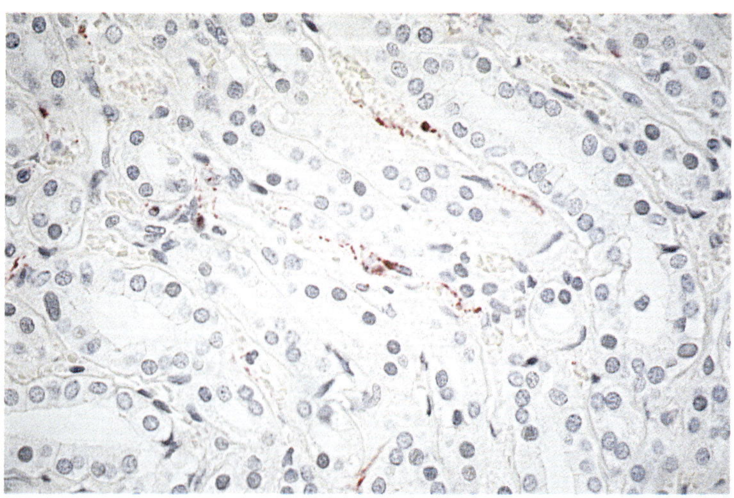

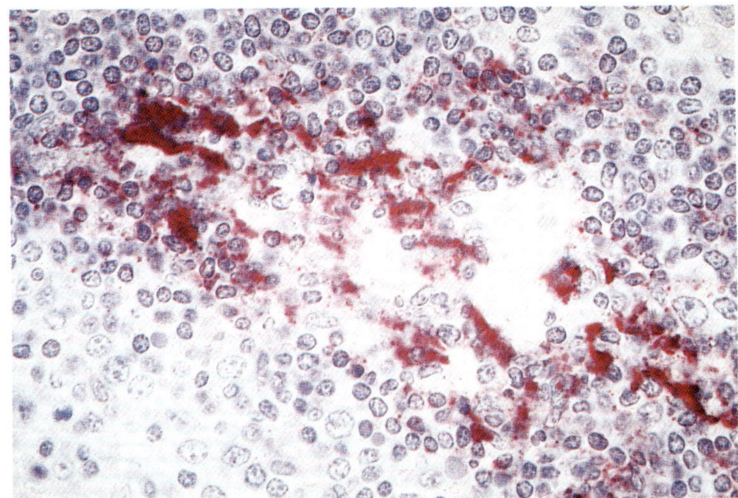

Figure 5.7 Localization of hantaviral antigens in follicular dendritic cells within a lymphoid follicle of spleen (rabbit anti-SNV serum; original magnification, ×158).

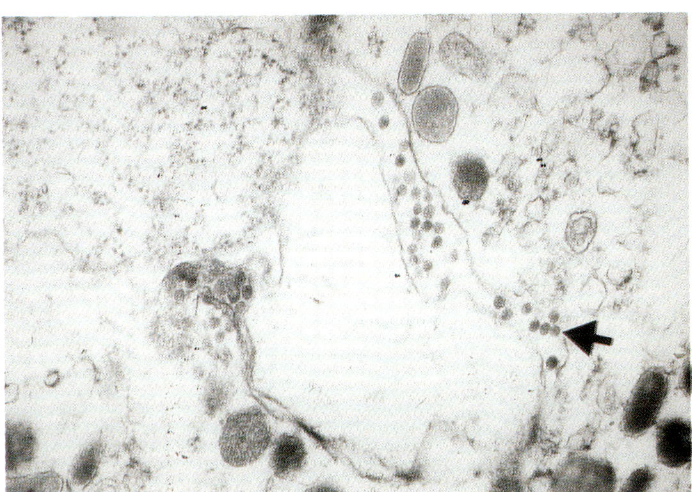

Figure 5.8 Collection of hantavirus-like particles in a pulmonary macrophage (arrow). Interstitial macrophage showing virus-like particles in association with a phagolysosome containing fragments of cellular debris (on right).

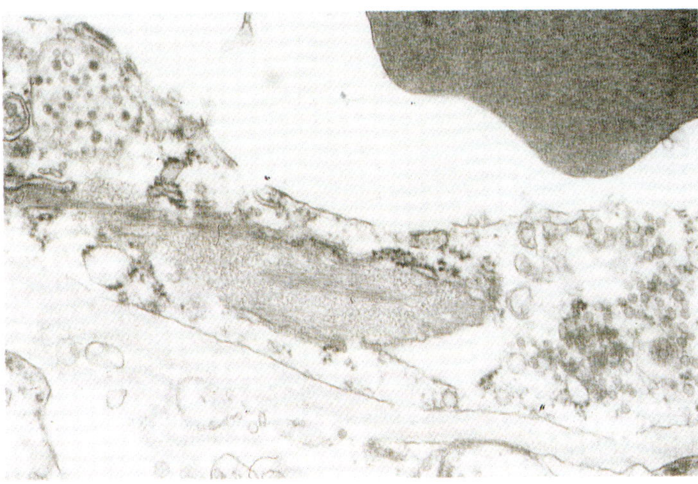

Figure 5.9 Electron micrograph showing typical hantaviral inclusions within the pulmonary microvasculature.

References

1a. **Burt, W. H., and R. P. Grossenheider.** 1980. *A Field Guide to the Mammals*, 3rd ed. Houghton Mifflin Co., New York.

1. **Centers for Disease Control and Prevention.** 1993. Update: hantavirus pulmonary syndrome—United States, 1993. *Morbid. Mortal. Weekly Rep.* **42:**816–820.

2. **Centers for Disease Control and Prevention.** 1993. Update: outbreak of hantavirus infection—southwestern United States, 1993. *Morbid. Mortal. Weekly Rep.* **42:**441–443.

3. **Centers for Disease Control and Prevention.** 1993. Outbreak of acute illness—southwestern United States, 1993. *Morbid. Mortal. Weekly Rep.* **42:**421–424.

4. **Centers for Disease Control and Prevention.** 1993. Update: outbreak of hantavirus infection—southwestern United States, 1993. *Morbid. Mortal. Weekly Rep.* **42:**477–479.

5. **Centers for Disease Control and Prevention.** 1994. Hantavirus pulmonary syndrome—northeastern United States. *Morbid. Mortal. Weekly Rep.* **43:**548–549, 555–556.

6. **Centers for Disease Control and Prevention.** 1994. Newly identified hantavirus—Florida, 1994. *Morbid. Mortal. Weekly Rep.* **43:**99–105.

7. **Chapman, L. E., and R. F. Khabbaz.** 1994. Etiology and epidemiology of the Four Corners hantavirus outbreak. *Infect. Agents Dis.* **3:**234–244.

8. **Childs, J. E., T. G. Ksiazek, C. F. Spiropoulou, J. W. Krebs, S. Morzunov, G. O. Maupin, K. L. Gage, P. E. Rollin, J. Sarisky, R. E. Enscore, J. K. Frey, C. J. Peters, and S. T. Nichol.** 1994. Serologic and genetic identification of *Peromyscus maniculatus* as the primary rodent reservoir for a new hantavirus in the southwestern United States. *J. Infect. Dis.* **169:**1271–1280.

9. **Chu, Y. K., C. Rossi, J. W. Leduc, H. W. Lee, C. S. Schmaljohn, and J. M. Dalrymple.** 1994. Serological relationships among viruses in the Hantavirus genus, family *Bunyaviridae*. *Virology* **198:**196–204.

10. **Duchin, J. S., F. T. Koster, C. J. Peters, G. L. Simpson, B. Tempest, S. R. Zaki, P. E. Rollin, S. Nichol, E. T. Umland, R. L. Moolenaar, S. E. Reef, K. B. Nolte, M. M. Gallagher, J. C. Butler, R. F. Breiman, and Hantavirus Study Group.** 1994. Hantavirus pulmonary syndrome: a clinical description of 17 patients with a newly recognized disease. *N. Engl. J. Med.* **330:**949–955.

11. **Elliott, L. H., T. G. Ksiazek, P. E. Rollin, C. F. Spiropoulou, S. Morzunov, M. Monroe, C. S. Goldsmith, C. D. Humphrey, S. R. Zaki, J. W. Krebs, G. Maupin, K. Gage, J. E. Childs, S. T. Nichol, and C. J. Peters.** 1994. Isolation of the causative agent of hantavirus pulmonary syndrome. *Am. J. Trop. Med. Hyg.* **51:**102–108.

12. **Goldsmith, C. S., C. D. Humphrey, L. H. Elliott, and S. R. Zaki..** 1994. Morphology of Muerto Canyon virus, causative agent of hantavirus pulmonary syndrome, p. 272–273. *In* G. W. Bailey and A. J. Garratt-Reed (ed.), *Proceedings of the Microscopy Society of America Fifty-Second Annual Meeting*, San Francisco.

13. **Hjelle, B., F. Chavez-Giles, N. Torrez-Martinez, T. Yates, J. Sarisky, J. Webb, and M. Ascher.** 1994. Genetic identification of a novel hantavirus of the harvest mouse *Reithrodontomys megalotis*. *J. Virol.* **68:**6751–6754.

14. **Hjelle, B., S. Jenison, N. Torrez-Martinez, T. Yamada, K. Nolte, R. Zumwalt, and G. Myers.** 1994. A novel hantavirus associated with an outbreak of fatal respiratory disease in the southwestern United States: evolutionary relationships to known hantaviruses. *J. Virol.* **68**:592–596.

15. **Ksiazek, T. G., C. J. Peters, P. E. Rollin, S. R. Zaki, S. Nichol, C. F. Spiropoulou, S. Morzunov, H. Feldman, A. Sanchez, A. Khan, B. Mahy, K. Wachsmuth, and J. Butler.** 1995. Identification of a new North American hantavirus that causes acute pulmonary insufficiency. *Am. J. Trop. Med. Hyg.* **52**:1017–1023.

16. **Leduc, J. W.** 1987. Epidemiology of Hantaan and related viruses. *Lab. Anim. Sci.* **37**:413–418.

17. **Lee, H. W.** 1989. World Health Organization (WHO) Collaborating Center for Virus Reference and Research, p. 11–18. *In* H. W. Lee and J. M. Dalrymple (ed.), *Manual of Hemorrhagic Fever with Renal Syndrome.* Korea University, Seoul.

18. **Nichol, S. T., C. F. Spiropoulou, S. Morzunov, P. E. Rollin, T. G. Ksiazek, H. Feldmann, A. Sanchez, J. Childs, S. R. Zaki, and C. J. Peters.** 1993. Genetic identification of a hantavirus associated with an outbreak of acute respiratory illness. *Science* **262**:914–917.

19. **Nolte, K. B., R. M. Feddersen, K. Foucar, S. R. Zaki, F. T. Koster, D. Madar, T. L. Merlin, E. T. Umland, P. J. McFeeley, and R. E. Zumwalt.** 1995. Hantavirus pulmonary syndrome in the United States: pathologic description of a disease caused by a new agent. *Hum. Pathol.* **26**:110–120.

20. **Rollin, P. E., T. G. Ksiazek, L. H. Elliott, E. V. Ravkov, M. L. Martin, S. Morzunov, W. Livingstone, M. Monroe, G. Glass, S. Ruo, A. S. Khan, J. E. Childs, S. T. Nichol, and C. J. Peters.** 1995. Isolation of Black Creek Canal virus, a new hantavirus from *Sigmodon hispidus* in Florida. *J. Med. Virol.* **46**:35–39.

21. **Schmaljohn, C. S.** 1990. Nucleotide sequence of the L genome segment of Hantaan virus. *Nucleic Acids Res.* **18**:6728.

22. **Schmaljohn, C. S., and J. M. Dalrymple.** 1983. Analysis of Hantaan virus RNA: evidence for a new genus of *Bunyaviridae. Virology* **131**:482–491.

23. **Spiropoulou, C. F., S. Morzunov, H. Feldmann, A. Sanchez, C. J. Peters, and S. T. Nichol.** 1994. Genome structure and variability of a virus causing hantavirus pulmonary syndrome. *Virology* **200**:715–723.

24. **Zaki, S. R.** 1995. Hantavirus pulmonary syndrome. *Microbiology* **38**:97–114.

25. **Zaki, S. R.** 1997. Hantavirus-associated diseases, p. 125–136. *In* D. H. Connor, F. W. Chandler, D. A. Schwartz, H. J. Manz, and E. E. Lack (ed.), *Pathology of Infectious Diseases.* Appleton and Lange, Stamford, Conn.

26. **Zaki, S. R., R. C. Albers, P. W. Greer, L. M. Coffield, L. R. Armstrong, A. S. Khan, R. Khabbaz, and C. J. Peters.** 1994. Retrospective diagnosis of a 1983 case of fatal hantavirus pulmonary syndrome. *Lancet* **343**:1037–1038.

27. **Zaki, S. R., P. W. Greer, L. M. Coffield, C. S. Goldsmith, K. B. Nolte, K. Foucar, R. M. Feddersen, R. E. Zumwalt, G. L. Miller, A. S. Khan, P. E. Rollin, T. G. Ksiazek, S. T. Nichol, B. W. J. Mahy, and C. J. Peters.** 1995. Hantavirus pulmonary syndrome: pathogenesis of an emerging infectious disease. *Am. J. Pathol.* **146**:552–579.

28. **Zaki, S. R., P. W. Greer, L. M. Coffield, K. B. Nolte, R. Zumwalt, E. Umland, R. M. Feddersen, K. Foucar, S. L. Ruo, P. Rollin, T. Ksiazek, S. Nichol, and C. J. Peters.** 1994. Outbreak of hantavirus-associated illness in the United States: immunohistochemical localization of viral nucleoproteins to endothelial cells in human tissues (abstract). *Lab. Invest.* **70:**129A.

29. **Zaki, S. R., A. S. Khan, R. A. Goodman, L. R. Armstrong, P. W. Greer, L. M. Coffield, T. G. Ksiazek, P. E. Rollin, C. J. Peters, and R. F. Khabbaz.** 1996. Retrospective diagnosis of hantavirus pulmonary syndrome, 1978–1993: implications for emerging infectious disease. *Arch. Pathol. Lab. Med.* **120:**134–139.

chapter 6

Kaposi's Sarcoma and Human Herpesvirus 8

Harold W. Jaffe and Sarah S. Frankel

Epidemiology

In 1872, Moritz Kaposi, a dermatologist working in Vienna, described five men over age 40 and one boy with "idiopathic multiple pigmented sarcomas" of the skin (21). Since that time, the disease described by Kaposi has become known as "classical" Kaposi's sarcoma (KS); epidemiologic studies have shown classical KS to be primarily a disease of elderly men, particularly men of southern European (especially Italian) and Ashkenazic Jewish ancestry (14, 43). Classical KS has been a rare disease in the United States; an estimated 300 to 400 cases occurred annually in this country during the mid-1970s (8). This form of KS is typically described as having an indolent clinical course, and lesions are usually limited to the skin, especially the skin of the lower legs or feet. Elderly men were said to die with KS rather than from KS. Persons with classical KS are at increased risk for a second malignancy, especially lymphomas (39).

Harold W. Jaffe, Division of AIDS, STD, and TB Laboratory Research, National Center for Infectious Diseases, Centers for Disease Control and Prevention, 1600 Clifton Road, N.E., Mailstop A-12, Atlanta, GA 30333. **Sarah S. Frankel,** Division of AIDS and Emerging Infectious Disease Pathology, Armed Forces Institute of Pathology, Washington, DC 20306, and Department of Vaccine Research, Division of Retrovirology, Walter Reed Army Institute of Research, 13 Taft Court, Suite 200, Rockville, MD 20850.

Pathology of Emerging Infections
Edited by C. Robert Horsburgh, Jr., and Ann Marie Nelson
© 1997 American Society for Microbiology, Washington, DC 20005-4171

A second epidemiologic form of KS was recognized in Africa. This endemic form of the disease occurs most commonly in equatorial Africa and accounted for 8% of all cancers among Ugandan men in the mid-1960s (41). Like classical KS, endemic KS occurs among men more often than women, and its incidence increases with age. Children also may be affected. The clinical course of KS among Africans may be more aggressive than that seen among Americans or Europeans.

A third epidemiologic form of KS is seen among persons with iatrogenic immunosuppression, most often in organ transplant recipients. In the Cincinnati Transplant Tumor Registry, KS accounted for 3 to 4% of all tumors reported (35). The incubation period for KS following transplantation was relatively short, a median of 16 months, versus 54 months for other tumors. In contrast to the other forms of KS, there is no clear male predominance in this form; rather, the sex distribution of cases is similar to that of transplant recipients. In about two-thirds of cases, the clinical course of disease is described as indolent, and complete remission of disease has been reported in some cases following cessation of immunosuppressive therapy.

The final epidemiologic form of KS is a disease seen among human immunodeficiency virus (HIV)-infected persons. The occurrence of KS among young, previously healthy homosexual men was one of the first indications of the AIDS epidemic in the United States (10), and KS in HIV-infected persons became an AIDS-defining condition. KS is by far the most common malignancy in HIV-infected persons (reported in almost 10% of all persons with AIDS). An analysis done in 1990 indicated that the incidence of KS among persons with AIDS was about 20,000 times that seen in the general population and about 300 times that seen in other immunosuppressed patients (7). The course of KS among HIV-infected persons is often aggressive, with multiple cutaneous lesions. Visceral disease, involving the lungs and gastrointestinal system, is common.

> *The occurrence of KS among young, previously healthy homosexual men was one of the first indications of the AIDS epidemic in the United States*

The proportion of HIV-infected persons who develop KS varies considerably among persons in different HIV transmission categories. Overall, the KS risk is highest for homosexual men, intermediate for persons infected through heterosexual contact and intravenous drug use, and lowest for persons with hemophilia (7). Although the incidence of KS as an initial AIDS-defining condition in the United States has been decreasing, KS continues to be seen later in the course of HIV infection. For example, following the initial diagnosis of AIDS, KS continues to occur at a rate approaching 10%/year among homosexual men (10a).

A number of the epidemiologic aspects of KS suggest that it may have an infectious cause. One group of studies concerns risk factors for KS among homosexual men. While the findings from these studies are not entirely consistent, they suggest that the KS risk for homosexual men is highest if they have multiple sex partners (2, 3, 19). Some studies indicate that sexual practices that lead to exposure to feces may additionally increase the KS risk (5). For homosexual men living in the United States, KS risk is highest for those living in areas of high AIDS incidence (7). For homosexual men living in the United Kingdom, KS risk is highest for those having sexual partners from the United States or Africa (6).

Additional epidemiologic data come from studies of KS among women with heterosexually acquired HIV infection. In the United States, the highest KS rates for HIV-infected women are seen in women born in Haiti or having sex partners from Haiti, an area of high KS incidence. Women whose male partners are bisexual have an intermediate KS risk, while the lowest risk is seen in women who acquired HIV through sex with heterosexual men (7). Finally, support for the infectious agent hypothesis comes from reports of KS among relatively young, HIV-uninfected homosexual men. These men, described mainly in New York City, have normal CD4+ T-lymphocyte counts and a clinically indolent course of KS disease (15).

Taken together, these observations suggest that if there is an infectious cause of KS, it is more common in homosexual men than other persons in the United States. Further, its primary route of transmission may be sexual, although fecal-oral exposure may play a role. This latter transmission route could be more important in developing parts of the world, such as Africa or Haiti, where sanitation may be poor. The occurrence of KS among HIV-uninfected homosexual men may represent the presence of the "KS agent" in the absence of HIV infection (4, 36, 37).

Human Herpesvirus 8 and KS

Despite the epidemiologic data that suggest an infectious cause of KS, no likely agent was identified until late 1994, when Chang et al. reported the detection of herpesvirus-like DNA sequences in AIDS-associated KS tissue (12). The sequences were found by the use of a molecular biologic technique called representational difference analysis, which allowed for amplification of DNA sequences present in the KS tissue but not the normal tissues of the same person. Although initially called KS-associated herpesvirus, this novel virus is now referred to as human herpesvirus 8 (HHV-8). Phylogenetic analyses indicate that HHV-8 is a gammaherpesvirus. Its closest known relative is herpesvirus saimiri, a virus that causes T-cell lymphoproliferative disorders in some New World monkeys. Among human herpesviruses, the closest relative of HHV-8 is Epstein-Barr virus (30). A number of subsequent reports described the detection of HHV-8 DNA in nearly all KS tissues tested, regardless of the epidemiologic form of the KS (1, 9, 13, 18, 29). There appears to be little variation among reported HHV-8 DNA sequences, and no subtype or strain of HHV-8 has been associated with any of the epidemiologic forms of KS. The sequences may be found in nontumor tissue from patients with KS, but they are rarely detected in other tumors from HIV-uninfected patients.

In support of the etiologic role of HHV-8 in KS, HHV-8 DNA has been detected in peripheral blood mononuclear cells preceding the onset of KS among HIV-infected patients (31, 44). One study of a cohort of HIV-infected persons found that over a median follow-up of 30 months, 6 (55%) of 11 persons with detectable HHV-8 infection developed KS in contrast with 12 (9%) of 132 persons without detectable HHV-8 (44). Other reported associations of HHV-8 include body cavity lymphomas in HIV-infected per-

HHV-8 DNA has been detected in peripheral blood mononuclear cells preceding the onset of KS among HIV-infected patients

sons and multicentric Castleman's disease (11, 40). The latter condition is an atypical lymphoproliferative disorder known to be associated with KS among both HIV-infected and -uninfected persons. A report of detection of HHV-8 sequences in both malignant and benign skin lesions among transplant recipients has not been confirmed (38).

The association of HHV-8 with KS also may have implications for the treatment and prevention of KS. Case reports have described KS remission among several HIV-infected patients following treatment with an antiherpesvirus compound, foscarnet (32). Several other studies have indicated a trend towards a decreased risk of developing KS among HIV-infected patients who received foscarnet for treatment of other herpesvirus infections (20, 27). One of these studies also found that another antiherpesvirus compound, ganciclovir, had a similar effect (27).

Current estimates of HHV-8 prevalence in specific populations vary widely, depending on the diagnostic test used

Current estimates of HHV-8 prevalence in specific populations vary widely, depending on the diagnostic test used. Available serologic tests use indirect immunofluorescence or immunoblot methods to detect antibodies to either latent or induced antigens expressed by HHV-8 in infected body cavity lymphoma cell lines. Initial reports of these tests indicated that HHV-8 antibodies are detected in between 65 and 88% of persons with HIV-associated KS. In contrast, 0 to 1% of HIV-negative U.S. blood donors have detectable HHV-8 antibodies, and between 18 and 35% of HIV-infected homosexual men without KS are seropositive (16, 22, 26). One study found HHV-8 antibodies in 4% of Italian blood donors and 51% of Ugandan patients who were HIV seronegative and without KS (17). Thus, the prevalence of HHV-8 antibodies appears to parallel the relative risk of KS in these populations. However, all of these antibody tests are somewhat insensitive, since none is reactive in all persons with HIV-associated KS.

More recently, an immunofluorescence test with increased sensitivity has been reported (23). When this test was used, HHV-8 seroprevalence was found to be 97% in persons with KS, 93% in HIV-infected homosexual men, 20% in HIV-uninfected blood donors, and 4% in children. These results suggest that HHV-8 may be sexually transmitted, but the detection of HHV-8 antibodies in children indicates the existence of other transmission routes as well.

Studies based on detection of HHV-8 DNA in semen samples also suggest that HHV-8 infection is relatively common and may be sexually transmitted. In an American study, a nested polymerase chain reaction (PCR) assay detected HHV-8 in 91% of semen specimens from HIV-infected homosexual men and 23% of specimens from healthy semen donors (25). In an Italian study, nested PCR detected HHV-8 in between 50 and 91% of semen samples from patients undergoing surgery for varicocele (28).

There is not yet a consensus regarding optimal diagnostic tests for HHV-8. No system for the reliable propagation of HHV-8 in tissue culture has been reported. Improved diagnostic tests will be needed to establish the modes of HHV-8 transmission, the prevalence of HHV-8 infection in sentinel populations, and the role of HHV-8 in the development of KS.

Clinical Manifestations

The initial presentation of KS is usually that of a painless erythematous macule, which may be asymptomatic. At this early stage, which correlates to patch stage histologically, the lesion resembles a bruise with discolored edges. As it progresses, this early lesion will enlarge, becoming scaly, violaceous or brown, and elevated. This lesion clinically resembles a melanocytic lesion or a papulosquamous eruption and correlates with the plaque stage histologically. Finally, the lesions become coalescent violaceous tumors which correlate to the tumor stage histologically (24).

The lesions tend to occur along lines of skin cleavage. In patients with AIDS-related KS, the lesions tend to occur on the face and trunk and within the oral cavity. Alternatively, lesions may occur in lymph nodes, viscerally and/or mucosally, without or long preceding cutaneous involvement. This is in contrast to the lesions of classical KS, which usually occur on the lower legs and feet. In AIDS patients the lesions also tend to be of smaller size and extensively distributed over the body and they tend to progress faster than the lesions of classical or endemic KS.

The initial presentation of KS is usually that of a painless erythematous macule, which may be asymptomatic

Histopathology

AIDS-related KS is not histopathologically distinct from classical, endemic, or transplant-associated KS. All four clinical forms of the disease progress through three histopathologic stages: patch, plaque, and nodular. Early patch stage lesions may resemble granulation tissue. The blood vessels of the dermis are dilated and increased in number. The endothelial cells which line the blood vessels may appear prominent or enlarged; they also may protrude into the vascular lumen. There is usually a diffuse cellular infiltrate, composed of lymphocytes, plasma cells, and some macrophages. There is also attempted new blood vessel formation. Hemosiderin deposition and extravasation of erythrocytes are also seen. Cytologic atypia is not a prominent feature of the lesion at this stage. The histopathologic findings at this stage of disease are frequently not diagnostic and often constitute a challenge to the surgical pathologist (24).

In the intermediate plaque and nodular (tumor) stages, groups of blood vessels with surrounding spindle cells are present. These spindle cells are peripheral to the endothelial cell layer. The spindle cells and often the dilated vessels are found within a stroma which contains both intra- and extracellular hemosiderin pigment as well as extravasated erythrocytes. There may also be associated spindle-cell proliferations of endothelial cells, as well as neoplastic proliferations of lymphatic channels. The spindle cell formations are composed of cells extending irregularly in haphazard directions. The nuclei of these cells may be elongated and may vary in size and shape. Periodic acid-Schiff-positive hyaline globules may frequently be seen within the spindle cells. In the later stages of the lesion, small numbers of mitotic figures may or may not be identified.

Pathogenesis

Electron microscopy and immunohistochemistry have failed to reveal definitive evidence for the cell of origin for KS

Electron microscopy and immunohistochemistry have failed to reveal definitive evidence for the cell of origin for KS. Much evidence supports endothelial cells as the progenitor cells of this tumor; however, there is evidence to support fibroblasts and pericytes as possibly playing a role in its etiology (24). This is currently being investigated. In addition to the cell of origin remaining in doubt, there is doubt as to whether KS is actually a true metastasizing malignancy. The observations that multiple lesions arise simultaneously and that there often is not a primary lesion seem to argue against it. Each lesion appears to act as an independent primary tumor. There is not a clear primary lesion with crops of metastatic daughters. Some lesions regress spontaneously. True monoclonality has yet to be established in a large cohort of tumors.

The growth of KS cell lines and the establishment of experimental tumors in mice are regulated by a variety of cytokines and angiogenic growth factors. These include transforming growth factor β, tumor necrosis factor α, interleukin 6, fibroblast growth factor, and endothelial growth factor, as well as the Tat protein of HIV (24, 42, 45). Not only do the cells respond to these molecules, they actually produce many of them in an autocrine manner. Robert Gallo and others have postulated that KS may be like Hodgkin's disease, in that a small number of malignant cells elicits a nodular tissue reaction. The tumor nodule is actually composed of a large number of reactive cells responding to the much smaller truly malignant clone. This is an attractive concept, though the potentially malignant clone has yet to be identified (34).

The identification of HHV-8 within the KS lesions has been a conundrum until very recently. Jan Marc Orenstein and colleagues presented complete and convincing data on the identification of HHV-8 in the skin, lymph node, and spleen of three HIV-1-infected patients with KS (33). All three tissues were PCR positive for the HHV-8 sequences. Spindle cells and immunoblast-like cells in residual lymphoid tissue were positive by in situ hybridization for the HHV-8 herpesvirus sequence. Transmission electron microscopy yielded the most convincing data: herpesvirus particles were identified in all of the tissues and vasoformative spindle cells that were productively infected with virus were seen. These investigators also described a distinctive eosinophilic intranuclear inclusion, visible by light microscopy, that correlates with the location of the viral particles as well as the location of the in situ signal within the nuclei of infected spindle cells (33). These findings strongly support the conclusion that HHV-8 is the causative infectious agent in KS.

Treatment and Prevention

There are no known effective treatment or prevention strategies.

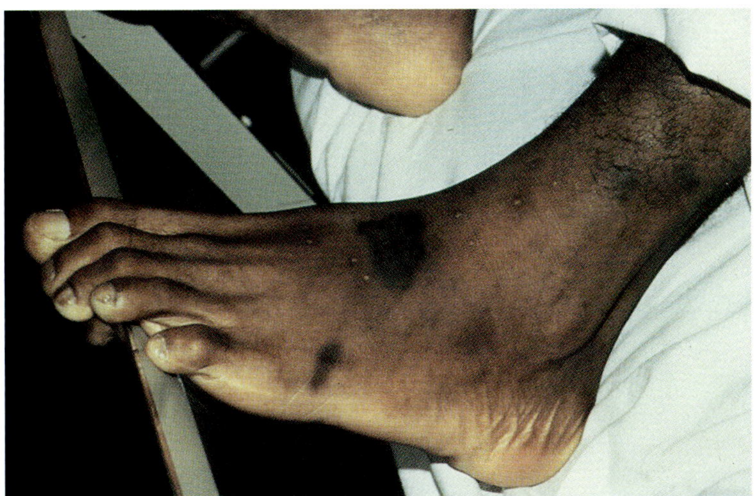

Figure 6.1　Gross photo of KS involving the skin of the foot. Note typical anatomical location of endemic (African) type.

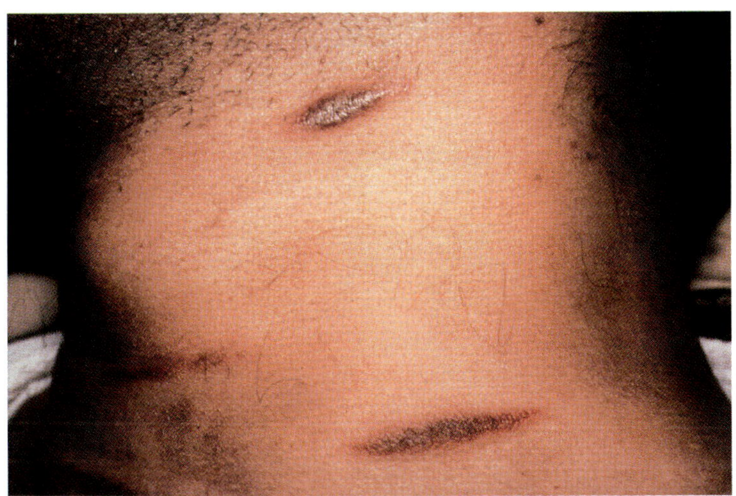

Figure 6.2　Gross photo of KS (patch and plaque stage) involving the skin of the neck. Note typical anatomical location of epidemic type.

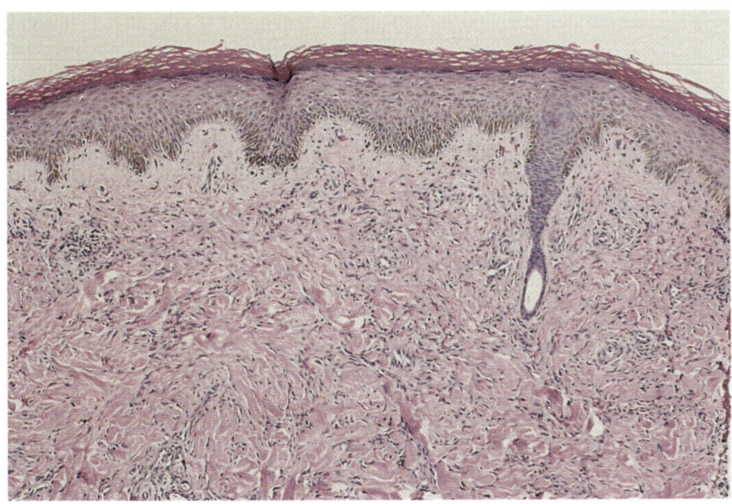

Figure 6.3　Low-power photomicrograph of early KS involving the skin. Proliferating cells intersect collagen bundles.

Figure 6.4 High-power photomicrograph of KS involving the skin. Note vascular promontories overlying a tumor stage lesion.

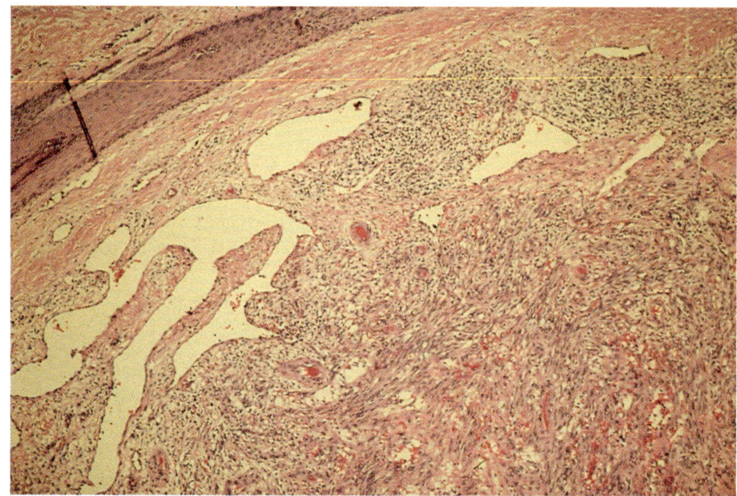

Figure 6.5 High-power photomicrograph of KS involving lymph node. Note typical sarcomatous pattern of spindle cells forming vascular slit-like spaces.

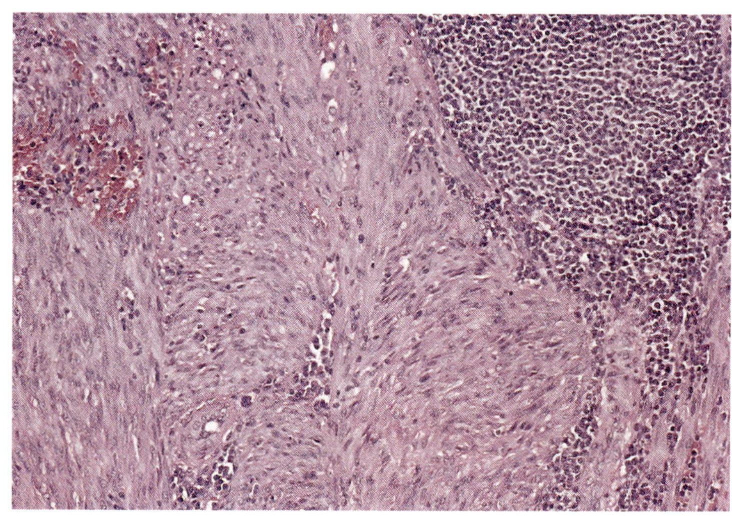

References

1. **Ambroziak, J. A., D. J. Blackbourn, B. G. Herndier, R. G. Glogau, J. H. Gullet, A. R. McDonald, E. T. Lennette, and J. A. Levy.** 1995. Herpes-like sequences in HIV-infected and uninfected Kaposi's sarcoma patients. *Science* **268:**582–583.

2. **Archibald, C. P., M. T. Schechter, T. N. Le, K. J. P. Craib, J. S. G. Montaner, and M. V. O'Shaughnessy.** 1992. Evidence for a sexually transmitted cofactor for Kaposi's sarcoma in a cohort of homosexual men. *Epidemiology* **3:**203–209.

3. **Armenian, H. K., D. R. Hoover, S. Rubb, S. Metz, R. Kaslow, B. Visscher, J. Chmiel, L. Kingsley, and A. Saah.** 1993. Composite risk score for Kaposi's sarcoma based on a case-control and longitudinal study in the multicenter AIDS cohort study (MACS) population. *Am. J. Epidemiol.* **138:**256–265.

4. **Beral, V.** 1991. Epidemiology of Kaposi's sarcoma. Cancer Surv. Ser. **10:**5–22.

5. **Beral, V., D. Bull, S. Darby, I. Weller, C. Carne, M. Beecham, and H. Jaffe.** 1992. Risk of Kaposi's sarcoma and sexual practices associated with faecal contact in homosexual or bisexual men with AIDS. *Lancet* **339:**632.

6. **Beral, V., D. Bull, H. Jaffe, B. Evans, N. Gill, H. Tillett, and A. J. Swerdlow.** 1991. Is risk of Kaposi's sarcoma in AIDS patients in Britain increased if sexual partners came from United States or Africa? *Br. Med. J.* **302:**624–625.

7. **Beral, V., T. A. Peterman, R. L. Berkelman, and H. W. Jaffe.** 1990. Kaposi's sarcoma among persons with AIDS: a sexually transmitted infection? *Lancet* **335:**123–128.

8. **Biggar, R. J., J. Horm, J. F. Fraumeni, Jr., M. H. Greene, and J. J. Goedert.** 1984. Incidence of Kaposi's sarcoma and mycosis fungoides in the United States including Puerto Rico. *J. Natl. Cancer Inst.* **73:**89–94.

9. **Boshoff, C., D. Whitby, T. Hatzioannou, C. Fisher, J. van der Walt, A. Hatzakis, R. Weiss, and T. Schulz.** 1995. Kaposi's-sarcoma-associated herpesvirus in HIV-negative Kaposi's sarcoma. *Lancet* **345:**1043–1044.

10. **Centers for Disease Control.** 1981. Kaposi's sarcoma and pneumocystis pneumonia among homosexual men—New York City and California. *Morbid. Mortal. Weekly Rep.* **30:**305–308.

10a. **Centers for Disease Control and Prevention.** Unpublished data.

11. **Cesarman, E., Y. Chang, P. S. Moore, J. W. Said, and D. M. Knowles.** 1995. Kaposi's sarcoma-associated herpesvirus-like DNA sequences in AIDS-related body-cavity-based lymphomas. *N. Engl. J. Med.* **332:**1186–1191.

12. **Chang, Y., E. Cesarman, M. S. Pessin, F. Lee, J. Culpepper, D. M. Knowles, and P. S. Moore.** 1994. Identification of herpesvirus-like DNA sequences in AIDS-associated Kaposi's sarcoma. *Science* **266:**1865–1869.

13. **Collandre, H., S. Ferris, O. Grau, L. Montagnier, and A. Blanchard.** 1995. Kaposi's sarcoma and new herpesvirus 1. *Lancet* **345:**1043.

14. **Digiovanna, J. J., and B. Safai.** 1981. Kaposi's sarcoma. Retrospective study of 90 cases with particular emphasis on the familial occurrence, ethnic background, and prevalence of other diseases. *Am. J. Med.* **71:**779–783.

15. **Friedman-Kien, A. E., B. R. Saltzman, Y. Z. Cao, M. S. Nestor, M. Mirabile, J. J. Li, and T. A. Peterman.** 1990. Kaposi's sarcoma in HIV-negative homosexual men. *Lancet* **335:**168–169.

16. **Gao, S.-J., L. Kingsley, D. R. Hoover, T. J. Spira, C. R. Rinaldo, A. Saah, J. Phair, R. Detels, P. Parry, Y. Chang, and P. S. Moore.** 1996. Seroconversion to antibodies against Kaposi's sarcoma-associated herpesvirus-related latent nuclear antigens before the development of Kaposi's sarcoma. *N. Engl. J. Med.* **335:**233–241.

17. **Gao, S.-J., L. Kingsley, M. Li, W. Zheng, C. Parravicini, J. Ziegler, R. Newton, C. R. Rinaldo, A. Saah, J. Phair, R. Detels, Y. Chang, and P. S. Moore.** 1996. KSHV antibodies among Americans, Italians and Ugandans with and without Kaposi's sarcoma. *Nat. Med.* **2:**925–928.

18. **Huang, Y. Q., J. J. Li, M. H. Kaplan, B. Poiesz, E. Katabira, W. C. Zhang, D. Feiner, and A. E. Friedman-Kein.** 1995. Human herpesvirus-like nucleic acid in various forms of Kaposi's sarcoma. *Lancet* **345:**759–761.

19. **Jacobson, L. P., A. Munoz, R. Fox, J. P. Phair, J. Dudley, G. I. Obrams, L. A. Kingsley, and B. F. Polk.** 1990. Incidence of Kaposi's sarcoma in a cohort of homosexual men infected with the human immunodeficiency virus type 1. *J. Acquired Immune Defic. Syndr.* **3**(Suppl. 1)**:**S24–S31.

20. **Jones, J. L., D. L. Hanson, S. Y. Chu, J. W. Ward, and H. W. Jaffe.** 1995. AIDS-associated Kaposi's sarcoma. *Science* **267:**1078–1079.

21. **Kaposi, M.** 1872. Idiopathisches multiples Pigmentsarkom der Haut. *Arch. Dermatol. Syphilis* **4:**265–273.

22. **Kedes, D. H., E. Operskalski, M. Busch, R. Kohn, J. Flood, and D. Ganem.** 1996. The seroepidemiology of human herpesvirus 8 (Kaposi's sarcoma-associated herpesvirus): distribution of infection in KS risk groups and evidence for sexual transmission. *Nat. Med.* **2:**918–924.

23. **Lennette, E. T., D. J. Blackbourn, and J. A. Levy.** 1996. Antibodies to human herpesvirus 8 in the general population and in Kaposi's sarcoma patients. *Lancet* **348:**858–861.

24. **Lever, W. F., and G. Schaumburg-Lever.** 1983. *Histopathology of the Skin.* J. B. Lippincott, Philadelphia.

25. **Lin, J.-C., S.-C. Lin, E.-C. Mar, P. E. Pellett, F. R. Stamey, J. A. Stewart, and T. J. Spira.** 1995. Is Kaposi's-sarcoma-associated herpesvirus detectable in semen of HIV-infected homosexual men? *Lancet* **346:**1601–1602.

26. **Miller, G., M.O. Rigsby, L. Heston, E. Grogan, R. Sun, C. Metroka, J. A. Levy, S. J. Gao, Y. Chang, and P. Moore.** 1996. Antibodies to butyrate-inducible antigens of Kaposi's sarcoma-associated herpesvirus in patients with HIV-1 infection. *N. Engl. J. Med.* **334:**1292–1297.

27. **Mocroft, A., M. Youle, B. Gazzard, J. Morcinek, R. Halai, and A. N. Phillips.** 1996. Anti-herpesvirus treatment and risk of Kaposi's sarcoma in HIV infection. *AIDS* **10:**1101–1105.

28. **Monini, P., L. De Lellis, M. Fabris, F. Rigolin, and E. Cassai.** 1996. Kaposi's sarcoma-associated herpesvirus DNA sequences in prostate tissue and human semen. *N. Engl. J. Med.* **334:**1168–1172.

29. **Moore, P. S., and Y. Chang.** 1995. Detection of herpesvirus-like DNA sequences in Kaposi's sarcoma in patients with and those without HIV infection. *N. Engl. J. Med.* **332:**1181–1185.

30. **Moore, P. S., S.-J. Gao, G. Dominguez, E. Cesarman, O. Lungu, D. M. Knowles, R. Garber, P. E. Pellett, D. J. McGeoch, and Y. Chang.** 1996. Primary characterization of a herpesvirus agent associated with Kaposi's sarcoma. *J. Virol.* **70:**549–558.

31. **Moore, P. S., L. A. Kingsley, S. D. Holmberg, T. Spira, P. Gupta, D. R. Hoover, J. P. Parry, L. J. Conley, H. W. Jaffe, and Y. Chang.** 1996. Kaposi's sarcoma-associated herpesvirus infection prior to the onset of Kaposi's sarcoma. *AIDS* **10:**175–180.

32. **Morfeldt, L., and J. Torsander.** 1994. Long-term remission of Kaposi's sarcoma following foscarnet treatment in HIV-infected patients. *Scand. J. Infect. Dis.* **26:**749.

33. **Orenstein, J. M., S. Alkan, A. Blauvelt, K.-T. Jeang, M. Weinstein, and B. Herndier.** 1997. Appearance of human herpes virus type 8 in Kaposis sarcoma, abstr. no. 735. In *4th International Conference on Retroviruses and Opportunistic Infections*, 22–26 January, Washington, D.C.

34. **Orfanos, C. E., R. Husak, U. Wolfer, and C. Garbe.** 1995. Kaposi's sarcoma: a reevaluation. *Recent Results Cancer Res.* **139:**275–296.

35. **Penn, I.** 1983. Kaposi's sarcoma in immunosuppressed patients. *J. Clin. Lab. Immunol.* 12:1–10.

36. **Peterman, T. A., H. W. Jaffe, and V. Beral.** 1993. Epidemiologic clues to the etiology of Kaposi's sarcoma. *AIDS* **7:**605–611.

37. **Peterman, T. A., H. W. Jaffe, A. E. Friedman-Kien, and R. A. Weiss.** 1991. The aetiology of Kaposi's sarcoma. *Cancer Surv. Ser.* **10:**23–37.

38. **Rady, P. L., A. Yen, J. L. Rollefson, I. Orengo, S. Bruce, T. K. Hughes, and S. K. Tyring.** 1995. Herpesvirus-like DNA sequences in non-Kaposi's sarcoma skin lesions of transplant patients. *Lancet* **345:**1339–1340.

39. **Safai, B., V. Mike, G. Giraldo, E. Beth, and R. A. Good.** 1980. Association of Kaposi's sarcoma with second primary malignancies. Possible etiopathogenic implications. *Cancer* **445:**1472–1479.

40. **Soulier, J., L. Grollet, E. Oksenhendler, P. Cacoub, D. Cazals-Hatem, P. Babinet, M. F. d'Agay, J. P. Clauvel, M. Raphael, and L. Degos.** 1995. Kaposi's sarcoma-associated herpesvirus-like DNA sequences in multicentric Castleman's disease. *Blood* **86:**1276–1280.

41. **Taylor, J. F., P. G. Smith, D. Bull, and M. C. Pike.** 1972. Kaposi's sarcoma in Uganda: geographic and ethnic distribution. *Br. J. Cancer* **26:**483–497.

42. **Valcuende-Cavero, F., M. I. Febrer-Bosch, and A. Castells-Rodellas.** 1994. Langerhans' cells and lymphocytic infiltrate in AIDS-associated Kaposi's sarcoma: an immunohistochemical study. *Acta Derm. Venereol.* **74:**183–187.

43. **Wahman, A., S. L. Melnick, F. S. Rhame, and J. D. Potter.** 1991. The epidemiology of classic, African and immunosuppressed Kaposi's sarcoma. *Epidemiol. Rev.* **13:**178–199.

44. **Whitby, D., M. R. Howard, M. Tenant-Flowers, N. S. Brink, A. Copas, C. Boshoff, T. Hatzioannou, F. E. Suggett, D. M. Aldam, and A. S. Denton.** 1995. Detection of Kaposi sarcoma associated herpesvirus in peripheral blood of HIV-infected individuals and progression to Kaposi's sarcoma. *Lancet* **346:**799–802.

45. **Williams, A. O., J. M. Ward, J. F. Li, M. A. Jackson, and K. C. Flanders.** 1995. Immunohistochemical localization of transforming growth factor-beta 1 in Kaposi's sarcoma. *Hum. Pathol.* **26:**469–473.

chapter 7

Buruli Ulcer

C. Robert Horsburgh, Jr., and Wayne M. Meyers

Mycobacterium ulcerans causes indolent, necrotizing, relatively nonpainful ulcers variously known as Buruli ulcer, Searles ulcer, Kumusi ulcer, Bairnsdale ulcer, or, most precisely, M. ulcerans infection. The geographic area in Uganda having the first large number of identified patients gave these lesions their more popular appellation, Buruli ulcer (21, 42). This name seems appropriate because Sir Albert Cook first described ulcers consistent with M. ulcerans infections in 1897 in Uganda (14). In 1948, MacCallum et al. published the first detailed description of M. ulcerans infection and established the etiology of the disease in a small group of patients in Australia (44); contact with their first patient dated to 1940. In 1950, van Oye and Ballion reported the first patient from Africa (Zaire) (91), but judging from personal interviews with local patients and medical workers and other circumstantial evidence, M. ulcerans infections in Zaire antedate 1935 (50).

C. Robert Horsburgh, Jr., Emory University School of Medicine, 69 Butler Street, S.E., Atlanta, GA 30303. **Wayne M. Meyers,** Mycobacteriology Branch, Division of Microbiology, Department of Infectious and Parasitic Disease Pathology, Armed Forces Institute of Pathology, Washington, DC 20306-6000.

Pathology of Emerging Infections
Edited by C. Robert Horsburgh, Jr., and Ann Marie Nelson
© 1997 American Society for Microbiology, Washington, DC 20005-4171

Reservoir and Mode of Transmission

The reservoir for human Buruli ulcer infection remains unknown

Despite the apparent widespread distribution of these organisms in the environment, the reservoir for human infection remains unknown. Koalas near Bairnsdale, Australia, are the only known naturally infected nonhuman hosts (48, 54), although a single isolation from a wild rat has been reported (32). Soil, plants, and water from areas in which M. *ulcerans* is endemic have been extensively cultured, and M. *ulcerans* has not been isolated (4, 5, 9, 64, 83).

Buruli ulcers occur most frequently in tropical areas that are marshy or near lakes or rivers (3, 4, 47, 88). However, no specific activities that bring persons in contact with water have been associated with the disease, leading to the conclusion that a riverine or lacustrine ecosystem provides the conditions necessary for the presence of the pathogen in the environment but that transmission is not through direct contact with contaminated water. Contact with soil in swampy areas has been associated with disease (47, 90), and it has been suggested that low soil pH is the environmental characteristic shared by such areas (26).

While precise and common modes of transmission remain unknown, direct inoculation into the skin seems the most likely route, both because single lesions are the rule and because infection in deep tissues is not observed. Most patients have ulcers that involve areas of the body less often clothed and more subject to trauma (e.g., upper and lower extremities, especially elbows, knees, and ankles). Meyers et al. reported that 8% of the patients studied at one focus in Bas-Zaire remembered an event of specific trauma (e.g., hypodermic injection, gunshot or land mine wound, thrown stone, etc.) at the ultimate site of the lesion (52), but the long incubation period of the infection makes recall of a specific inoculation event unlikely. In one patient, a lesion developed at the site of a hypodermic injection (vaccination) in the deltoid area, approximately 3 months postinoculation (52). Documentation and ancillary circumstances favored the concept that the needle puncture introduced M. *ulcerans* from overlying contaminated skin.

Hofer et al. reported M. *ulcerans* in disseminated osteomyelitic lesions that followed a snake bite in a child from Benin (34). Others have proposed inoculation by an insect as the mode of transmission (8, 42, 72, 73). Experimentally, M. *ulcerans* infects a variety of animals by intradermal inoculation, including mice, rats, hamsters, phalangers, armadillos, and lizards (7, 39, 45, 58, 59, 92), but not guinea pigs, rabbits, or chickens (58); lizards can also be infected by the oral route (46).

Alternatively, Portaels suggested, on the basis of an unpublished hypothesis by Pattyn, that aerosols may carry M. *ulcerans* and enter the host via the nasorespiratory path with subsequent hematogenous spread to cool body sites, in a manner reminiscent of the generally accepted mode of transmission and pathogenesis of leprosy (65, 66). However, this novel and plausible explanation seems less likely than transmission by direct inoculation of M. *ulcerans*. Epidemiologic studies have not supported a role for person-to-person transmission (71).

Epidemiology

Buruli ulcers have been reported from many tropical locations, largely in central and west Africa, where cases have been reported from Benin (29, 36), Cameroon (6, 73), Gabon (9), Ghana (90), the Ivory Coast (16, 17, 47), Liberia (55), Nigeria (57), Togo (53), Uganda (86–88), and Zaire (50). Cases have been seen in both tropical and temperate areas of Australia (26, 27, 35, 44, 72), Papua New Guinea (71, 75), Malaysia (61), and the Pacific Islands (10); an unconfirmed report of disease in India has been noted (70). Occasional reports have appeared from South America, including cases from Mexico (40), French Guyana (68, 69), and possibly Peru and Bolivia (70); the extent of the disease in South America remains to be determined. This wide geographic distribution has led Hayman to conclude that the organism was present in prior geologic eras (25). In recent years there have been marked increases in disease prevalence, especially in west Africa (36, 47, 53, 90) and Australia (35). Disease rates in Uganda have been estimated at 2 to 5% of the population (2, 86), while in the Ivory Coast, some villages have rates as high as 16% (47).

Children between the ages of 2 and 14 years are the most highly affected age group (47, 85, 90); among children, boys and girls have similar rates of disease. Some studies have shown higher rates among adult women than among adult men (2, 47, 85). No racial predilection is apparent. Seasonality has been observed in some studies (26, 71, 73, 76, 85) but not in others (47, 90). When seasonality is observed, disease is more frequent during the dry season; however, increased access to medical attention during the dry season and the variable incubation period of the disease make these observations difficult to interpret. Revill and Barker suggested that seasonality of Buruli ulcers in males is obscured by year-round incidence in females (76). Ulcers on the trunk and head accounted for only 8% of lesions in one large series (47); lower extremity lesions were twice as common as upper extremity lesions. Two studies found leg lesions to be more common on the right leg (26, 47), while another found left leg lesions to be more common (72, 90).

Human immunodeficiency virus (HIV)-infected persons do not appear to be at increased risk for Buruli ulcers (17): in a study in the Ivory Coast, 20 of 20 persons with Buruli ulcers tested were HIV seronegative (47). In addition, those at highest risk for HIV infection (infants and sexually active adults) were at the lowest risk for Buruli ulcer. Positive serologic tests for HIV in patients with mycobacterial infection must be interpreted cautiously, especially when only enzyme-linked immunosorbent assay results are available, because of apparent cross-reactivity between mycobacterial antigens and HIV (37).

Children between the ages of 2 and 14 years are the most highly affected age group; boys and girls have similar rates of disease

Pathogenesis and Pathology

M. *ulcerans* is strongly acid fast, stains well with Ziehl-Neelsen stains, and has an optimal growth temperature of 30 to 32°C on routine mycobacteriologic media, such as Löwenstein-Jensen medium. Primary isolation often requires incubation for 6 to 12 weeks or longer. The phenolic mycoside of M. ulcerans is identical to that of M. marinum, and the gene sequences for 16S rRNA are identical, except that at position 1248 of the 16S rRNA gene, M. ulcerans has a guanine and M. marinum has an adenine base (15, 78, 79). Preliminary observations employing 16S rRNA sequence data suggest that strains of M. ulcerans from various areas divide geographically into at least three groups: African, American, and Australian (67).

The pathologic changes that characterize early M. ulcerans infections depend in large measure on two distinct properties of the etiologic agent: (i) M. ulcerans grows optimally at temperatures lower than central body temperatures, i. e., at 30 to 33°C, and (ii) M. ulcerans produces a toxin. This temperature growth requirement largely limits the infection to body surfaces, and the toxin destroys tissue and suppresses local immune responses. Primarily on the basis of histopathologic findings in the preulcerative or early ulcerative stages of M. ulcerans infection, Connor and colleagues at the Armed Forces Institute of Pathology postulated that M. ulcerans produced a toxin. This hypothesis arose from their observation that necrosis extended far beyond the microcolonies of acid-fast bacilli (AFB) in the central area of the lesion and on the striking absence of inflammatory exudates. To test this conjecture, Read et al. (74), Krieg et al. (38), and Hockmeyer et al. (33) determined the effect of filtrates of M. ulcerans grown in liquid media on monolayers of cultured fibroblasts and responses in animals. They found that these sterile filtrates had a strong cytotoxic effect, even at low concentrations, and reproduced some of the clinical and histopathologic changes of M. ulcerans disease when injected into experimental animals. With these findings giving at least a partial explanation for the tissue necrosis, Pimsler et al. (63) turned to the question of the relative lack of inflammatory exudates in lesions and the absence of regional lymphadenopathy. They established that a toxin-containing preparation from M. ulcerans possessed immunosuppressive properties against murine T-lymphocytes and suppressed phagocytosis by macrophages. Mechanisms of immunosuppression have not been established, but the toxin at high concentrations, such as may accumulate in lesions, may be directly toxic to inflammatory cells or may inhibit cytokine production, release, or activity. Toxin that drains into regional lymph nodes may prevent regional lymphadenopathy.

On the basis of these findings and speculations, the pathogenesis of Buruli ulcer may proceed as follows. After introduction of M. ulcerans into the dermis or subcutaneous tissue, there is a latent phase during which this slowly growing organism gradually proliferates sufficiently to elaborate minute amounts of toxin that gradually destroy tissues. The necrosis, especially of fatty tissue, may provide a favorable milieu for the more rapid proliferation of M. ulcerans, accelerating necrosis and eventually producing a clinically apparent nodule. During the ensuing extensive necrotic phase of the disease, there is virtually no host cellular response (12, 13, 20) and the burulin skin test remains negative (81). There is no experimental evidence for the development of humoral antibodies to the M. ulcerans toxin, but it is likely that either the toxin is neutralized or the organisms cease to produce toxin, at which time the healing phase ensues. When healing com-

> M. ulcerans produces a toxin that destroys tissue; the necrosis, especially of fatty tissue, may provide a favorable milieu for more rapid proliferation of M. ulcerans

mences, the skin test becomes positive, suggesting immunologic host response to antigenic components of M. *ulcerans* and development of granulomas that destroy the etiologic agent, leading eventually to fibrosis and healing. Pimsler suggested that M. *ulcerans* may cease to proliferate and die because of nutrient depletion in the isolated pool of necrotic components in the lesion, setting off the above events that lead to healing (62).

Microscopically, the preulcerative lesion is a circumscribed area of necrosis containing numerous AFB, which are confined largely to the center of the lesion. The lesion is symmetrical, with contiguous coagulation necrosis of the deep dermis and panniculus and sometimes of the fascia. Ulcers seldom penetrate beyond the fascia, but rarely, underlying muscle may be damaged. Patients may present with osteomyelitis, either locally or at distant sites. Smears from osteomyelitic lesions may contain AFB (12, 34, 41, 43); Hofer et al. have demonstrated M. *ulcerans* in lesions of bone by molecular methods (34). Necrosis extends well beyond the areas containing bacilli. At the edge of the necrotic area there is interstitial edema but few or no inflammatory exudates. Conspicuously, fat cells enlarge and die, but they retain their ghost outlines for variable periods. Specimens from Africa studied at the Armed Forces Institute of Pathology often show significant endogenous mineral deposits, while those from Australia reveal only slight mineralization (29). Capillaries and larger vessels are destroyed or damaged, perhaps contributing to the striking necrosis of fat. Hayman tends to attribute the fat necrosis more to infarction than to a direct effect of a toxin (29); however, in even the most minimal lesions, necrosis of fat seems to be a primary event. Thus, it is reasonable to attribute this necrosis to action of a bacterial toxin. The entire process, as lesions advance, could represent the combined direct effect of a cytotoxin and infarction that in the panniculus leads to wide undermining of the overlying skin. Necrosis of the dermis and damage to the epidermis eventually lead to ulceration, beginning most often at the center of the lesion.

AFB in Ziehl-Neelsen-stained sections are confined almost exclusively to the necrotic slough in the bed of the ulcer and in the surrounding necrotic fat. The surrounding tissue and dermis seldom reveal large numbers of AFB, if any. As Hayman noted, clusters of M. *ulcerans* in no way resemble globi of *Mycobacterium leprae* (29). Furthermore, in view of the vast differences in the histopathologic findings with leprosy and Buruli ulcers, application of the terms "lepromatous" and "tuberculoid" to describe responses in M. *ulcerans* infections, as some investigators have proposed, seems unwarranted (30). As the ulcer enlarges, the undermining proceeds most actively in the panniculus, with at least partial sparing of the overlying dermis. This overhanging flap often extends 10 cm or more and gradually reepithelializes, with granulation tissue developing in the base of the ulcer. Hypersensitivity granulomas, probably stimulated by mycobacterial antigens, and possibly granulomas responding to necrotic fat develop in the dermis and tissues surrounding the lesions. Healing follows this granulomatous phase.

Several observations suggest that patients develop immunity to M. *ulcerans* after healed infection. Reinfection is uncommon (47, 88), although this could be due to limited reexposure. During the course of disease, granuloma

Necrosis of the dermis and damage to the epidermis eventually lead to ulceration, beginning most often at the center of the lesion

formation suggests the onset of cell-mediated immunity. After healing, patients have delayed hypersensitivity skin reactions to extracts of M. *ulcerans* (47, 85); antibody responses to M. *ulcerans* have not been well characterized (85).

Differential Diagnosis

The unique undermining, necrotic slough, and surrounding edema often make clinical diagnosis straightforward. Large numbers of AFB in Ziehl-Neelsen-stained smears from the base of the ulcer or in the drainage from the ulcer constitute further evidence. Cultivation of the slowly growing M. *ulcerans* from the lesion confirms the diagnosis but is frequently unsuccessful. Isolation must be performed by culturing at 30 to 33°C. Where available, molecular techniques can provide direct identification of M. *ulcerans* (34). Histopathologic features of preulcerative or active ulcerated lesions are usually distinctive and sufficient for diagnosis. Biopsy specimens should include the base and surrounding necrotic tissue at the edge of an undermined area. Specimens from the edge of the overlying flap are seldom diagnostic. Microscopic changes in long-standing or healing ulcers are usually nonspecific.

The differential diagnosis includes tropical phagedenic ulcer, stasis ulcer, decubitus ulcer, trophic and trophoneurotic ulcers, cancrum oris, anthrax, and cutaneous diphtheria. Hayman and Smith suggested that necrotizing arachnidism may simulate Buruli ulcer (31). After rupturing, pyogenic abscesses in the scalp of neonates are also widely undermined and can be mistaken for M. *ulcerans* infection in areas in which M. *ulcerans* is endemic. In immunosuppressed patients, BCG vaccination sites and *Mycobacterium marinum* infection may imitate Buruli ulcer.

Clinical Presentation

The incubation period of M. ulcerans infection seems highly variable, but it is usually under 3 months

The incubation period of M. *ulcerans* infection seems highly variable, but it is usually under 3 months (85). Among one group of 180 patients in Zaire, lesions in 14 patients developed at sites of trauma to the skin from 2 weeks to 3 years posttrauma (52). In 10 of these patients, the ulcers appeared within 3 months posttrauma. These observations are supported by results of animal studies, which indicate that the time to development of disease depends on the size of the inoculum (22). Muelder and Nourou (56) proposed a clinical staging system for M. *ulcerans* infections that is similar to the informal histopathologic staging system of Connor et al. (13). In the Muelder-Nourou system, the disease is divided into four stages: stage I, subcutaneous nodule; stage II, cellulitis; stage III, ulceration; and stage IV, scarring. This may prove useful; however, the overlapping of stages seen in most patients may limit its general application (28). In practice, stages I and II are rarely recognized (less than 5% of cases in our experience); most cases are recognized in the ulcerative stage. This is due both to the brevity typical of stages I and II and to preferential presentation of persons with ulcers for medical attention. Subclinical infection has not been documented; it has been suggested that subclinical infection may be common because of the high rate of reactions to the Burulin skin test (2), but other mycobacterial diseases were not excluded as the cause of the reactivity.

Ulcers of M. *ulcerans* are only minimally painful, a fact that helps distinguish them from other tropical ulcerative conditions. It has been hypothesized that the extensive tissue necrosis impairs afferent pain fibers, resulting in less pain than would be expected for the size and depth of the lesions. Systemic signs and symptoms, such as fevers or weight loss, are also rare and, when present, should suggest an alternative diagnosis. Buruli ulcers are often purulent, but significant bacterial superinfection is rare, perhaps as a result of a bacteriostatic activity of the toxin or the host inflammatory response. Erythema and induration predominate in stages I and II, but they subside rapidly with the onset of ulceration and are rarely appreciated clinically at this stage.

Healing is slow, with a median time to healing of 4 to 6 months. The disease often follows a waxing and waning course, with shrinking of lesions followed by further local extension. Distant satellite lesions are extremely uncommon, and deep tissue disease is seen only as a result of local extension. Healing occurs by secondary intention after sloughing of the epidermis and subcutaneous fat, with later reepithelialization. Scars are depressed and extensive, with a characteristic stellate pattern. Considerable deformity results from this mode of healing, particularly because lesions are usually on the extremities of children, in whom scarring often leads to contractures, subluxation, disuse atrophy, and distal lymphedema. Circumferential cicatrization may lead to stunting of limb growth. In one series, 26% of patients were left with functional disability of a limb (47). Loss of vision due to scarring in the orbital area has also been reported (89).

Death due to Buruli ulcer has only rarely been observed. Three deaths have been reported in Zaire: one was a malnourished mother in the early postpartum period (her infant was not affected), another was a child with fatal measles ("postmeasles syndrome"), and the third patient had a recurrence of Buruli ulcer 19 months after successful heat therapy. The recurrence was at a site far distant from the heat-treated lesion. Shortly after the Buruli ulcer recurrence, this 45-year-old woman died in a hepatic coma, probably from a hepatoma. Autopsy permission was not obtained for any of these three patients. In the Ivory Coast, only 14 of 326 (4%) patients with Buruli ulcers died over an 8-year period (47).

Association with other diseases has not been extensively investigated. Meyers and Connor found six patients with both leprosy and M. *ulcerans* infection among 1,061 leprosy patients and 180 patients with Buruli ulcer from the same area of endemicity (49). All six of these patients had borderline or borderline-tuberculoid leprosy. While there was no laboratory proof, it was speculated that the high levels of antibodies to mycobacterial antigens in lepromatous patients may neutralize M. *ulcerans* toxin and hence help them resist Buruli ulcer disease.

Studies in animals have demonstrated worsening of M. *ulcerans* infection after pharmacologic immunosuppression (19). In humans, altered clinical course due to immunosuppression has only rarely been documented; multiple lesions suggesting disseminated M. *ulcerans* disease were reported in one

Healing is slow, with a median time to healing of 4 to 6 months. The disease often follows a waxing and waning course, with shrinking of lesions followed by further local extension

patient who was diagnosed with leukemia soon afterwards (26). M. *ulcerans* infection has been documented in four HIV-infected patients, but no apparent worsening of the mycobacterial infections was reported (1, 18). However, other immunosuppressive factors, such as malnutrition, may have a substantial impact on the clinical course of M. *ulcerans* infection.

Treatment and Prevention

M. *ulcerans* is susceptible to dapsone, rifampin, clofazimine, streptomycin, ethambutol, minocycline, cycloserine, kanamycin, and viomycin in vitro (6, 43, 59, 60, 80, 82). Moreover, therapy of experimental M. *ulcerans* infection in animals with rifampin, clofazimine, streptomycin, and dapsone has been successful (43, 59, 82, 84). Unfortunately, results of clinical trials give less cause for optimism; a double-blind, randomized controlled trial of clofazimine showed that the drug was not useful for treatment of M. *ulcerans* infection (77). A case series from the Ivory Coast showed better results when using streptomycin, but patients were not randomized (16); this contrasts with the results of Clancey et al., who administered streptomycin to patients with Buruli ulcer "without clear evidence of clinical improvement," while dapsone therapy for 3 months showed that lesions "seemed to improve" (11). Moreover, daily therapy with an injectable agent such as streptomycin is not practical in most areas where Buruli ulcer is prevalent. A pilot study of rifampin therapy for Buruli ulcers also failed to show efficacy (51). The failure of antibiotic regimens has been attributed both to difficulty in administering therapy before the disease is in advanced stages and to poor penetration of antibiotic agents into areas of necrotic tissue. However, a case of successful therapy with rifampin and clarithromycin was recently reported (18).

The preferential growth of the organism at 30 to 32°C has led some investigators to apply local heat to the lesions to aid healing

The preferential growth of the organism at 30 to 32°C has led some investigators to apply local heat to the lesions to aid healing. Such therapy has been successful in animal models and in case series (23, 39, 51, 75). However, these investigators employed constant heat application in an inpatient setting, sometimes supplemented by antibiotics; intermittent, self-administered heat therapy has been less successful (24, 26). Surgical excision is the standard treatment; when performed at the nodular stage, it is usually curative. However, as noted above, patients rarely present at this stage of disease. For ulcerated lesions, wide surgical excision is the treatment of choice (11, 23, 75). Adjunctive skin grafting is usually required (16, 23).

Prevention of M. *ulcerans* infection would be best accomplished by avoidance of exposure to the pathogen, but unfortunately, such a strategy must wait until the reservoir is identified. A randomized, controlled trial of BCG vaccination demonstrated 18 to 74% protection, but this protection waned dramatically after 6 months (86). One study has suggested that wearing protective clothing might reduce the risk of disease, but this strategy has not been evaluated (47).

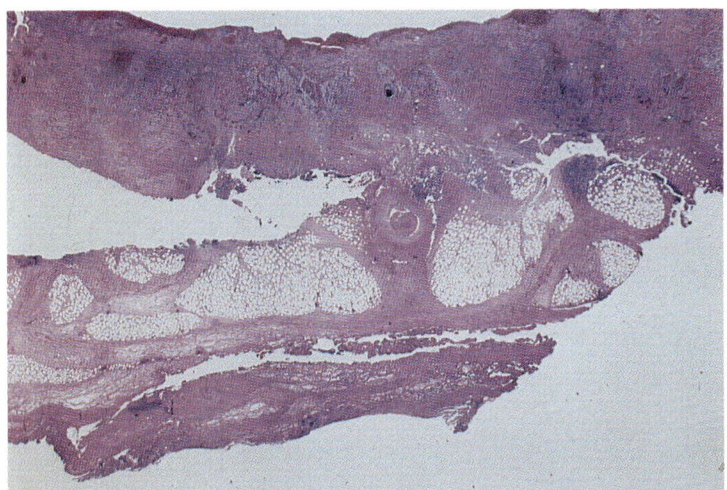

Figure 7. 1   Biopsy specimen of skin from the edge of an ulcer (hematoxylin and eosin stain; original magnification, ×2.5). Note undermining of dermis and massive coagulation necrosis of skin, subcutitis, and underlying fascia.

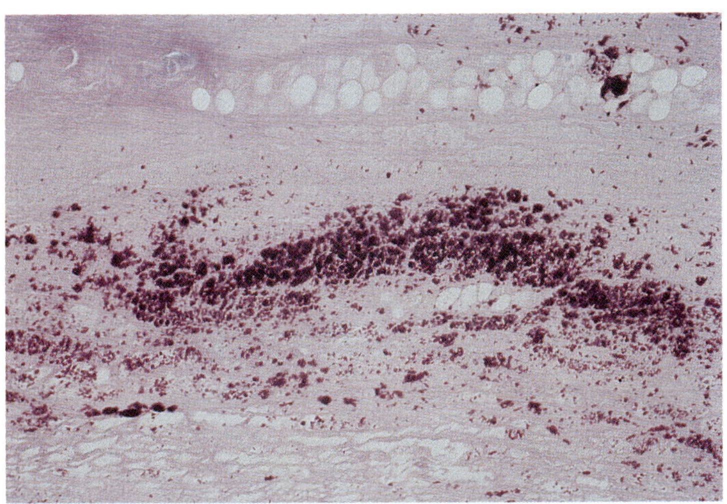

Figure 7.2   Biopsy specimen of skin from the edge of an ulcer (Ziehl-Neelsen stain; original magnification, ×250). Clumps of acid-fast bacilli in necrotic fascia at the base of the ulcer depicted in Fig. 7. 1 are shown.

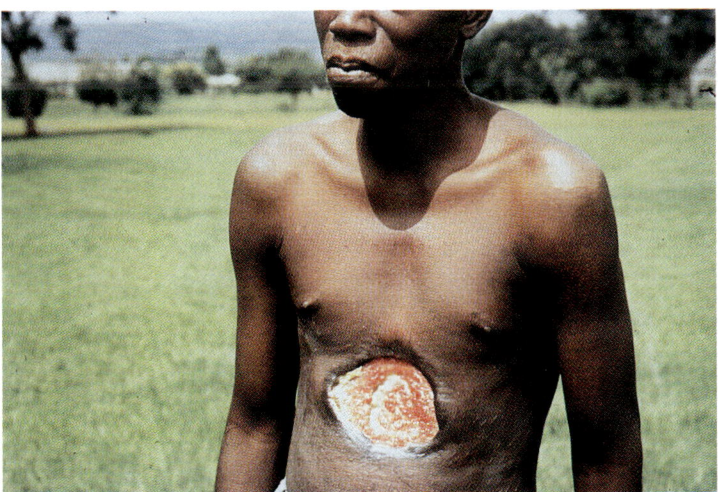

Figure 7. 3   Primary ulcerative lesion of M. *ulcerans* on the abdomen. Note the deep erosion in the center of the ulcer.

Figure 7.4 *M. ulcerans* lesion of the face involving the eye. Enucleation was required because of destruction of the eyelids.

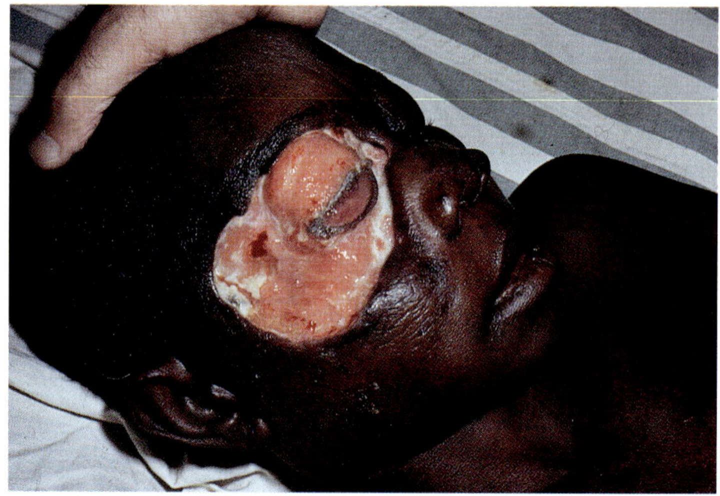

Figure 7.5 View of a leg lesion after surgical debridement. Wide surgical margins were necessary to achieve control of the infection. Active disease remains at the edge of debridement on the thigh.

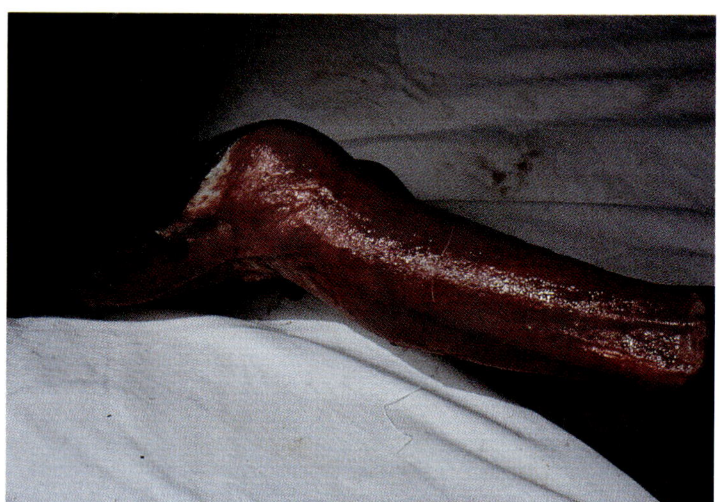

Figure 7.6 Healed lesion showing contracture deformity. The area received a skin graft; the characteristic scar is stellate and depressed.

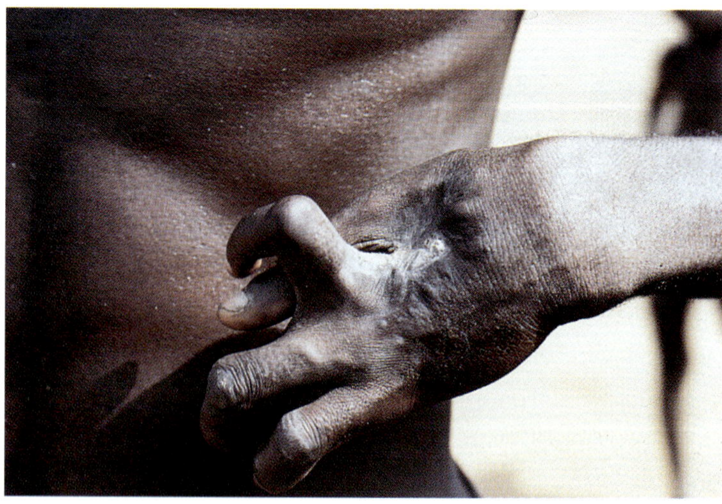

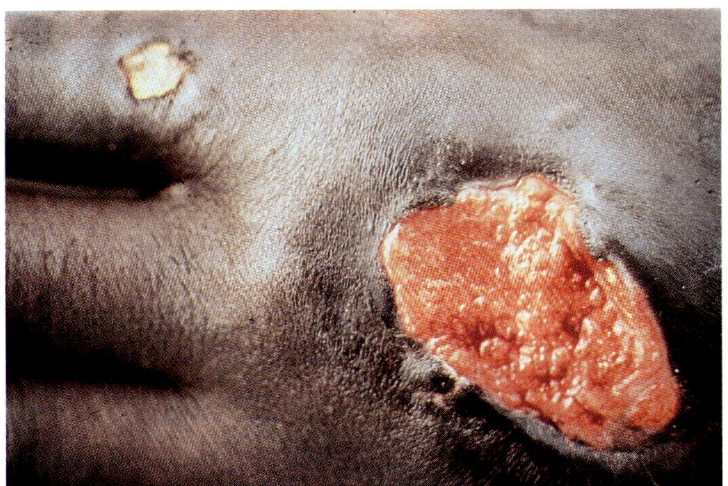

Figure 7. 7 Early ulcerative lesion on the dorsum of the hand. The two ulcers communicated subcutaneously.

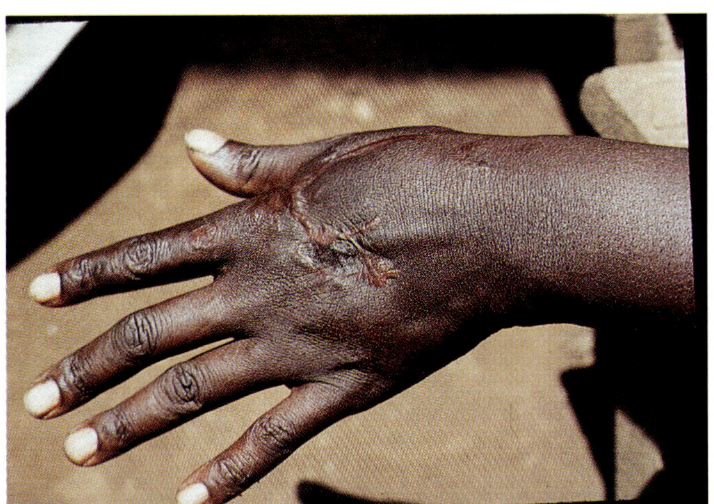

Figure 7. 8 Healed lesion (shown in Fig. 7.7). Patient was treated with local heat without antibiotics or surgical excision.

References

1. **Allen, S.** 1992. Buruli ulcer and HIV infection. *Int. J. Dermatol.* **31:**744–745.

2. **Barker, D. J. P.** 1973. Epidemiology of *Mycobacterium ulcerans* infection. *Trans. R. Soc. Med. Hyg.* **67:**43–47.

3. **Barker, D. J. P., and J. W. Carswell.** 1973. *Mycobacterium ulcerans* infection among tsetse control workers in Uganda. *Int. J. Epidemiol.* **2:**161–165.

4. **Barker, D. J. P., J. K. Clancey, R. H. Morrow, and S. K. Rao.** 1970. Transmission of Buruli disease. *Br. Med. J.* **2:**558.

5. **Barker, D. J. P., J. K. Clancey, and S. K. Rao.** 1972. Mycobacteria on vegetation in Uganda. *East Afr. Med. J.* **49:**667–671.

6. **Boisvert, H.** 1977. L'ulcère cutané à *Mycobacterium ulcerans* au Cameroun. II. Etude bactériologique. *Bull. Soc. Pathol. Exot.* **70:**125–131.

7. **Bollanger, A., B. R. V. Forbes, and W. B. Kirkland.** 1950. Transmission of a recently isolated mycobacterium to phalangers (Trichosorus vulpecula). *Aust. J. Med. Sci.* **12:**146–147.

8. **Buckle, G.** 1972. Notes on *Mycobacterium ulcerans*. *Aust. N. Z. J. Surg.* **41:**320–322.

9. **Burchard, G. D., and M. Bierther.** 1986. Buruli ulcer: clinical pathological study of 23 patients in Lambaréné, Gabon. *Trop. Med. Parasitol.* **37:**1–8.

10. **Christie, M.** 1987. Suspected *Mycobacterium ulcerans* disease in Kiribati. *Med. J. Aust.* **146:**600–604.

11. **Clancey, J. K., O. G. Dodge, H. F. Lunn, and M. L. Oduori.** 1961. Mycobacterial skin ulcers in Uganda. *Lancet* **ii:**951–954.

12. **Connor, D. H., and F. Lunn.** 1966. Buruli ulceration: a clinicopathologic study of 38 Ugandans with *Mycobacterium ulcerans* infection. *Arch. Pathol.* **81:**183–189.

13. **Connor, D. H., W. M. Meyers, and R. E. Krieg.** 1976. Infection by *Mycobacterium ulcerans*, p. 226–235. *In* C. H. Binford and D. H. Connor (ed.), *Pathology of Tropical and Extraordinary Disease*. Armed Forces Institute of Pathology, Washington, D.C.

14. **Cook, A.** 1970. Mengo hospital notes, Makarere Medical School Library, Kampala, Uganda. *Br. Med. J.* **2:**378–379.

15. **Daffe, M., A. Varnerot, and V. V. Levy-Frebault.** 1992. The phenolic mycoside of *Mycobacterium ulcerans*: structure and taxonomic implications. *J. Gen. Microbiol.* **138:**131–137.

16. **Darie, H., S. Djakeaux, and A. Cautoclaud.** 1994. Approche thérapeutique des infections à *Mycobacterium ulcerans*. *Bull. Soc. Pathol. Exot.* **87:**19–21.

17. **Darie, H., T. le Guyadec, and J. Touze.** 1993. Aspects épidémiologiques et cliniques de l'ulcère de Buruli en Côte d'Ivoire. *Bull. Soc. Pathol. Exot.* **86:**272–276.

18. **Delaporte, E., S. Alfandari, and F. Piette.** 1994. *Mycobacterium ulcerans* associated with infection due to the human immunodeficiency virus. *Clin. Infect. Dis.* **18:**839.

19. **Dhople, A. M., and N. E. Morrison.** 1967. Effect of immunosuppression in the multiplication of *Mycobacterium ulcerans* in the mouse foot pad. *Int. J. Lepr.* **35:**194–197.

20. **Dodge, O. G.** 1964. Mycobacterial skin ulcers in Uganda: histopathological and experimental aspects. *J. Pathol. Bacteriol.* **88:**167–174.

21. **Dodge, O. G., and H. F. Lunn.** 1962. Buruli ulcer: a mycobacterial skin ulcer in a Uganda child. *J. Trop. Med. Hyg.* **65:**139–142.

22. **Fenner, F.** 1957. Homologous and heterologous immunity in infection of mice with *Mycobacterium ulcerans* and *Mycobacterium balnei. Am. Rev. Tuberc.* **76:**76–89.

23. **Glynn, P. J.** 1972. The use of surgery and local temperature elevation in *Mycobacterium ulcerans* infection. *Aust. N. Z. J. Surg.* **41:**312–317.

24. **Goutzamanis, J. J., and G. L. Gilbert.** 1995. *Mycobacterium ulcerans* infection in Australian children: report of eight cases and review. *Clin. Infect. Dis.* **21:**1186–1192.

25. **Hayman, J.** 1984. Mycobacterium ulcerans: an infection from Jurassic time? *Lancet* **ii:**1015–1016.

26. **Hayman, J.** 1985. Clinical features of *Mycobacterium ulcerans* infection. *Aust. J. Dermatol.* **26:**67–73.

27. **Hayman, J.** 1991. Postulated epidemiology of *Mycobacterium ulcerans* infection. *Int. J. Epidemiol.* **20:**1093–1098.

28. **Hayman, J.** 1991. *Mycobacterium ulcerans* infection. *Lancet* **337:**124.

29. **Hayman, J.** 1993. Out of Africa: observations on the histopathology of *Mycobacterium ulcerans* infection. *J. Clin. Pathol.* **46:**5–9.

30. **Hayman, J., and A. McQueen.** 1985. The pathology of *Mycobacterium ulcerans* infection. *Pathology* **17:**594–600.

31. **Hayman, J., and I. M. Smith.** 1991. Necrotising arachnidism in Australia. *Med. J. Aust.* **155:**351.

32. **Hayman, J. A., and H. J. Huygens.** 1982. *Mycobacterium ulcerans* infection across Lake Victoria. *Med. J. Aust.* **i:**138.

33. **Hockmeyer, W. T., R. E. Krieg, M. Reich, and R. D. Johnson.** 1978. Further characterization of *Mycobacterium ulcerans* toxin. *Infect. Immun.* **21:**124–128.

34. **Hofer, M., B. Hirschel, P. Kirschner, M. Beghetti, A. Kaelin, C. A. Siegrist, S. Suter, A. Teske, and E. C. Bottger.** 1993. Brief report: disseminated osteomyelitis from *Mycobacterium ulcerans* after a snakebite. *N. Engl. J. Med.* **328:**1007–1009.

35. **Johnson, P. D. R., M. G. K. Veitch, D. E. Leslie, P. E. Flood, and J. A. Hayman.** 1996. The emergence of *Mycobacterium ulcerans* infection near Melbourne. *Med. J. Aust.* **164:**76–78.

36. **Josse, R., L. Andrè, C. Zinsou, S. Anagonou, A. Guedenon, M. Botineau, J. Catraye, J. Foundohou, and J.-É. Touzé.** 1992. Etude clinique et épidémiologique de ulcère de Buruli chez le jeune au Bénin. *Cahiers Santé* **2:**23–27.

37. **Kashala, O., R. Marlink, M. Ilunga, M. Diese, B. Gormus, K. Xu, P. Mukeba, K. Kasongo, and M. Essex.** 1994. Infection with human immunodeficiency virus type 1 (HIV-1), human T cell lymphotropic virus type 1 (HTLV-1), and type 2 (HTLV-2) among leprosy patients and their contacts: correlation between HIV-1 cross-reactivity and antibodies to lipoarabinomannan (LAM). *J. Infect. Dis.* **169:**296–304.

38. **Krieg, R. E., W. T. Hockmeyer, and D. H. Connor.** 1974. Toxin of *Mycobacterium ulcerans*: production and effects in guinea pig skin. *Arch. Dermatol.* **110:**783–788.

39. **Krieg, R. E., J. H. Wolcott, and W. M. Meyers.** 1979. *Mycobacterium ulcerans* infections: treatment with rifampin, hyperbaric oxygenation, and heat. *Aviat. Space Environ. Med.* **50:**888–892.

40. **Lavalle Aguillar, R., F. M. Iturribarria, and G. Middlebrook.** 1950. Un cas de infeccion humana par *Mycobacterium ulcerans* en el hemiferio occidental (nota previa). *Int. J. Lepr.* **21:**469–476.

41. **Lunn, H. F.** 1963. Mycobacterial lesions in bone. *East Afr. Med. J.* **40:**113–117.

42. **Lunn, H. F., D. H. Connor, N. E. Wilks, G. R. Barnley, F. Kamunvi, J. K. Clancey, and J. D. A. Bee.** 1965. Buruli (mycobacterial) ulceration in Uganda—a new focus of Buruli ulcers in Madi district, Uganda. *East Afr. Med. J.* **42:**275–288.

43. **Lunn, H. F., and R. J. W. Rees.** 1964. Treatment of mycobacterial skin ulcers in Uganda with a riminophenazine derivative (B663). *Lancet* **i:**247–249.

44. **MacCallum, P., J. C. Tolhurst, G. Buckle, and H. A. Sissons.** 1948. A new mycobacterial infection in man. *J. Pathol. Bacteriol.* **60:**93–122.

45. **Marcus, L. C., K. D. Stottmeier, and R. H. Morrow.** 1975. Experimental infection of anole lizards (Anolis carolinensis) with *Mycobacterium ulcerans* by the subcutaneous route. *Am. J. Trop. Med. Hyg.* **24:**649–655.

46. **Marcus, L. C., K. D. Stottmeier, and R. H. Morrow.** 1976. Experimental alimentary infection of anole lizards (Anolis carolinensis) with *Mycobacterium ulcerans. Am. J. Trop. Med. Hyg.* **25:**630–632.

47. **Marston, B. J., M. O. Diallo, C. R. Horsburgh, Jr., I. Diomande, M. Z. Saki, J. Kanga, P. Gbery, H. B. Lipman, S. M. Ostroff, and R. C. Good.** 1995. Emergence of Buruli ulcer disease in the Daloa region of Côte d'Ivoire. *Am. J. Trop. Med. Hyg.* **52:**219–224.

48. **McOrist, S., I. V. Jerrett, M. Anderson, and J. Hayman.** 1985. Cutaneous and respiratory tract infection with *Mycobacterium ulcerans* in two koalas (Phascolarctos cinereus). *J. Wildlife Dis.* **21:**171–173.

49. **Meyers, W. M., and D. H. Connor.** 1975. *Mycobacterium ulcerans* infections in leprosy patients. *Lepr. Rev.* **46:**21–27.

50. **Meyers, W. M., D. H. Connor, B. McCullough, J. Bourland, R. Moris, and L. Proos.** 1974. Distribution of *Mycobacterium ulcerans* infections in Zaire, including the report of new foci. *Ann. Soc. Belge Med. Trop.* **54:**147–157.

51. **Meyers, W. M., W. M. Shelly, and D. H. Connor.** 1974. Heat treatment of *Mycobacterium ulcerans* infections without surgical excision. *Am. J. Trop. Med. Hyg.* **23:**924–929.

52. **Meyers, W. M., W. M. Shelly, D. H. Connor, and E. K. Meyers.** 1974. Human *Mycobacterium ulcerans* infections developing at sites of trauma to skin. *Am. J. Trop. Med. Hyg.* **23:**919–923.

53. **Meyers, W. M., N. Tignokpa, G. B. Priuli, and F. Portaels.** 1996. *Mycobacterium ulcerans* infection (Buruli ulcer): first reported patients from Togo. *Br. J. Dermatol.* **134:**1116–1121.

54. **Mitchell, P. J., I. V. Jerrett, and K. J. Slee.** 1984. Skin ulcers caused by *Mycobacterium ulcerans* in koalas near Bairnsdale, Australia. *Pathology* **16:**256–260.

55. **Monson, M. H., D. W. Gibson, D. H. Connor, R. Kappes, and H. A. Heinz.** 1984. *Mycobacterium ulcerans* in Liberia: a clinicopathologic study of 6 patients with Buruli ulcer. *Acta Tropica* **41:**165–172.

56. **Muelder, K., and A. Nourou.** 1990. Buruli ulcer in Benin. *Lancet* **336:**1109–1111.

57. **Oluwasanmi, J. O., T. F. Solanke, E. O. Olurin, S. O. Itayemi, G. O. Alabi, and A. O. Lucas.** 1976. *Mycobacterium ulcerans* (Buruli) skin ulceration in Nigeria. *Am. J. Trop. Med. Hyg.* **25:**122–128.

58. **Pattyn, S. R.** 1965. Bactériologie et pathologie humaine et expérimentale des ulcères à *Mycobacterium ulcerans. Ann. Soc. Belge Med. Trop.* **45:**121–130.

59. **Pattyn, S. R., and J. Royackers.** 1965. Traitement de l'infection expérimentale de la souris par *Mycobacterium ulcerans* et *Mycobacterium balnei. Ann. Soc. Belge Med. Trop.* **45:**31–38.

60. **Pattyn, S. R., and J. van Ermengem.** 1968. DDS sensitivity of mycobacteria. *Int. J. Lepr.* **36:**427–431.

61. **Pettit, J. H. S., N. J. Marchette, and R. J. W. Rees.** 1966. *Mycobacterium ulcerans* infection: clinical and bacteriological study of the first case recognized in southeast Asia. *Br. J. Dermatol.* **78:**187–197.

62. **Pimsler, M.** 1994. Personal communication.

63. **Pimsler, M., T. A. Sponsler, and W. M. Meyers.** 1988. Immunosuppressive properties of the soluble toxin from *Mycobacterium ulcerans. J. Infect. Dis.* **157:**577–580.

64. **Portaels, F.** 1973. Contribution a l'étude des mycobactéries de l'environnement au Bas-Zaire. *Ann. Soc. Belge Med. Trop.* **53:**373–387.

65. **Portaels, F.** 1989. Epidémiologie des ulcères à *Mycobacterium ulcerans. Ann. Soc. Belge Med. Trop.* **69:**91–103.

66. **Portaels, F.** 1992. Mycobactèrioses, p. 1207–1224. *In* P. G. Janssens, M. Kivits, and J. Vuylsteke (ed.), *Médecine et Hygiène en Afrique Centrale de 1885 à Nos Jours.* Fondation Roi Baudoin, Brussels.

67. **Portaels, F., P.-A. Fonteyne, H. De Beenhouwer, P. de Rijk, A. Guédénon, J. Hayman, and W. M. Meyers.** 1996. Variability of 3′ end of 16S rRNA sequence of *Mycobacterium ulcerans* is related to geographic origin of isolates. *J. Clin. Microbiol.* **34:**962–965.

68. **Pradinaud, R., A. Basset, and E. Grosshans.** 1974. Vingt cas de mycobactérioses cutanées en Guyane française. *Castellania* **2:**273–274.

69. **Pradinaud, R., and E. Grosshans.** 1972. Le problème des mycobactérioses cutanées en Guyane française. *Bull. Soc. Fr. Derm. Syph.* **79:**684–686.

70. **Radford, A. J.** 1974. *Mycobacterium ulcerans:* a review. I. Epidemiology. *Papua New Guinea Med. J.* **17:**129–133.

71. **Radford, A. J.** 1974. *Mycobacterium ulcerans* infection in Papua New Guinea. *Papua New Guinea Med. J.* **17:**145–149.

72. **Radford, A. J.** 1975. *Mycobacterium ulcerans* in Australia. *Aust. N. Z. J. Med.* **5:**162–169.

73. **Ravisse, P.** 1977. L'ulcère cutané à *Mycobacterium ulcerans* au Cameroun. I. Etude clinique, épidémiologique, et histologique. *Bull. Soc. Pathol. Exot.* **70:**109–129.

74. **Read, R. G., C. M. Heggie, W. M. Meyers, and D. H. Connor.** 1974. Cytotoxic activity of *Mycobacterium ulcerans. Infect. Immun.* **9:**1114–1122.

75. **Reid, I. S.** 1967. *Mycobacterium ulcerans* infection: a report of 13 cases at the Port Moresby General Hospital, Papua. *Med. J. Aust.* **1:**427–431.

76. **Revill, W. D. L., and D. J. P. Barker.** 1972. Seasonal distribution of mycobacterial skin ulcers. *Br. J. Prev. Soc. Med.* **26:**23–27.

77. **Revill, W. D. L., M. C. Pike, R. H. Morrow, and J. Ateng.** 1973. A controlled trial of the treatment of *Mycobacterium ulcerans* infection with clofazimine. *Lancet* **ii:**873–877.

78. **Rogall, T., T. Flohr, and E. C. Böttger.** 1990. Differentiation of Mycobacterium species by direct sequencing of amplified DNA. *J. Gen. Microbiol.* **136:**1915–1920.

79. **Rogall, T., J. Wolters, T. Flohr, and E. C. Böttger.** 1990. Towards a phylogeny and definition of species at the molecular level within the genus *Mycobacterium. Int. J. Syst. Bacteriol.* **40:**323–330.

80. **Schroder, K. H.** 1975. Investigation into the relationship of M. *ulcerans* to M. *buruli* and other mycobacteria. *Am. Rev. Respir. Dis.* **111:**559–562.

81. **Stanford, J. L.** 1983. Immunologically important constituents of mycobacteria: antigens, p. 113. *In* C. Ratledge and J. L. Stanford (ed.), *Biology of the Mycobacteria.* Academic Press, New York.

82. **Stanford, J. L., M. S. R. Hutt, I. Phillips, and W. D. L. Revill.** 1974. Antibiotic treatment in *Mycobacterium ulcerans* infection. *Ain Shams Med. J.* **25**(Suppl.):258–261.

83. **Stanford, J. L., and R. C. Paul.** 1973. A preliminary report on some studies of environmental mycobacteria from Uganda. *Ann. Soc. Belge Med. Trop.* **53:**389–393.

84. **Stanford, J. L., and I. Phillips.** 1972. Rifampicin in experimental *Mycobacterium ulcerans* infection. *J. Med. Microbiol.* **5:**39–45.

85. **Stanford, J. L., W. D. L. Revill, W. J. Gunthorpe, and J. M. Grange.** 1975. The production and preliminary investigation of Burulin, a new skin test reagent for *Mycobacterium ulcerans* infection. *J. Hyg. Camb.* **74:**7–16.

86. **Uganda Buruli Group.** 1969. BCG vaccination *Mycobacterium ulcerans* infection (Buruli ulcer). *Lancet* **i:**111–114.

87. **Uganda Buruli Group.** 1970. Clinical features and treatment of pre-ulcerative Buruli lesions (*Mycobacterium ulcerans* infection). *Br. Med. J.* **2:**390–393.

88. **Uganda Buruli Group.** 1971. Epidemiology of *Mycobacterium ulcerans* infection (Buruli ulcer) at Kinyara, Uganda. *Trans. R. Soc. Trop. Med. Hyg.* **65:**763–775.

89. **van der Werf, T. S., and W. T. A. van der Graaf.** 1990. Buruli ulcer in west Africa. *Lancet* **ii:**1440.

90. **van der Werf, T. S., W. T. A. van der Graaf, D. G. Groothuis, and A. J. Knell.** 1989. *Mycobacterium ulcerans* infection in Ashanti region, Ghana. *Trans. R. Soc. Trop. Med. Hyg.* **83:**410–423.

91. **van Oye, E., and M. Ballion.** 1950. Faudra-t-il tenir compte d'une nouvelle affection à bacilles acido-résistants en Afrique? (Note préliminaire). *Ann. Soc. Belge Med. Trop.* **30:**619–627.

92. **Walsh, G. P., R. E. Krieg, and E. M. Meyers.** 1995. Personal communication.

chapter 8

Viral Hepatitis

Craig N. Shapiro, Eric E. Mast, and Kamal G. Ishak

At least five human hepatitis viruses have been characterized to date (Table 8.1). In the United States, an estimated 32% of acute viral hepatitis is due to hepatitis A virus (HAV), 43% is due to hepatitis B virus (HBV), 21% is due to hepatitis C virus (HCV), and 4% is due to other possible viral agents (Fig. 8.1)(16). These agents account for substantial morbidity and mortality in the United States (Table 8.2) and worldwide. The clinical presentation of acute infection with each of these viruses is similar, and diagnosis therefore depends on the use of specific serologic tests. The epidemiology of these viruses is determined by a variety of factors, including their modes of transmission, which are in turn determined by the body fluids in which each virus is found in infected persons.

Craig N. Shapiro, Hepatitis Branch, Division of Viral and Rickettsial Diseases, National Center for Infectious Diseases, Centers for Disease Control and Prevention, 1600 Clifton Road, N.E., Mailstop G-37, Atlanta, GA 30333. **Eric E. Mast,** Hepatitis Branch, Division of Viral and Rickettsial Diseases, National Center for Infectious Diseases, Centers for Disease Control and Prevention, 1600 Clifton Road, N.E., Mailstop G-37, Atlanta, GA 30333. **Kamal G. Ishak,** Department of Hepatic and Gastrointestinal Pathology, Armed Forces Institute of Pathology, Washington, DC 20306-6000.

Pathology of Emerging Infections
Edited by C. Robert Horsburgh, Jr., and Ann Marie Nelson
© 1997 American Society for Microbiology, Washington, DC 20005-4171

Table 8.1 Viral hepatitis: an overview

Hepatitis virus	Source of virus	Route of transmission	Chronic infection	Prevention
A	Feces	Fecal-oral	No	Pre- and postexposure immunization
B	Blood and blood-derived body fluids	Percutaneous/ permucosal	Yes	Pre- and postexposure immunization
C	Blood and blood-derived body fluids	Percutaneous/ permucosal	Yes	Blood donor screening; risk behavior modification
D	Blood and blood-derived body fluids	Percutaneous/ permucosal	Yes	Pre- and postexposure immunization; risk behavior modification
E	Feces	Fecal-oral	No	Ensure safe drinking water

Epidemiology

HAV is shed in the feces, and peak titers occur during the 2 weeks before and 1 week after onset of illness. Virus is also present in serum and saliva during this period, although in concentrations several orders of magnitude less than those in feces. Therefore, the most common mode of HAV transmission is fecal-oral, with the virus being transmitted by person-to-person contact or by contaminated food or water. HAV transmission through blood or blood products occurs relatively rarely, and saliva has not been demonstrated to play a role in transmission.

HAV infection is distributed globally, but disease patterns differ and correlate with the hygienic and sanitary conditions of a given geographic region (33). In countries with very poor sanitary and hygienic conditions, most persons are infected as young children, at an age when HAV infection is often asymptomatic; reported disease rates in these areas are low and outbreaks are rare. In countries with variable sanitary conditions, infection can predominate in children, adolescents, or adults, depending on the geographic region. Paradoxically, because infections in these areas often occur in age groups in which infection is symptomatic and because conditions

> *HAV infection is distributed globally, but disease patterns differ and correlate with the hygienic and sanitary conditions of a given geographic region*

Table 8.2 Estimates of acute and chronic disease burden for viral hepatitis, United States

Hepatitis virus	Acute infections $(10^3/\text{yr})^a$	Fulminant deaths/yr	Chronic infections (10^5)	Chronic liver disease deaths/yr
HAV	125–200	100	0	0
HBV	140–320	150	10–12.5	5,000
HCV	35–180	?	35	8,000–10,000
HDV	6–13	35	0.7	1,000

[a] Range is based on estimated annual incidence from 1984 to 1994.

which promote transmission are common, disease rates can be higher than in countries with very poor sanitary conditions. Community-wide epidemics contribute significantly to the burden of disease in regions with variable sanitation. In countries with very good sanitation and hygienic conditions, infection rates in children are generally low. In these countries, disease tends to occur among specific risk groups, such as travelers to areas where hepatitis A is endemic, and intravenous drug users, among whom hygienic practices may be poor.

In the United States, hepatitis A has occurred in large nationwide epidemics approximately every 10 years (80). The highest disease rates are in children aged 5 to 14 years old. Community-wide outbreaks, with children often playing an important role in disease transmission, account for a large number of cases. In 1993, among cases reported to the Centers for Disease Control and Prevention (CDC), the most frequently reported risk factor was household or sexual contact with a person with hepatitis (22%), which was followed by day care attendance or employment (15%), recent international travel (6%), and association with a suspected food- or water-borne outbreak (2%) (Fig. 8.2). Many persons with hepatitis A do not identify risk factors; their source of infection may be other infected persons who are asymptomatic.

On the basis of the National Health and Nutrition Examination Survey (NHANES III), a population-based sample which tested approximately 10,100 serum samples from 1989 to 1991, the overall prevalence of antibodies to HAV in the general U.S. population is 33% (80). This represents a decrease since NHANES II, conducted from 1978 to 1980, which found the overall prevalence to be 38%.

Recent events involving the epidemiology of hepatitis A include the recognition of outbreaks among hemophiliacs receiving solvent-detergent-treated factor VIII concentrates in Europe in 1992 and 1993 and in the United States in 1995 (15). Contamination of the factor VIII concentrates presumably was due to plasma donors who were incubating HAV at the time of donation and was substantial enough that the virus purified along with factor VIII during the preparation process. The solvent-detergent step used in factor VIII preparation to inactivate lipid-containing viruses is ineffective against HAV.

HBV is present in high titers in blood and exudates (e.g., from skin lesions) of acutely and chronically infected persons. Moderate viral titers are found in semen, vaginal secretions, and saliva. Other body fluids that do not contain blood or serous fluid, such as feces or urine, are not a source of HBV. Therefore, the three principal modes of HBV transmission are percutaneous (injection drug use, blood or body fluid exposures among health care workers, and blood transfusions), sexual (heterosexual or male homosexual), and perinatal (through blood exposure at the time of birth) (29). Transmission between siblings and others household contacts readily occurs, through transmission from skin lesions, such as eczema or impetigo; through sharing of potentially blood-contaminated objects, such as toothbrushes and razor blades; and occasionally through bites. Nosocomial outbreaks, although rare, have occurred from improper use or disinfection of medical devices

HBV is present in high titers in blood and exudates of acutely and chronically infected persons

(e.g., finger-stick devices, acupuncture needles) or from infected health care workers to patients during invasive procedures.

HBV infection occurs worldwide. Approximately 45% of the world's population live in geographic areas with high HBV endemicity (8% or more of the general population are chronically infected), 43% live in areas of moderate endemicity (2 to 7% are chronically infected), and 12% live in areas of low endemicity (<2% are chronically infected). Overall, an estimated 300 million persons worldwide are HBV carriers. On the basis of testing from the NHANES III survey, the overall prevalence of chronic HBV infection among the general U.S. population is 0.3%, (0.08% among whites and 1.1% among blacks) (18).

After correcting for underreporting and asymptomatic infections, an estimated 200,000 new HBV infections have occurred annually in the United States during the past 10 years (54). Since the mid-1980s, however, the number of cases of acute hepatitis B reported to the CDC annually has decreased by approximately 50%. This decrease is believed to be due to behavior changes among drug users and homosexual men in response to the AIDS epidemic. In more recent years, hepatitis B vaccination may also have had an impact in lowering disease rates. Currently, heterosexual transmission accounts for more cases than any other mode of transmission. Among cases reported during 1992 and 1993 in the Sentinel Counties Study, a surveillance system operated by CDC in four U.S. counties, the most frequent risk factor was heterosexual exposure to a contact with hepatitis or to multiple partners (41%), which was followed by injection drug use (15%), homosexual activity (9%), household contact (2%), and health care employment (1%) (18).

Perinatal transmission and transmission to young children in households, while not reflected in surveillance data because acute infection at these ages is largely asymptomatic, account for a substantial proportion of chronic disease due to HBV infection. In the United States, 8% of acute cases occur among children 10 years of age, but infections among this age group account for an estimated 36% of chronic infections. Therefore, vaccination targeted to children and adolescents is important in preventing chronic HBV infection. Vaccination of children will also prevent HBV infection at older ages, when they may engage in behaviors which put them at risk for HBV infection.

HCV is the primary agent of parenterally transmitted non-A, non-B hepatitis. HCV circulates in low titers in the blood of infected persons and is detected inconsistently in other body fluids. Transmission via parenteral, sexual, and perinatal exposures has been identified; however, many patients with hepatitis C do not report such exposures. The most efficient mode of HCV transmission is direct percutaneous blood exposure, such as through needle sharing among drug users or through transfusion of blood or blood products. The risk of HCV transmission following a needle-stick exposure to blood from a source positive for antibody to HCV (anti-HCV) is 3 to 10% (60).

Studies examining the risk of sexual and perinatal HCV transmission have been limited by small sample size and variable types of serologic test-

> *An estimated 200,000 new HBV infections have occurred annually in the United States during the past 10 years*

ing, and in some cases, they have provided conflicting results. Some studies of sexual contacts and spouses of anti-HCV-positive persons have found HCV infection rates, determined by detection of anti-HCV or detection of HCV by the polymerase chain reaction (PCR), as high as 32%, whereas other studies of similar contacts and of homosexual men have found little or no HCV infection (26, 41, 69, 70). Studies of infants born to HCV-infected human immunodeficiency virus (HIV)-negative women have found the risk of transmission, determined by persistent anti-HCV positivity, to be from 0 to 13%. Several recent HCV studies have suggested the importance of viral titer in determining the risk of transmission. For example, in one study of perinatal transmission, transmission occurred only from mothers with titers of 10^6 genome copies per ml; in another study of 15 anti-HCV-positive mothers, transmission occurred from only one woman with a titer of 10^{10} genome copies per ml (50, 67).

Anti-HCV seroprevalence studies have characterized the risk of HCV infection in other groups. Studies of health care workers have shown anti-HCV prevalence to be around 1%; one study showed an association of anti-HCV positivity with a history of accidental needle-sticks. The prevalence of anti-HCV among U.S. dialysis patients ranges from 10 to 30%. Some of these studies have shown an association between anti-HCV positivity and years on dialysis, independent of a history of blood transfusion.

Results from the NHANES III serosurvey indicate that the prevalence of anti-HCV in the general U.S. population is 1.8%, which corresponds to 3.9 million anti-HCV-positive persons nationwide (18). On the basis of surveillance data for community-acquired hepatitis C, 150,000 acute HCV infections have been estimated to occur annually in the United States during the past decade. The number of new infections has decreased significantly since 1989, largely because of a decrease in cases associated with injection drug use. Still, injection drug use is the most commonly reported risk factor (4). In the Sentinel Counties Study during 1990 to 1993, 36% of patients with acute hepatitis C reported a history of injection drug use, 13% of patients with acute hepatitis C had exposure to a household or sexual contact with hepatitis or had multiple sexual partners, 5% had a history of a blood transfusion, 3% were health care workers, and 1% were dialysis patients. Forty-two percent did not report a source of infection; these persons may have denied risk factors or may have unrecognized exposures (e.g., sexual contact with a person who is asymptomatically infected).

Recent events involving the epidemiology of hepatitis C include reports from the United States and abroad of hepatitis C associated with receipt of intravenous immune globulin (IVIG) (10). Cases were associated with IVIG from a specific manufacturer and began occurring in October 1993, corresponding to the time when IVIG had been prepared using second-generation anti-HCV-screened plasma. It is possible that institution of second-generation anti-HCV screening of source plasma affected the safety of IVIG by affecting the removal of HCV during the preparation process or by removing potential neutralizing antibody. Studies to date do not indicate a risk of HCV infection from intramuscular IG.

Recent reports from the United States and abroad have associated hepatitis C infection with receipt of intravenous immune globulin

Because hepatitis delta virus (HDV) is transmitted only as a coinfection with HBV or as a superinfection in a person who is already HBV infected, the modes of transmission of HDV are similar to those of HBV (73). The global prevalence of HDV infection also corresponds to the prevalence of HBV infection, with some distinct features. Most countries with low endemic chronic HBV infection have low prevalence of HDV infection among HBV-infected persons. In countries with high endemic HBV infection, the prevalence of HDV infection can vary greatly. Regions with moderate to high HDV prevalence include Italy, Spain, Turkey, Egypt, and the Amazon Basin in South America. Asia and Africa, although having high prevalence of HBV infection, have relatively low prevalence of HDV infection.

In the United States, an estimated 4% of acute HBV infections are coinfections with HDV (3). Among blood donors who are hepatitis B surface antigen (HBsAg) positive, the prevalence of HDV infection is 2 to 8%. Seroepidemiologic studies indicate that HDV transmission in the United States occurs mostly through injection drug use and less commonly through sexual transmission. The seroprevalence of antibody to HDV among HBV-infected injection drug users ranges from 20 to 53%. A large outbreak of fulminant hepatitis associated with hepatitis delta among injection drug users was observed in the northeastern United States in the mid-1980s.

Hepatitis E virus (HEV), the causative agent of hepatitis E (or enterically transmitted non-A, non-B hepatitis), is excreted in feces, and fecally contaminated drinking water has been the most frequently documented vehicle of transmission. Person-to-person HEV transmission is not believed to commonly occur, as low rates of secondary household transmission among patients are observed. Case-fatality rates among pregnant women are high compared with case-fatality rates among other patients (15 to 20% versus 0.5 to 3%, respectively). Hepatitis E occurs in large outbreaks in areas with extremely poor sanitary conditions, such as refugee camps in developing countries. Since the 1950s, outbreaks have been reported in many countries, including India, Pakistan, Burma, Indonesia, China, Mexico, and many countries in Africa. Sporadic endemic transmission also occurs in many developing countries, but few studies have addressed how such transmission occurs. Hepatitis E has been reported in the United States only occasionally, primarily among travelers returning from regions in which HEV is endemic, and no secondary transmission has been observed (55).

Hepatitis G virus (HGV) from a patient with transfusion-associated non-A, non-B hepatitis was recently cloned and sequenced (52, 81). Experimental transmission of HGV to nonhuman primates has been demonstrated, but these animals had no evidence of liver pathology. The genomic organization of HGV is consistent with those of viruses in the *Flaviviridae* family. It has a positive-sense RNA genome of approximately 9,300 nucleotides that encodes a single polyprotein. HGV has a high degree of nucleotide homology (86%) with GBV-C, another recently discovered hepatitis virus, and is distantly related to HCV (27% nucleotide homology).

HGV is associated with approximately 0.3% of all acute viral hepatitis reported in the United States, and approximately 20% of patients with HCV

Hepatitis E has been reported in the United States only occasionally, primarily among travelers returning from regions in which HEV is endemic, and no secondary transmission has been observed

infection are also infected with HGV. In one study of patients with community-acquired HGV infection, none of five patients with HGV infection developed biochemical evidence of chronic hepatitis during a follow-up period of 2 to 9 years. In contrast, chronic hepatitis developed in more than 60% of the patients with HCV infection, and rates seen with HCV infection alone were similar to those seen with dual HCV-HGV infections. However, even in the absence of biochemical evidence of chronic liver disease, persistent HGV infection developed in 100% of the HGV alone group and in 90% of the dual infection group. HGV is transmitted by blood transfusion, but the incidence of posttransfusion hepatitis G appears to be extremely low. Other risk factors for acquisition of HGV infection remain to be determined.

Evidence for the presence of viruses causing acute and chronic hepatitis other than the five characterized viruses includes the lack of detection of HCV in patients with posttransfusion and community-acquired non-A, non-B hepatitis. For example, in the CDC Sentinel Counties Study, among 130 patients with acute non-A, non-B hepatitis who were followed for at least 6 months and tested both with anti-HCV and by the polymerase chain reaction, 18% did not have detectable HCV infection (5). Parenteral, sexual, or household exposures were less likely to be reported by these patients than by patients who were HCV positive. They also developed chronic hepatitis at a significantly lower rate than HCV-positive patients (29 versus 58%, respectively). The etiologic agents in these patients remain to be identified, and more extensive characterization of the epidemiology awaits the development of diagnostic assays.

Pathology of Acute Viral Hepatitis

The appearance of the liver under the scanning objective of the light microscope is one of acinar disarray caused by the sum total of the changes to be described. Two degenerative changes predominantly affect hepatocytes in viral hepatitis, namely, ballooning and apoptosis (Fig. 8.3 and 8.4) (36, 37). These are seen throughout the acinus in various combinations, and not all hepatocytes in a given acinus are affected. In some cases of hepatitis B, however, ballooning tends to be more severe in zone 3.

Apoptosis is a type of cell death that leads to elimination of dead cells; it results in fragmentation of the injured hepatocyte (79). Recent studies have shown that it is induced by transforming growth factor-β1 (66). In ultrastructural studies of apoptosis, the nuclear outline becomes convoluted and the chromatin aggregates in dense, sharply circumscribed masses that abut on the nuclear membrane (79). At the same time, the condensed cytoplasm of the liver cell develops protuberances which separate and are released into the spaces of Disse and sinusoids, while the nucleus breaks up into discrete masses. Microscopically, the larger cell fragments, which may contain parts of the nucleus, are generally referred to as "acidophilic" or "hyaline" bodies (Fig. 8.3). The apoptotic bodies are quickly phagocytosed by Kupffer cells or adjoining liver cells, where they undergo degeneration and are reduced to residual bodies.

HGV is transmitted by blood transfusion, but the incidence of posttransfusion hepatitis G appears to be extremely low

Ballooning degeneration refers to the swelling of hepatocytes, often to several times the normal size (Fig. 8.4). Affected cells have an indistinct cell membrane, and sometimes the membranes between adjacent hepatocytes disintegrate. The cytoplasm is rarefied, often with perinuclear condensation of a small quantity of cytoplasmic remnants. There may be bile retention in some ballooned hepatocytes. Karyolysis is the typical nuclear degenerative change. The fate of ballooned hepatocytes is lysis, with disappearance or "dropping out." The remnants of these cells attract lymphocytes and, less often, other types of inflammatory cells (focal necrosis), as well as hypertrophied and focally hyperplastic Kupffer cells. Regenerative activity, both amitotic and mitotic, may be seen shortly after the onset of viral hepatitis. The number of regenerating cells gradually increases as the patient recovers. Cholestasis is not a significant component of the histopathology of acute viral hepatitis, with the exception of hepatitis E. When present, it is usually seen as an occasional, haphazardly distributed canalicular bile plug.

In addition to hepatocellular degeneration and regeneration, the acute phase of viral hepatitis is characterized by marked hypertrophy and hyperplasia of Kupffer cells. These cells also contain a light brown, finely granular pigment presumed to be phagocytosed from necrotic hepatocytes, in addition to apoptotic bodies of various sizes. The portal areas in viral hepatitis are usually heavily infiltrated with inflammatory cells; lymphocytes predominate, but a small number of plasma cells, eosinophilic leukocytes, and neutrophils may be present (Fig. 8.5). The inflammatory response often extends beyond the confines of the portal areas, leading to some blurring of outline of the limiting plate. Vessels in the portal areas show no noticeable changes in acute viral hepatitis. Occasional cases may reveal abnormalities of the bile ductal epithelium, such as swelling, necrosis, and infiltration by lymphocytes.

There is still controversy about histopathologic differences between the various types of viral hepatitis. Some investigators believe that there are no significant differences between acute viral hepatitis A, B, or C (47, 68). Other investigators believe that hepatitis A differs from hepatitis B and hepatitis C in the periportal predominance of the injury (Fig. 8.6) (1, 38, 83). In one recent study, bile duct degenerative changes were considered diagnostic of acute viral hepatitis C (53). Hepatitis E, as well as some cases of hepatitis A, is associated with a cholestatic type of acute hepatitis. It is characterized by marked cholestasis, pseudoglands, and only mild necroinflammatory changes. The comparative histopathology of acute hepatitis caused by HAV, HBV, HDV, HCV, and HEV is listed in Table 8.3. The recently cloned HGV is an RNA virus that can cause both acute and chronic hepatitis (52). The virus is distantly related to HCV. Clinically, the acute hepatitis caused by HGV cannot be differentiated from that caused by HCV. The histopathology of acute HGV hepatitis has not been described to date.

The subsiding phase of viral hepatitis is characterized by diminution of degenerative changes and increased regeneration. The differences between this and the active phase are, however, mainly quantitative. Acinar disarray diminishes or disappears, and the hepatic parenchyma gradually reverts to a normal appearance, though various degrees of unrest are still evident. The

In addition to hepatocellular degeneration and regeneration, the acute phase of viral hepatitis is characterized by marked hypertrophy and hyperplasia of Kupffer cells

Table 8.3 Comparison of histopathology of different types of acute viral hepatitis

Histopathologic change	Type of hepatitis				
	A	B	D[a] Epidemic/endemic	C Parenteral/sporadic	E Epidemic/sporadic
Spotty necrosis[b]	+	+	+	+	+
Zone 3 ballooning necrosis	−	±	+	±	−
Zone 1 ballooning necrosis	+	−	−	−	−
Panacinar ballooning	−	+[3]	−	−	−
Massive necrosis	+	+	+	+	?
Steatosis[c]	±	+	+	−	±
Marked cholestasis and/or pseudoglands	±	−	−	−	+
Kupffer cell hypertrophy plus iron and/or lipofuscin	+	+	+	+	−
Kupffer cell hypertrophy plus bile accumulation	±	−	−	−	+
Portal inflammation	+	+	+	+	+
Types of inflammatory cells[d]	L, P	L, P	L, P	N, L	
Ductular proliferation	±	±	±	±	±
Bile duct degeneration	−	−	−	±	−
Fibrosis	−	+[3]	−	−	−

[a] Thus far reported from South America and Africa.
[b] Includes apoptosis, unicellular acidophilic and ballooning degeneration, and focal necrosis.
[c] Microvesicular steatosis; seen only in posttransplant reinfection.
[d] L, lymphocytes; P, plasma cells; N, neutrophils; E, eosinophils.

liver cell plates display some irregularity of alignment, and any slight damage that may have affected the reticulin network has been repaired. Only occasional degenerating cells and small foci of necrosis are evident. A minimal degree of cholestasis in zone 3 is often noted in subsiding hepatitis. One of the striking features is the continuing hypertrophy and focal hyperplasia of Kupffer cells and portal macrophages. They become relatively more conspicuous, because the hepatocytes are less swollen. These cells now contain hemosiderin in addition to lipofuscin, and characteristically, these two pigments are admixed in various proportions in sections from the same biopsy specimen (36, 37). The portal area inflammatory response gradually diminishes and becomes spotty. Uncomplicated viral hepatitis is not followed by any significant periportal or intra-acinar fibrosis. Rarely, the features of acute hepatitis may persist for many months or even years, and the histologic changes may not differ from those of acute hepatitis on light or electron microscopy. The term "chronic lobular hepatitis" has been used for this infection, which is characterized clinically by relapses and remissions. There is no fibrosis, and recovery eventually occurs, with or without therapy.

Severe acute viral hepatitis is associated with submassive necrosis. When necrosis occurs in hepatitis B it involves zone 3, sometimes with extension into zone 2 of the hepatic acini, but cases of severe viral hepatitis A are characterized by necrosis predominantly involving zone 1 (45). The zones of necrosis with the collapsed reticulin framework may be linked together ("bridging necrosis"). In patients with a subacute course who subsequently die, regenerative nodules, often having a tumor-like appearance, may be seen grossly. These have an irregular alignment of reticulin fibers, plates of hepatocytes that are two cells thick, and various degrees of cholestasis. The surrounding reticulin framework of the necrotic parenchyma is progressively compressed as the nodules enlarge, and it may eventually become collagenized.

The most severe cases of acute viral hepatitis are associated with massive necrosis (Fig. 8.7). Sections from the liver show uniform disappearance (dropping out) of hepatocytes, but occasionally, haphazardly distributed cells can survive, as can a cuff of cells around portal areas. The reticulin framework is usually intact but frequently collapsed because of the loss of liver cells, with resultant approximation of portal areas. The sinusoids can be empty or engorged with blood.

Variable numbers of inflammatory cells are present in the spaces of Disse and sinusoids. They include lymphocytes and plasma cells, as well as a lesser number of eosinophilic leukocytes and neutrophils. Central vein endophlebitis may be present. Kupffer cells reveal marked hypertrophy and hyperplasia, and their cytoplasm is packed with lipofuscin. Zone 1 of the hepatic acinus shows a characteristic neocholangiolar proliferation, with neutrophilic infiltration. The portal areas are variably infiltrated with inflammatory cells similar to those in the acini, as well as with pigment-laden macrophages; the inflammatory cells may infiltrate the periportal areas. This spillover can be distinguished from piecemeal necrosis of chronic hepatitis by the lack of separation of liver cells from the limiting plate and by the absence of periportal fibrosis.

Pathology of Chronic Hepatitis

The histopathology of chronic hepatitis, regardless of etiology, is characterized by several lesions, the most important of which is piecemeal necrosis (6, 8). Other changes, such as bile duct lesions, portal inflammation, intraacinar degeneration and necrosis, and periportal and bridging fibrosis, are present to a variable extent. Additional specific features may be present, depending on the etiology (e.g., ground-glass cells of the HBV carrier state) (39).

Piecemeal Necrosis

This necroinflammatory change, sometimes referred to as "lymphocytic" piecemeal necrosis, initially destroys the limiting plate of liver cells (i.e., is periportal) (Fig. 8.8 and 8.9). In the untreated patient there is continuous erosion of the hepatic parenchyma with closer and closer approximation of expanded portal areas. The necroinflammatory changes are succeeded by fibrosis. Piecemeal necrosis may not involve all portal areas equally in a given case and can affect either a segment or the entire perimeter of a portal area. It can continue unabated in the cirrhotic liver, complicating chronic hepatitis and thus contributing to the activity of the cirrhotic process.

Degenerative changes affecting liver cells in piecemeal necrosis include cytoplasmic dissociation (a change characterized by swelling of liver cells with cytoplasmic rarefaction, coarse clumping of cytoplasmic organelles, and, eventually, lysis of nuclei and cell membranes) and apoptosis (2, 79). The latter change results in the formation of variably sized, often rounded fragments of liver cells that are located in the liver plates or sinusoids. The larger apoptotic bodies, sometimes containing nuclear fragments, are often referred to as acidophilic bodies. Within the sinusoids, the apoptotic bodies are hardly ever free but are usually phagocytosed and ultimately digested by Kupffer cells.

There is a very intimate relationship between lymphocytes and liver cells in chronic hepatitis that is apparent even on cursory examination. The degenerating hepatocytes and inflammatory cells are closely apposed, the lymphocytes often being located in the spaces of Disse, with indentation of the cytoplasm of liver cells (polesis). Sometimes the hepatocyte completely encircles a lymphocyte or plasma cell (emperipolesis). There is loss of microvilli of the plasma membrane of the liver cell facing the lymphocyte. It should be noted that the processes of polesis and emperipolesis that can be seen in chronic hepatitis are seen not only in the areas of periportal piecemeal necrosis but also throughout the hepatic acini, at various distances from the leading edge of the piecemeal necrosis.

A recent study of apoptosis has shown that it is mediated by the Fas antigen, a cell surface antigen which belongs to the receptor family that induces tumor necrosis factor receptor, nerve growth factor receptor, B-cell CD40 antigen, and T-cell OX40 antigen. Hiramatsu et al. studied the immunohistochemical expression of Fas antigen and hepatitis C core antigen in chronic hepatitis C (34). Fas antigen was expressed in the cytoplasm of liver cells among infiltrating lymphocytes at the advancing edge of piecemeal necrosis; more expression was observed in areas of active inflammation than in areas with no inflammation. The prevalence of Fas antigen was higher in the patients expressing HCV core antigen than in those that did not. These investigators suggested that Fas expression could be triggered directly by HCV infection or indirectly through the immune system, with resultant cytotoxic T lymphocyte-induced DNA fragmentation. Regardless of the mechanism, these observations have demonstrated an important role for Fas antigen expression in the inflammatory response and piecemeal necrosis in chronic hepatitis C and possibly other types of chronic hepatitis.

Portal Area Lesions

In chronic hepatitis, the portal area connective tissue is variably infiltrated by lymphocytes and plasma cells. Lymphoid aggregates or follicles with reactive centers may be present (Fig. 8.10A). They are now considered typical, though not pathognomonic, of chronic hepatitis C. Immunohistochemical studies of these aggregates show functional lymphoid follicles containing activated B cells in germinal centers surrounded by a follicular dendritic cell network. A mantle zone of B cells surrounds the activated B cells. The B-cell follicle in turn is surrounded by a T-cell zone. Some of the plasma cells in chronic hepatitis B may contain antibodies against HBsAg (anti-HBs) and hepatitis B core antigen (anti-HBc). Portal macrophages are

In chronic hepatitis, the portal area connective tissue is variably infiltrated by lymphocytes and plasma cells.

often hypertrophied and contain periodic acid-Schiff-positive (but diastase-resistant) granular material.

A histopathologic feature that is highly characteristic, if not pathognomonic, of chronic hepatitis, is the isolation and entrapment of single or groups of liver cells in the expanded portal areas. Bile duct lesions have been reviewed recently by Vyberg (87). He recognized three types of hepatitis-associated bile duct lesions. The type 2 lesion is the one most frequently seen with chronic hepatitis. It involves bile ducts with an outer diameter of 15 to 40 μm. The abnormal ducts are frequently surrounded by a lymphoid aggregate or follicle. Some represent preexisting ducts undergoing degeneration with swelling, cytoplasmic vacuolization, nuclear pyknosis, or karyorrhexis and infiltration by inflammatory cells, typically mononuclear (Fig. 8.10B). The basement membrane is usually not destroyed, and actual destruction of ducts is rare. Some of the abnormal ducts are actually composed of cells with an abundant eosinophilic cytoplasm, suggesting metaplasia of duct cells to hepatocytes. Such metaplasia of bile duct cells to hepatocytes has recently been documented ultrastructurally and immunohistochemically by Nomoto et al. (65).

Periportal Fibrosis and Associated Changes

The usually progressive necroinflammation of piecemeal necrosis in chronic hepatitis is associated with collagenization of the spaces of Disse and deposition of basement membrane material, a process of "capillarization" that was described many years ago by Schaffner and Popper. Central to this process is the extracellular matrix (interstitial and basement membrane collagens, glycoproteins, and proteoglycans) that is markedly increased as a result of synthesis by fat-storing (Ito) cells and transitional cells. Initially, the fibrosis has a characteristic stellate or arachnoidal appearance. Capillarization of sinusoids around regenerated, two-cell-thick plates of liver cells leads to rosette formation. A typical rosette consists of four to six hepatocytes resting on a basement membrane and fibrous tissue that surround a small, centrally located canaliculus. Marked rosetting is more characteristic of autoimmune than viral chronic hepatitis.

As the fibrosis progresses, portal-to-portal fibrous bridges are formed. "Central"-to-portal (and even central-to-central) fibrous bridges can develop from superimposed episodes of necrosis involving zone 3, as described later. Broad areas of fibrosis can result from the healing of bouts of multiacinar necrosis. Elastic fibers are deposited during healing, in addition to collagen fibers; their presence can be demonstrated by the same stains used for identification of HBsAg in tissue sections, i.e., orcein, aldehyde fuchsin, and Victoria blue. The end result is the development of cirrhosis, in which the necroinflammatory changes of piecemeal necrosis (now periseptal) often continue unabated.

Intra-Acinar Lesions

Most instances of chronic hepatitis reveal intra-acinar necroinflammatory changes of variable severity, in addition to periportal piecemeal necrosis. In the typical case they are focal ("spotty") and consist mainly of apoptosis.

Scattered apoptotic bodies of various sizes are observed, as well as focal necrosis with aggregates of lymphocytes and plasma cells and polesis and emperipolesis. Hypertrophied Kupffer cells that have scavenged the apoptotic bodies and other granular debris are also present in the foci of necrosis. Steatosis, mild to moderate and generally macrovesicular, is now considered typical of chronic hepatitis C, as will be noted later. It is an infrequent finding in chronic hepatitis B or autoimmune chronic hepatitis (unless the patient had been treated with corticosteroids).

Hepatocellular Injury in Exacerbations and Relapses

More severe intra-acinar injury is generally seen in exacerbations and relapses of chronic hepatitis. In chronic hepatitis B these may be spontaneous, secondary to withdrawal of cytotoxic or immunosuppressive therapy, or associated with HDV or HIV infection. In addition to spontaneous exacerbations and relapses after interferon therapy, there are recent reports of reactivation of chronic hepatitis C after withdrawal of immunosuppressive therapy (32, 85).

More severe intra-acinar injury is generally seen in exacerbations and relapses of chronic hepatitis

Spontaneous flare-ups of chronic hepatitis C may be related to sequence variations of the hypervariable region of HCV. In addition to the clinical and biochemical findings, acute exacerbations of chronic hepatitis B are characterized by increases in serum HBV DNA and immunoglobulin M (IgM) anti-HBc titers. In our experience, one or more of the following additional changes can be observed in exacerbations or relapses: (i) an increase in the degree of spotty necrosis, (ii) ballooning degeneration, often most severe in zone 3, with dropout of hepatocytes and central-to-central and central-to-portal bridging necrosis that is subsequently followed by fibrosis (ballooning degeneration may be associated with variable cholestasis; in such cases there is significant periportal cholangiolar proliferation, with infiltration of the cholangioles by neutrophils [acute cholangiolitis]), and (iii) multi-acinar necrosis, which is followed eventually by the formation of irregularly shaped, multiacinar scars.

Until recently, the pathogenesis of the exacerbations in chronic hepatitis had remained unclear. Murayama et al. (62) studied 19 patients with chronic hepatitis B for alterations in HBV DNA, HBsAg, anti-HBc, and HBsAg-specific immune complex formation before, during, and after spontaneous acute exacerbations of liver injury. They found significant correlations between increasing levels of these serum markers and liver injury and suggested that the cyclic injury may reflect increases in HBV replication which are followed by an increase in the immune responses which mediate the liver injury.

Regeneration

Regeneration is typically seen in the form of two-cell-thick plates (periportal and periseptal) and an increased number of bi- and trinucleated cells. Mitoses may be present in patients with recent exacerbations or relapses. A high proliferative rate of liver cells was demonstrated by immunohistochemistry for proliferating cell nuclear antigen in chronic viral hepatitis (both B and C) by Nakamura et al. (63).

The continuous piecemeal necrosis with resultant periportal fibrosis and the bridging and multi-acinar necrosis with healing by fibrous bridges and irregular scars eventually lead to cirrhosis

Cirrhosis

The continuous piecemeal necrosis with resultant periportal fibrosis and the bridging and multi-acinar necrosis with healing by fibrous bridges and irregular scars eventually lead to cirrhosis. Variable degrees of continuing necroinflammatory changes are usually present, and their extent should be noted by the histopathologist. Episodes of gastrointestinal hemorrhage can result in anoxic (coagulative) necrosis. HDV superinfection of HBV cirrhosis can lead to extensive necrosis with decompensation and liver failure.

The cirrhosis following chronic hepatitis is either macronodular or mixed macro- and micronodular in type. Liver cell dysplasia (large or small cell type), adenomatoid hyperplasia, and macroregenerative nodules, when present, should be noted in the histopathologic diagnosis because of their putative preneoplastic significance.

The specific markers of HBV infection, demonstrable by light or electron microscopy or immunohistochemically, are of paramount importance in differential diagnosis. Ground-glass cells that contain HBsAg can be positively identified by special stains (orcein, Victoria blue, or aldehyde fuchsin) (Fig. 8.11 and 8.12). The differential diagnosis of ground-glass cells is listed in Table 8.4. Sanded liver cell nuclei due to excess HBcAg accumulation are difficult to recognize histopathologically. Furthermore, similar nuclei have been seen in delta hepatitis. Both HBsAg and HBcAg are readily demonstrable immunohistochemically in liver cells in paraffin sections, as well as in ductular cells, by using commercially available antibodies (Fig. 8.13 and

Table 8.4 Ground-glass cells in viral hepatitis and other conditions

Location	PAS[a]	Orcein, Victoria blue	Ultrastructure	Diagnosis
Non-neoplastic liver				
Haphazard	−	+	SER[b] proliferation plus tubular or round HBsAg particles	HBsAg carrier without clinical disease or with chronic hepatitis or cirrhosis
Acinar zone 3 or panacinar	−	−	SER proliferation	Drug-induced change (e.g., phenobarbital, diphenylhydantoin, chlorpromazine)
Acinar zone 1	+	−	Non-membrane-bound secondary lysosomes, degenerating organelles, glycogen, and lipid droplets	Drug-induced injury due to cyanamide
	+	−	Fibrillar non-membrane-bound material plus glycogen	Type IV glycogenesis
	+	−	Large aggregates of SER and glycogen	Lafora's disease
Neoplastic liver				
Haphazard	−	−	Amorphous cytoplasmic material (fibrinogen) type	Hepatocellular carcinoma, fibrolamellar
	−	+	SER proliferation plus tubular or round HBsAg particles	Hepatocellular carcinoma

[a] PAS, periodic acid-Schiff.
[b] SER, smooth endoplasmic reticulum.

8.14). The expression of pre-S1 and pre-S2 in 44 patients with chronic hepatitis B was studied by Chu and Liaw (19). All had synthesis and display of the two antigens. Their distribution and quantitative expression were closely related to the status of HBV replication but not to the histological activity. Concurrent HDV superinfection did not appear to modulate the synthesis and expression of the pre-S peptides in the liver.

Delta antigen can be demonstrated in tissue sections immunohistochemically. The antigen is located mainly in the nuclei of liver cells, but there may be occasional cytoplasmic antigen. In situ hybridization studies for HBV and HDV have been reviewed recently by Negro et al. (64) and will not be discussed further. Routine assays for serum HBV DNA or liver HBcAg are more sensitive and reliable and less time-consuming than in situ hybridization of tissue HBV nucleic acids.

A number of viruses have been implicated in superinfections of patients with chronic hepatitis B. They include HAV, HDV, HCV, cytomegalovirus, and HIV. Superimposed hepatitis A appears to have no adverse effect on the course of chronic hepatitis B. Superinfection with HDV, on the other hand, is associated with acute exacerbations, with a sudden worsening and a fatal outcome or with more severe and progressive chronic liver disease. However, in one study of 30 patients with chronic B hepatitis from Taiwan, HDV superinfection was not particularly different from spontaneous acute exacerbations and the progression of the disease was slow (51). In general, most experts agree that the degree of degeneration and necrosis is greater in delta-hepatitis-positive than in delta-hepatitis-negative chronic hepatitis B. The prognosis appears to depend to some extent on the individual immune response; it is much poorer in drug addicts than in nonaddicts. Occasionally, some patients may clear both hepatitis B and delta hepatitis infections after HDV superinfection.

Double infections with HBV and HCV have been reported by several groups of investigators. Chronic infections with the two viruses can be acquired simultaneously or at different times. Coinfection with both viruses has been documented in at least one study of posttransfusion hepatitis (59). An inverse relationship between HBV and HCV replication in a study of 55 patients with double infections was found by Pontisso et al. (74). Liver disease activity was generally milder in patients with an active HCV infection and inactive HBV status, suggesting that HBV replication might be more harmful than HCV replication in that particular subgroup of patients. Cytomegalovirus infection superimposed on HBsAg-positive chronic hepatitis can lead to a fatal outcome.

As already noted, HIV infection can result in reactivation of hepatitis B. In HIV and HBV coinfection, the liver disease (biochemically and histologically) tends to be less severe, with less fibrosis than in HIV-negative HBV carriers. HIV superinfection of an HBV carrier is also associated with less liver inflammation and decreased aminotransferase values, although viral replication is increased. Immunohistochemically, many more hepatitis B e antigen (HBeAg)- and HBcAg-positive hepatocytic nuclei are seen, which is similar to the findings in patients on immunosuppressive drugs; there is a negative correlation with histopathologic disease activity.

Chronic infections with HBV and HCV can be acquired simultaneously or at different times

The histopathologic features of chronic hepatitis C have been delineated in a recent flurry of publications. The studies leading to these publications were made possible by the commercial availability of serologic tests for diagnosis of HCV infection. Earlier reports of detailed studies of non-A, non-B hepatitis in hemophiliacs and other patients, however, had accurately described most of the changes now considered characteristic of chronic hepatitis C. Steatosis, sinusoidal inflammatory infiltrates, prominence of Kupffer cells, lymphoid follicle formation, and bile duct epithelial changes are all histologic features favoring chronic non-A, non-B hepatitis. Various degrees of all of these features are described in Table 8.5 (7, 30, 49, 76, 78). Bile duct loss was reported in only one study, and the presence of Mallory-body-like material was reported in another. Of all the lesions in chronic hepatitis C, the most characteristic (though not always present or pathognomonic) are the lymphoid aggregates/follicles, bile duct damage, and steatosis. It must be emphasized at this juncture that the fundamental lesions of chronic hepatitis, as described in an earlier section, i.e., the diffuse portal inflammation, piecemeal necrosis, spotty necrosis and apoptosis, and the sequelae of the necroinflammation (periportal fibrosis, bridging fibrosis, and cirrhosis), are all an integral part of the morphologic spectrum of chronic hepatitis C. Indeed, it is these features that must be relied on for the diagnosis of chronic hepatitis C, since bile duct lesions and lymphoid aggregates have been described in acute hepatitis C. A recent study has shown an interesting correlation between the mode of transmission of HCV and the severity of the chronic hepatitis. Transfusion-acquired hepatitis C was found to be associated with more aggressive histological inflammatory activity than hepatitis resulting from intravenous drug use. In this context, it is worth noting that in another recent study the prevalence of hepatitis C in injection drug abusers was 86%.

Immunohistochemical studies of the lymphoid aggregates/follicles in chronic hepatitis C have been noted in an earlier section. HLA-DR expression in bile ducts undergoing damage was studied by Danque et al. (23). In that study, HLA-DR was not detected in any of 30 liver biopsies from patients with chronic hepatitis C, 90% of whom had histologic evidence of bile duct damage. It was concluded that the mechanism of bile duct injury in chronic hepatitis C must be different from that of other liver diseases with bile duct damage that do express HLA-DR antigen, such as primary biliary

Transfusion-acquired hepatitis C is associated with more aggressive histological inflammatory activity than hepatitis resulting from intravenous drug use

Table 8.5 Histopathology of chronic hepatitis C

Lesion	% Change				
	Scheuer (78)	Bach et al. (7)	Gerber et al. (30)	Lefkowitch et al. (49)	Roberts et al. (76)
Bile duct damage	22.2	91.0	76.0	31.2	25.4
Bile duct loss	0.0	91.0	0.0	0.0	0.0
Lymphoid aggregates/follicles	78.0	49.0	45.0	49.4	68.2
Steatosis	53.7	72.0	31.0	68.9	42.9
Mallory bodies	0.0	0.0	0.0	17.6	0.0

cirrhosis, primary sclerosing cholangitis, graft-versus-host disease, and allograft rejection. Similar conclusions were arrived at in another study by Broomé et al. (11), who found HLA-DR expression on the biliary epithelium in patients with primary biliary cirrhosis and primary sclerosing cholangitis but not in patients with chronic hepatitis C or alcoholic cirrhosis or normal controls. In a study by Chu et al. (20), the genomic and replicative HCV RNA sequences were correlated with the histologic activity of chronic hepatitis C. It was concluded that a direct viropathic effect is less important than other mechanisms (such as the host immune response) in the pathogenesis of hepatocyte and bile duct injury in chronic hepatitis C.

PCR has been used to detect HCV RNA in sera and/or liver tissue (fresh or paraffin embedded) by several groups of investigators. Immunohistochemistry has been successfully utilized to detect HCV antigens in fresh frozen or paraffin-embedded tissue. HCV RNA has been demonstrated in liver tissue by in situ hybridization and more recently by in situ PCR. In all cases the HCV antigens have been located in the cytoplasm of liver cells. In one study, immunoelectron microscopy revealed HCV-N35 antigen along the endoplasmic reticulum.

Immunohistochemistry has been successfully utilized to detect HCV antigens in fresh frozen or paraffin-embedded tissue

Differential Diagnosis (Table 8.6)

Autoimmune Chronic Hepatitis

A classification of autoimmune hepatitis proposed by Stechemesser et al. (82) includes four different subgroups: type 1a, lupoid hepatitis (antinuclear antibody positive, with or without actin antibody); type 1b, only actin antibody positive; type 2, liver-kidney microsomal antibody positive; and type 3, liver-pancreas antibody positive (with or without other autoantibodies).

Table 8.6 Etiology and histologic features of chronic hepatitis

Etiology	Distinctive histologic features
Hepatitis B	Ground-glass cells; "sanded" nuclei; positive immunohistochemical stains for HBsAg and HBcAg; core and surface antigen particles in liver cell nuclei and cytoplasm, respectively (electron microscopy)
Hepatitis C	Bile duct degeneration; lymphoid aggregates/follicles; steatosis
Drug injury[a]	None
Wilson's disease	Copper accumulation in liver cells; Mallory bodies (zone 1); steatosis; glycogenated nuclei; heterogeneity of mitochondria with separation of inner and outer membranes and membranes of cristae (electron microscopy)
α_1-Antitrypsin deficiency	Eosinophilic periodic acid-Schiff-positive globules in liver cells; positive immunocytochemical stains for α_1-antitrypsin; amorphous inclusions in endoplasmic reticulum (electron microscopy)
Autoimmune	Rosettes; many plasma cells; giant hepatocytes
Idiopathic	None

[a] Isoniazid, methyldopa, oxyphenisatin, nitrofurantoin, dantrolene, diclofenac, and others.

There are no histologic features that reliably distinguish autoimmune chronic hepatitis from chronic hepatitis B, other than the specific markers of HBV infection in the latter (such as ground-glass cells and the demonstration of HBsAg or HBcAg by various techniques). Other investigators believe that hypocellular areas of collapse and microacinus formation (rosettes) are suggestive of autoimmune chronic hepatitis. A predominance of plasma cells in portal areas is characteristic of autoimmune chronic hepatitis, being most helpful in distinguishing it from chronic hepatitis C, in which the predominant cell is the lymphocyte. However, an abundance of plasma cells can be found in chronic hepatitis B and some cases of drug-induced chronic hepatitis. Bach et al. (7) recently compared autoimmune chronic hepatitis with chronic hepatitis C. They found that severe intra-acinar necrosis and inflammation, piecemeal necrosis, multinucleated hepatocytes, and broad areas of parenchymal collapse were seen more often in autoimmune chronic hepatitis than in chronic hepatitis C (in which bile duct damage, steatosis, and lymphoid aggregates were more common).

It is important to briefly mention that anti-HCV has been detected in one subtype of autoimmune chronic hepatitis, type 2, which is characterized by liver-kidney-microsomal (LKM-1) antibodies. Autoantibodies to cytosol antigen type 1 appear to be a more specific marker for autoimmune chronic hepatitis type 2 than are anti-LKM-1 autoantibodies. Several groups of investigators have concluded that HCV might be directly responsible for the development of type 2 (anti-LKM-1 positive) autoimmune chronic hepatitis in genetically predisposed persons. To date, no histopathologic differences between the various subtypes of autoimmune chronic hepatitis have emerged.

Multinucleated giant cells have been reported in some cases of autoimmune chronic hepatitis, other disorders with autoimmune features, and a number of hepatotropic viral infections. The terms "postinfantile giant-cell hepatitis," "syncytial giant-cell hepatitis," and "postinfantile giant-cell transformation in hepatitis" have been used to identify such cases. Phillips et al. (71) reported 10 patients, 4 with subacute hepatic failure and 6 with severe chronic hepatitis. Electron microscopy revealed structures resembling paramyxovirus nucleocapsids, and it was suggested that this virus could be the etiological agent of the liver disease.

Cryptogenic Chronic Hepatitis

The label "cryptogenic chronic hepatitis," as well as its end stage, cryptogenic cirrhosis, has been used in the past as a wastebasket for chronic necroinflammatory disease of unknown etiology. Many such cases now have been shown to be related to hepatitis C. In a study from the United Kingdom, 67% of patients with cryptogenic chronic liver disease had hepatitis C nucleocapsid antibodies (12). In a study from Spain, 82% of patients with cryptogenic chronic hepatitis were anti-HCV positive (77). Cases not due to HCV are infrequently associated with autoantibodies, suggesting that cryptogenic cirrhosis is distinct from autoimmune liver disease. However, in a recent comparative study of 12 patients with cryptogenic hepatitis and 94 patients with autoimmune hepatitis, Czaja et al. (22) found no differences

HCV might be directly responsible for the development of type 2 autoimmune chronic hepatitis in genetically predisposed persons

in clinical expression, genetic phenotype, and corticosteroid responsiveness between the two groups. They concluded that cryptogenic hepatitis may be an autoimmune disorder that has escaped detection by conventional immunoserological markers. Histopathologically, there are no characteristic features of true cryptogenic hepatitis or cirrhosis; the cirrhosis is generally inactive with little inflammation.

Cryptogenic hepatitis may be an autoimmune disorder that has escaped detection by conventional immunoserological markers

Chronic Hepatitis and Alcohol

The combined effects of alcoholism and infection with either HBV or HCV have interested clinical investigators for many years. The subject of HCV and alcoholic liver disease was reviewed recently (57), as was the association between HBV and alcoholism (86). Space does not permit more than a few comments about this important topic. The morphologic changes of chronic alcoholic hepatitis are distinctive and are not likely to be confused with those seen with chronic hepatitis. Changes that should implicate a viral etiology for chronic hepatitis in the alcoholic who is HBsAg-positive or anti-HCV-positive include piecemeal necrosis and lymphoplasmacytic portal and parenchymal inflammation. In patients with HCV infection, there is close contact of T-cytotoxic cells to hepatocytes expressing class I HLA in areas of periportal and intra-acinar necrosis. Needless to say, the serologic tests for hepatitis B and C markers and the biochemical findings (in particular the gamma-glutamyl transferase and the aspartate aminotransferase/alanine aminotransferase [ALT] ratio) are critical in differential diagnosis.

Drug-Induced Chronic Hepatitis

A number of drugs have been incriminated in causing chronic hepatitis. They include acetaminophen, aspirin, amineptine, clometacine, dantrolene, diclofenac, fenofibrate, glafenine, isoniazid, isoxonine, methyldopa, nitrofurantoin, oxyphenisatin, papaverine, pemoline, perhexilene maleate, propylthiouracil, sulfonamides, ticrynafen, and tolazamide. While the list appears lengthy, only one or two instances were reported with some of these drugs. Furthermore, many of the older reports antedated the discovery of HCV, making at least some suspect. Histopathologic differences between drug-induced and other types of chronic hepatitis (other than the specific or distinctive features of chronic hepatitis B or C) have not been forthcoming. In the case of some drugs, e.g., nitrofurantoin, serologic autoimmune markers may be demonstrable, raising the possibility that the drugs could have triggered an autoimmune chronic hepatitis.

Chronic Hepatitis Associated with Inherited Metabolic Diseases

Chronic hepatitis is a recognized stage in the evolution of the liver disease in Wilson's disease. This should always be considered in differential diagnosis of chronic hepatitis in a young person. Helpful histopathologic clues include steatosis, glycogenated nuclei in zone 1, cytochemically demonstrable copper accumulation, presence of Mallory bodies in periportal liver cells (in the absence of other features of cholestasis), and clusters of oxyphil hepatocytes; these changes are in addition to the other features that are found in all cases of chronic hepatitis (piecemeal necrosis, portal inflammation, etc.), regardless of etiology. The ultrastructural changes, particularly the pleomorphism of mitochondria and widening of their intercristal spaces, are pathognomonic of Wilson's disease.

Chronic hepatitis is also seen in heterozygotes (MZ phenotype) with α_1-antitrypsin deficiency. Recently, Propst et al. (75) found that most instances of chronic hepatitis in adults with homozygous and heterozygous α_1-antitrypsin deficiency that they studied were related to hepatotropic viruses (80% had HCV infection) or other risk factors (e.g., autoimmune hepatitis).

Nomenclature of Chronic Hepatitis

Several recent editorials and reviews have called for abandoning the widely used division of chronic hepatitis into chronic persistent hepatitis, chronic active hepatitis, and chronic lobular hepatitis and instead using one designation for chronic necroinflammatory disease: chronic hepatitis, with various degrees of activity and emphasis on the etiology. The need for reassessment of the existing classification is a result of the extensive experience gained from morphologic studies of all types of chronic hepatitis, in particular hepatitis C; the availability of new drugs (such as interferon) for treatment of chronic viral hepatitis; and the long-term follow-up studies that have shown a discordance between the prognosis and the histologic subtype of chronic necroinflammatory disease of the liver. The histopathology at any given time in the course of a patient's illness is no more than a snapshot that can change from chronic persistent hepatitis to chronic lobular hepatitis to chronic active hepatitis, depending on the natural course of the disease (quiescent phase versus reactivations or relapses), therapy, superinfection with other viral agents, underlying genetic diseases (e.g., α_1-antitrypsin deficiency and hepatitis C), or modifying disorders (e.g., alcoholism). Sampling error may also lead to an erroneous subcategorization of the chronic liver disease in different biopsy specimens, even when they are obtained at the same time or within close intervals of time. Scheuer (78) has commented that from the point of view of treatment, the separation of chronic persistent hepatitis from mild chronic active hepatitis is fundamentally unsound and ethically unacceptable; it betrays a misunderstanding of the evolution of chronic hepatitis and may deprive patients of effective treatment. Scoring systems for the degree of activity of chronic hepatitis and the stage of the disease (resulting from fibrosis and cirrhosis) are listed in Tables 8.7 and 8.8.

Table 8.7 Degree of activity in chronic hepatitis

Category	Lesion and degree of injury			
	Portal area inflammation	Piecemeal necrosis	Spotty necrosis	Bridging and/or multi-acinar necrosis
Mild	Mild, patchy	Absent or mild	Mild	Absent
Moderate	Moderate	Moderate	Moderate	Absent
Marked	Marked	Marked	Marked	Absent
Very marked	Marked	Marked	Marked	Present

Table 8.8 Degree of fibrosis in chronic hepatitis

Category	Component lesion		
	Fibrous expansion of portal areas	Bridging fibrosis[a]	Bridging with nodules (cirrhosis)
Mild	Absent or mild	Absent	Absent
Moderate	Moderate	Absent[b]	Absent
Marked	Marked	Marked	Absent[c]
Very marked	Marked	Marked	Present

[a] Bridging can be portal to portal, portal to zone 3 (central), or zone 3 to zone 3.
[b] Occasional bridging may be present.
[c] Occasional nodule may be present ("incomplete cirrhosis").

Clinical Manifestations

The incubation period of hepatitis A is 15 to 50 days, with an average of 28 days. The illness caused by HAV infection typically has an abrupt onset of signs and symptoms that include fever, malaise, anorexia, nausea, abdominal discomfort, dark urine, and jaundice (48). Hepatitis A usually does not last longer than 2 months, although some persons may have prolonged or relapsing signs and symptoms for up to 6 months. The likelihood of having symptoms with HAV infection is directly related to age. In children younger than 6 years of age, most infections are asymptomatic; among older children and adults, infection is usually symptomatic. HAV infection occasionally produces fulminant hepatitis A. The case-fatality rate among reported patients of all ages is approximately 0.3%, but it can be higher among older persons (approximately 2% among persons >40 years of age). HAV infection does not result in chronic infection or chronic liver disease.

The incubation period of hepatitis B ranges from 6 weeks to 6 months (average, 4 months). Onset of symptoms is gradual and may include skin rashes and arthralgias in addition to the usual symptoms of viral hepatitis. Symptoms of acute hepatitis generally last 2 to 4 weeks, but fatigue and other symptoms may persist for several months. The clinical manifestations of hepatitis B are highly age dependent. Infection rarely produces symptoms in infants, produces typical illness in only 5 to 15% of young children, and is symptomatic in 33 to 50% of adolescents and adults. Fatality from acute infection is low (case fatality, <1%).

Acute HBV infection usually resolves with the development of protective antibodies but may develop into chronic infection (the carrier state). Among the most serious consequences of hepatitis B are the sequelae associated with chronic HBV infection, including chronic hepatitis, cirrhosis, and liver cancer. The risk of development of chronic HBV infection is inversely associated with the age at which infection is acquired. Children under the age of 5 have a 20 to 50% risk of becoming carriers of the virus after acute infection, while older children and adults have a 5 to 10% risk of becoming carriers after acute infection. Persons with chronic infection have an estimated 15 to 25% lifetime risk of dying prematurely from cirrhosis or

Hepatitis A usually does not last longer than 2 months, although some persons may have prolonged or relapsing signs and symptoms for up to 6 months

liver cancer (58). A number of other clinical entities are associated with chronic hepatitis B. These include polyarteritis nodosa and glomerulonephritis. The pathogenesis of these diseases is thought to be due to deposition of circulating HBsAg-antibody complexes in affected organs.

Acute HCV infection is generally mild, with 25% or fewer of infected persons having a recognized illness. When symptoms do occur with acute HCV infection, the incubation period is 6 to 7 weeks on average (range, 2 weeks to 24 weeks) and the symptoms are indistinguishable from other types of viral hepatitis.

The most important feature of hepatitis C is the high frequency with which acute disease progresses to chronic infection. Follow-up studies of patients with acute hepatitis C show that an average of 67% (range, 58 to 81%) have persistently elevated ALT levels more than 6 months after illness, indicating chronic hepatitis. The risk of development of chronic hepatitis appears to be independent of the source of infection. Chronic active hepatitis or cirrhosis has been found in 29 to 76% of patients who have undergone liver biopsy within several years after acute hepatitis C. Seroprevalence studies showing high anti-HCV rates among patients with hepatocellular carcinoma and case-control studies finding a strong association of anti-HCV positivity with hepatocellular carcinoma suggest that HCV infection may also be a contributing cause of this disease. Several extrahepatic manifestations have been reported with HCV infection. In several studies, approximately 50% of patients with mixed cryoglobulinemia were anti-HCV positive. HCV infection has also been reported to be associated with membranous glomerulonephritis.

In general, the symptoms of acute delta hepatitis (either coinfection or superinfection) are similar to those of acute hepatitis due to other viruses; however, the liver injury with acute delta hepatitis tends to be more severe. The incubation period for coinfection ranges from 6 to 12 weeks, and for superinfection it ranges from 3 to 4 weeks. Coinfection with HBV and HDV does not usually result in chronic HBV or HDV infection, but it is associated with a risk of fulminant hepatitis that is higher than that associated with HBV infection alone. In contrast, HDV superinfection almost always results in chronic HDV infection, and the risk of development of chronic hepatitis and the rate at which cirrhosis develops with chronic HDV infection are greater than those seen with HBV infection alone. The clinical features of delta superinfection differ by geographic region. Large outbreaks of fulminant delta virus infection have occurred in several countries in South America, but they have not been described elsewhere. In Europe, persons with long-term delta infection but without liver enzyme abnormalities or histopathologic changes on liver biopsy have been described. It has not been determined whether this is due to viral or host factors.

Incubation periods of 15 to 60 days (mode, 40 days) during hepatitis E outbreaks have been reported (9). Clinical signs and symptoms in patients with symptomatic HEV infection are similar to those of other types of viral hepatitis, with a prodromal phase of about 1 week that is generally followed by an icteric phase. The most commonly reported signs and symptoms include malaise (95 to 100%), anorexia (66 to 100%), nausea/vomiting (29 to

100%), abdominal pain (37 to 82%), fever (23 to 97%), and hepatomegaly (10 to 85%) (42, 61). Other less frequent signs and symptoms include diarrhea, arthralgia, pruritus, and urticarial rash. Laboratory findings in patients with hepatitis E are also similar to findings in patients with other forms of viral hepatitis and include elevated serum bilirubin, ALT, aspartate aminotransferase, alkaline phosphatase, and gamma-glutamyl transferase. Resolution of hyperbilirubinemia and elevated aminotransferase levels generally occurs within 3 weeks (range, 1 to 6 weeks) after illness onset. Fulminant hepatitis is common among pregnant women, in whom hepatitis E case-fatality rates of 5 to 26% have been reported (40). Case-fatality rates have generally been highest among pregnant women infected during the third trimester. No evidence of chronic hepatitis has been detected among patients followed up clinically and with liver biopsies following acute hepatitis E (21, 44).

Diagnosis

Virtually all patients with acute hepatitis A have detectable IgM antibodies to HAV (IgM anti-HAV). The diagnosis of acute HAV infection (25) is therefore confirmed during the acute or early convalescent phase of infection by the presence of IgM anti-HAV. IgM anti-HAV generally disappears within 6 months after onset of symptoms. IgG anti-HAV, which appears during the convalescent phase of infection, remains detectable in serum for the lifetime of the individual and confers enduring protection against disease. Commercial diagnostic tests for the detection of IgM and total anti-HAV in serum are available.

Because the clinical manifestations of acute hepatitis B are similar to those of other types of viral hepatitis, serologic testing is necessary to establish a diagnosis. Commercial assays to detect acute HBV infection, chronic HBV infection, susceptibility, and vaccine response are widely available. In acute hepatitis B, HBsAg is the first serologic marker to become detectable, usually between 2 and 11 weeks after exposure. IgM antibody to hepatitis B core antigen (IgM anti-HBc) and IgG anti-HBc (measured as total anti-HBc) appear shortly after HBsAg, as does hepatitis B e antigen (HBeAg). In persons who recover from infection, HBsAg and HBeAg persist for up to several months and then gradually become undetectable. Subsequently, IgM anti-HBc gradually disappears, after which antibody to HBsAg (anti-HBs) develops, indicating recovery with lifelong immunity to reinfection. IgG anti-HBc persists for life. In some persons with acute HBV infection, there is a period, referred to as the window, between the disappearance of HBsAg and the appearance of anti-HBs when only IgM and total anti-HBc are detectable.

In patients with chronic HBV infection, HBsAg remains detectable and can persist for life. The diagnosis of chronic HBV infection is made by detecting HBsAg in two serum specimens taken at least 6 months apart or by detecting the presence of HBsAg and IgG anti-HBc in the absence of IgM. In chronic HBV infection, total anti-HBc is detectable, but IgM anti-HBc and anti-HBs are generally not detectable. HBeAg may be pre-

Commercial assays to detect acute HBV infection, chronic HBV infection, susceptibility, and vaccine response are widely available

sent, and it is associated with active viral replication and higher circulating viral titers.

The presence of HBsAg in persons with acute infection and with chronic infection indicates that the person is infectious, regardless of the HBeAg status. Anti-HBs, but not anti-HBc, is elicited in persons who receive hepatitis B vaccine. Therefore, immunity from hepatitis B vaccine can be distinguished from immunity from natural infection by the presence of anti-HBs in the absence of total anti-HBc.

HCV RNA is the earliest marker of HCV infection and is detectable by PCR testing as early as 2 weeks after exposure. However, PCR testing for HCV RNA is not licensed for use in the United States, and the diagnosis of HCV infection is dependent on the detection of anti-HCV. The currently available second-generation enzyme immunoassays for anti-HCV detect antibody to three recombinant proteins: two expressed from the nonstructural region of the HCV genome and one from the structural (core) region. On the basis of these assays, anti-HCV has been detected in an average of 70 to 90% of patients with parenterally transmitted non-A, non-B hepatitis (4). Anti-HCV is detectable by 5 to 6 weeks after onset of hepatitis in 80% of patients and by 12 weeks in 90% (4). As with any screening test, the proportion of repeatedly reactive enzyme immunoassay results that are falsely positive varies depending on the prevalence of infection in the population screened. Although no true confirmatory test has been developed, supplemental tests for specificity, such as the recombinant immunoblot assay, are available and should be used to verify the results of specimens found to be positive by enzyme immunoassay. Because the appearance of anti-HCV may be delayed in patients with acute HCV infection, if acute hepatitis C is suspected in a patient and initial testing is negative for anti-HCV, repeat testing should be done after at least 1 month, and possibly later. Diagnosis of chronic hepatitis C is made by the detection of anti-HCV and the persistence of elevated liver enzymes for 6 months. To evaluate the severity and extent of liver damage and whether specific treatment is indicated, a liver biopsy is usually necessary.

Patients with current or resolved HDV infection have antibody to the HDV antigen (anti-HDV) (73). Patients with chronic delta hepatitis and active HDV replication have very high levels of anti-HDV. Patients with HBV-HDV coinfection may have only low levels of anti-HDV and IgM anti-HDV. In acute hepatitis, HDV-HBV coinfection can usually be distinguished from HDV superinfection by the presence or absence, respectively, of IgM anti-HBc. HDV infection can also be diagnosed by the presence of HDV antigen or HDV RNA in serum (determined by using either hybridization or PCR). In addition, specialized assays to detect HDV antigen or HDV RNA in liver biopsies exist. In general, serologic and liver assays for infection are not widely available or used, and therefore HDV infection may be underdiagnosed. Testing for HDV infection should be considered for patients with acute and chronic hepatitis B, particularly for those patients with fulminant hepatitis. Knowledge of a patient's HDV infection status may help in counseling about prognosis and prevention of transmission to others.

No serologic tests to diagnose HEV infection are commercially available in the United States. However, several diagnostic tests, including enzyme immunoassays and Western blot assays based on recombinant HEV proteins to detect IgM and IgG anti-HEV in serum, an immunofluorescent-antibody blocking assay to identify anti-HEV reacting to native HEV antigen in serum, and PCR to detect HEV RNA in serum and stool, are available in research laboratories (24, 28, 46, 56, 84). Both IgM and IgG anti-HEV are generally detectable at the time of illness onset. The titer of IgM anti-HEV declines rapidly during early convalescence but can be detected in some patients for 5 to 6 months. IgG anti-HEV can be detected in most patients for at least 1 year after acute infection, in approximately 50% of persons at least 14 years following infection, and for up to 10 years in experimentally infected chimpanzees (18, 43). The natural history of protective immunity has not been determined. However, in one study, the presence of IgG anti-HEV appeared to provide short-term protection against disease (13).

Treatment

Because HAV infection is self-limited and does not result in chronic infection or chronic liver disease, treatment is generally supportive. Hospitalization may be necessary in patients who are dehydrated from nausea and vomiting or who have fulminant hepatitis A. Medications that might cause liver damage or that are metabolized by the liver should be used with caution. No specific diet or activity restrictions are necessary. In patients with fulminant hepatitis A, agents such as prostaglandin E and interferon have been studied with inconclusive results; liver transplantation is successful in some persons (88).

As with hepatitis A, symptoms of acute hepatitis B are generally self-limited, and initial treatment of acutely infected patients is supportive. Liver transplantation has been used to treat patients who have fulminant acute hepatitis B, with favorable survival rates (<50%). For chronically infected persons, treatment resulting in clearance of HBV is expected to reduce the risk of development of cirrhosis and liver cancer and the transmission of HBV to others. Numerous agents, including prednisone, interleukin-2, thymosin, ribavirin, and azidothymidine, for the treatment of chronic HBV infection have been studied. To date, alpha interferon is the agent shown to be most effective, and it is the only treatment for chronic HBV infection licensed in the United States (35).

Symptoms of acute hepatitis B are generally self-limited, and initial treatment of acutely infected patients is supportive

The most important factors associated with a favorable response to alpha interferon include high pretreatment serum ALT levels, low pretreatment serum HBV DNA levels, and adult-acquired HBV infection. The treatment course for alpha interferon is 5×10^6 U daily or 10×10^6 U three times a week, for 12 to 24 weeks, with monitoring of HBsAg, HBeAg, HBV DNA, and ALT before and after therapy to assess response. With this regimen, approximately 40% of persons have loss of viral replication (as measured by disappearance of HBeAg and/or HBV DNA), and 10 to 20% lose HBsAg. The response is sustained after treatment, with <10% of patients having a relapse of hepatitis within a year of treatment. Among those in whom HBeAg disappeared, nearly 70% also lost HBsAg after 4 years of follow-up.

Evaluation of therapy in patients with hepatitis C has generally focused on persons with chronic HCV infection. The only agent found to be effective is alpha interferon, but it generally suppresses infection and is rarely curative. Standard therapy is recombinant alpha-2b interferon administered at a dose of 3×10^6 U subcutaneously three times a week for 6 months (35). With this regimen, approximately 50% of persons will respond with normalization of ALT levels; however, 50 to 70% of these patients will relapse, with elevated ALT levels and detection of HCV RNA in serum. For patients who do not respond initially, therapeutic options are limited. For patients who relapse after therapy, most will respond with repeated interferon treatment, but long-term treatment is not well tolerated because of the side effects of interferon, including bone marrow suppression and emotional lability and depression. Studies are underway to determine the best way to maintain remission in patients who respond initially to interferon.

Since long-term response is limited, most clinicians treat HCV-infected patients who have persistently elevated liver enzymes and/or have moderate to severe inflammation on liver biopsy, because they are most likely to benefit from therapy. Because hepatitis C is slowly progressive and prolonged therapy is difficult and costly, treatment of HCV-infected patients without symptoms and with minimal disease on liver biopsy is controversial.

Only alpha interferon has been shown to have any benefit in the treatment of chronic HDV infection (27). In general, 25 to 60% of patients respond with normalized ALT values after 3 to 4 months of treatment; however, most relapse with elevated ALT values and detectable HDV RNA when treatment is stopped. Prolonged treatment with alpha interferon (6 to 12 months) may result in long-term resolution of biochemical abnormalities and clearance of HDV RNA; successful clearance of HDV RNA is associated with clearance of HbsAg.

Treatment for hepatitis E is supportive. No studies evaluating the efficacy of antiviral agents or other specific therapies for treatment of hepatitis E have been done.

Prevention

General measures for hepatitis A prevention include maintenance of good personal hygiene, with attention to hand washing before preparing food; provision of safe drinking water; and adequate disposal of sanitary waste. To help control and prevent hepatitis A in communities experiencing hepatitis A outbreaks among homosexual and bisexual men, health education messages should stress the modes of HAV transmission and the measures which can be taken to reduce the risk of transmission of any sexually transmitted disease, including enterically transmitted agents such as HAV.

Two types of products are available for the prevention of hepatitis A, immune globulin (IG) and hepatitis A vaccine (17). IG is a solution of antibodies prepared from human plasma. It is made by using a serial ethanol precipitation procedure which has been shown to inactivate HBV and HIV. When administered intramuscularly prior to exposure to HAV or within 2 weeks after exposure, IG is >85% effective in preventing hepatitis A. IG administration is recommended for persons in a variety of exposure situations, including sexual or household contacts of persons with hepatitis A, staff and children at a day care center where a child or employee is recognized to have acute hepatitis A, patrons of food establishments with an infected food handler with poor hygiene who handled uncooked foods or foods after cooking, and persons in selected settings where HAV transmission is occurring (hospitals, institutions). IG may also be used for preexposure prophylaxis, e.g., for persons traveling to countries with endemic hepatitis A. The duration of protection is dependent on dose. Persons traveling for less than 3 months should receive 0.02 ml/kg of body weight. Those traveling for 3 months or longer should receive 0.06 ml/kg, and the dose should be repeated if continued exposure occurs.

Within the past several years, inactivated hepatitis A vaccines which have the potential to provide long-term protection against hepatitis A have been developed. These vaccines have been shown to be safe, highly immunogenic, and highly efficacious. Immunogenicity studies indicate that between 99 and 100% of persons respond to one dose of hepatitis A vaccine, and after two doses of vaccine, antibodies persist for at least several years. Efficacy studies show that inactivated hepatitis A vaccines are 94 to 100% effective in preventing hepatitis A.

Within the past several years, inactivated hepatitis A vaccines which have the potential to provide long-term protection against hepatitis A have been developed.

The two hepatitis A vaccines licensed in the United States are HAVRIX, manufactured by SmithKline Beecham Pharmaceuticals, and VAQTA, manufactured by Merck & Co. (17). The dose of HAVRIX is quantified in ELISA units (ELU), and HAVRIX is currently licensed in two formulations for children and adolescents (2 to 18 years of age): 360 ELU per dose (0.5 ml) in a three-dose schedule (0, 1, and 6 to 12 months) and 720 ELU per dose (0.5 ml) in a two-dose schedule (0 and 6 to 12 months). For adults (>18 years of age), the vaccine is licensed as 1,440 ELU per dose (1.0 ml), given in a two-dose schedule (0 and 6 to 12 months). The dose of VAQTA is quantified as units (U). The dose and schedule for children and adolescents (2 to 17 years of age) is 25 U per dose in a two-dose schedule (0 and 6 to 18 months), and that for adults (>17 years of age) is 50 U per dose in a two-dose schedule (0 and 6 months). Hepatitis A vaccine is recommended for persons with documented risk of HAV infection, including international travelers, children living in communities with high rates of hepatitis A and periodic outbreaks (e.g., Native American reservations, Alaska Native villages), homosexual men, illegal drug users, patients with clotting factor disorders, persons who work with the virus in research settings, and persons who have chronic liver disease, because of their increased risk of fulminant hepatitis A should they acquire HAV infection (17).

Prevention of HBV infection relies upon three general measures: (i) behavior modification to reduce the risk of infection, (ii) preexposure immunization with hepatitis B vaccine, and (iii) postexposure prophylaxis of contacts of infected persons with hepatitis B vaccine and hepatitis B immune globulin (HBIG).

The most effective measure to prevent HBV infection is use of the hepatitis B vaccine. Hepatitis B vaccine is safe and highly effective. Three doses of vaccine induce protective levels of antibody in 90% or greater of vaccine recipients, and studies of long-term protection indicate that protective efficacy lasts at least 12 years.

When the hepatitis B vaccine became available in 1982, initial recommendations involved targeting adult groups at high risk of infection (e.g., health care workers, injection drug users, homosexually active men). In 1988, recommendations for HBsAg screening of pregnant women and vaccination and HBIG administration to infants born to infected mothers were issued. With the realization of the limited effectiveness of a targeted vaccination approach, vaccine advisory groups in 1991 and 1992 recommended routine infant immunization with hepatitis B vaccine (14). In 1994, the Armed Forces Institute of Pathology recommended that all children aged 11 to 12 years should be given hepatitis B vaccine if they have not previously received it. The components of the current recommendations therefore include (i) screening of pregnant women for HBsAg and administration of hepatitis B vaccine and HBIG to infants of HBsAg-positive women, (ii) routine infant vaccination, (iii) routine vaccination of previously unvaccinated children aged 11 to 12 years, and (iv) vaccination of all other persons (e.g., children, adolescents, adults) who are at high risk of HBV infection.

In specific exposure situations to HBV, because of the high risk of transmission, unvaccinated exposed persons should receive a single dose of HBIG (0.06 ml/kg), which should be followed by the hepatitis B vaccine series (14). Persons in these exposure situations include infants born to HBsAg-positive women, sexual contacts of persons with acute HBV infection, and persons with percutaneous exposure (e.g., needle-stick) to blood from persons who are HBV infected.

No effective vaccine to prevent HCV infection exists. Furthermore, recent studies indicate that postexposure administration of intramuscular IG does not protect against HCV infection. Therefore, prevention of HCV infection must rely upon routine anti-HCV screening of blood donors, to prevent transfusion-related hepatitis C, and modification of high-risk behaviors. Safer sex practices, including use of condoms and reduction of the number of sexual partners, and safer needle-using practices may lower the risk of acquiring HCV infection.

> *Prevention of HCV infection must rely upon routine anti-HCV screening of blood donors, to prevent transfusion-related hepatitis C, and modification of high-risk behaviors*

Persons who are anti-HCV positive should be counseled to prevent transmission to others. They should be informed of the potential for sexual transmission. For persons in a stable monogamous relationship, there are insufficient data to recommend changes in current sexual practices. For persons with multiple sexual partners, the number of partners should be reduced and measures should be taken to reduce the risk of acquiring sexually transmitted diseases in general, including the use of condoms. Consideration should be given to testing exposed sexual partners for hepatitis C and, if positive, evaluating them for the presence of chronic liver disease.

Preexposure hepatitis B vaccine and postexposure prophylaxis with both HBIG and hepatitis B vaccine can prevent HBV-HDV coinfection. Therefore, primary prevention of HDV infection relies upon hepatitis B vaccination. No effective vaccine exists to prevent HDV infection in persons who are chronically HBV infected. Persons who are HBV infected should be educated regarding measures to reduce their risk of acquiring HDV infection, including avoiding unprotected intercourse and not sharing needles.

No products to prevent hepatitis E are available. IG prepared from plasma collected in areas in which HEV is not endemic is not effective in preventing clinical disease during hepatitis E outbreaks, and the efficacy of IG prepared from plasma collected in areas in which HEV is endemic is unclear. In studies conducted to date with prototype vaccines in animals, vaccine-induced antibody attenuated HEV infection, but it did not prevent virus excretion in stools. If a vaccine is developed, the epidemiology of hepatitis E needs to be further defined in order to determine whether vaccination strategies could be effectively used to prevent this disease. Prevention of hepatitis E relies primarily on the provision of clean drinking water. Epidemiologic data suggest that boiling water may inactivate HEV; however, no data regarding the efficacy of chlorination of water in inactivating HEV are available, and studies are needed to determine other appropriate environmental control measures. Until such prevention measures are determined, prudent hygienic practices that may prevent hepatitis E and other enterically transmitted diseases among travelers to developing countries include avoiding drinking water (and beverages with ice) of unknown purity, eating uncooked shellfish, and eating uncooked fruits or vegetables that are not peeled or prepared by the traveler.

Figure 8.1 Acute viral hepatitis by type, United States, 1982 to 1993.

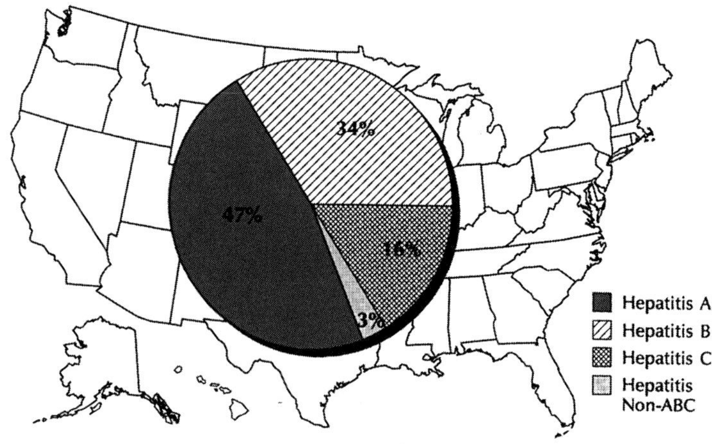

Figure 8.2 Sources of hepatitis A virus infection by mutually exclusive groups, United States, 1983 to 1993.

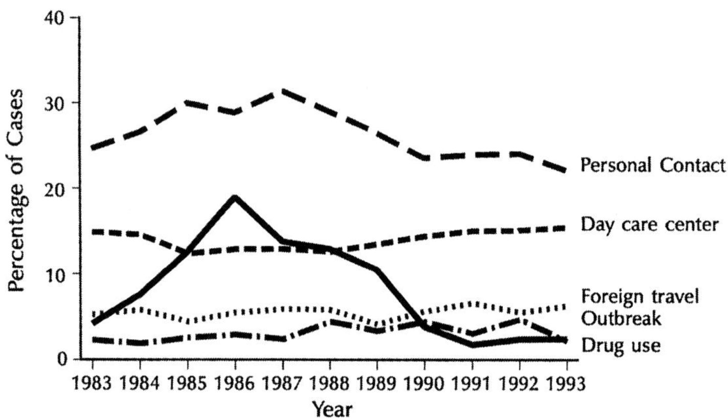

Figure 8.3 Acute viral hepatitis B. Apoptotic (acidophilic) body (arrowheads) and focal necrosis (hematoxylin and eosin stain; magnification, ×450). Armed Forces Institute of Pathology photograph.

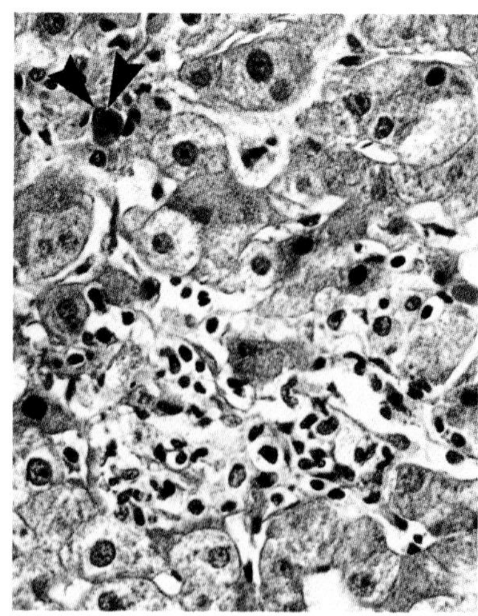

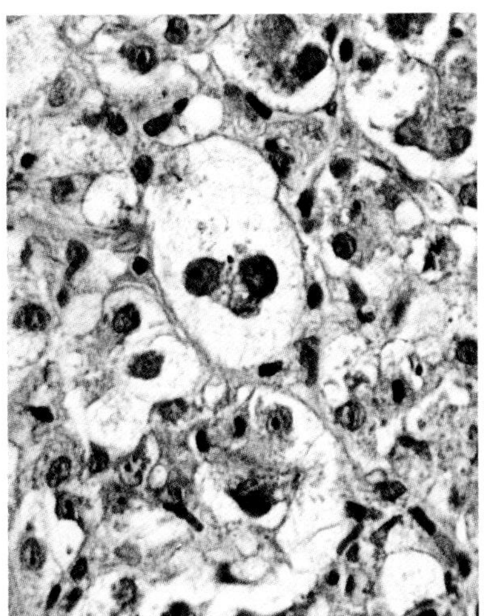

Figure 8.4 Same case as in Fig. 8.3. Ballooning degeneration of liver cell (hematoxylin and eosin stain; magnification, ×450). Armed Forces Institute of Pathology photograph.

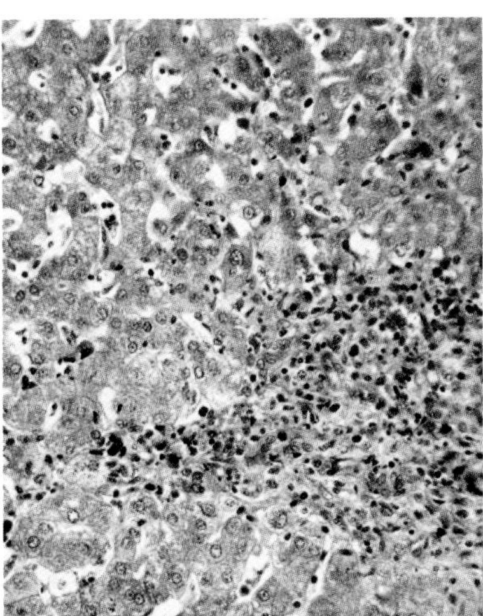

Figure 8.5 Same case as in Fig. 8.3 and 8.4. Portal area shows moderate inflammation (hematoxylin and eosin stain; magnification, ×250). Armed Forces Institute of Pathology photograph.

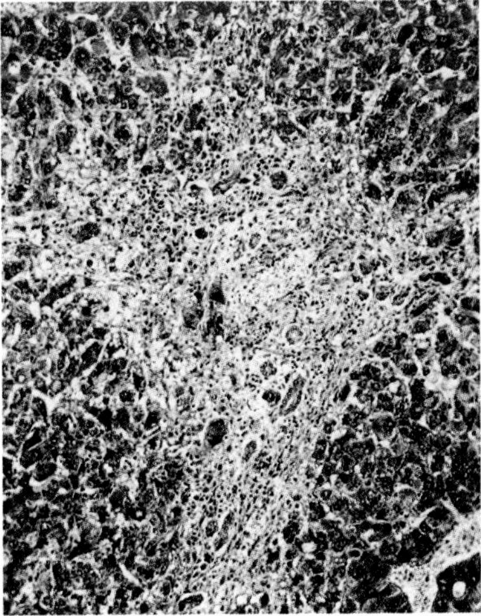

Figure 8.6 Acute hepatitis A with necrosis and drop out in zone 1 (Masson stain; magnification, ×100). Armed Forces Institute of Pathology photograph.

Figure 8.7 Acute fulminant non-A, non-B hepatitis showing massive necrosis (hematoxylin and eosin stain; magnification, ×25). Armed Forces Institute of Pathology photograph.

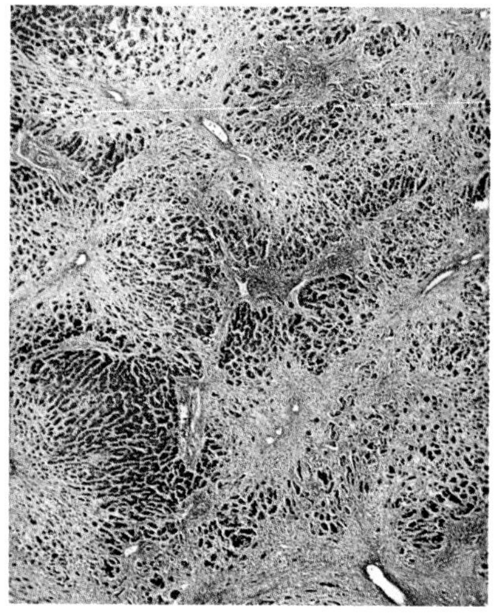

Figure 8.8 Chronic autoimmune hepatitis showing marked portal inflammation, expansion of the portal area, and piecemeal necrosis (hematoxylin and eosin stain; magnification, ×150). Armed Forces Institute of Pathology photograph.

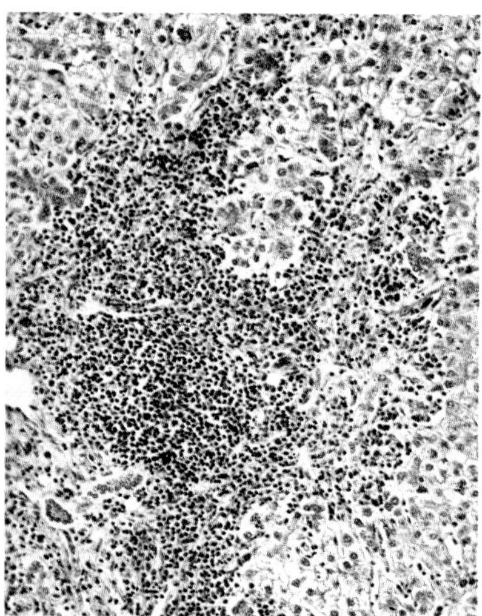

Figure 8.9 High-power view of case illustrated in Fig. 8.8, showing piecemeal necrosis; note apoptotic body (arrowhead) (hematoxylin and eosin stain; magnification, ×300). Armed Forces Institute of Pathology photograph.

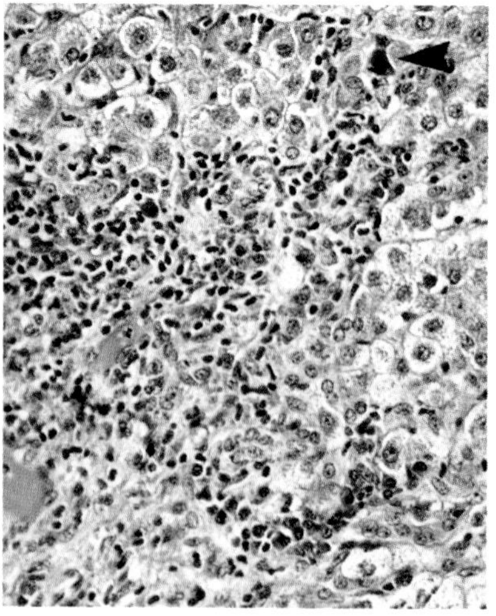

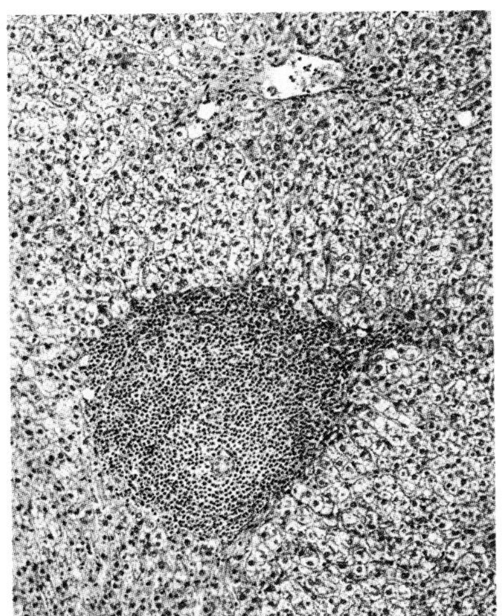

Figure 8.10A Chronic hepatitis C with a lymphoid follicle, lymphocytic portal inflammation, and piecemeal necrosis (hematoxylin and eosin stain; magnification, ×120). Armed Forces Institute of Pathology photograph.

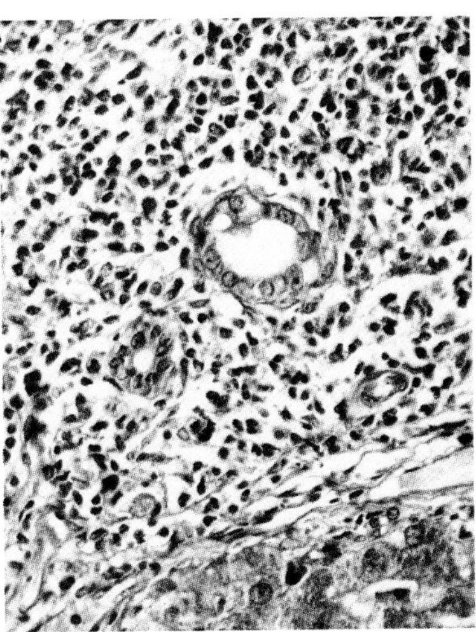

Figure 8.10B Degenerating bile duct with a slightly dilated lumen and shrunken or vacuolated cells (hematoxylin and eosin stain; magnification, ×450). Armed Forces Institute of Pathology photograph.

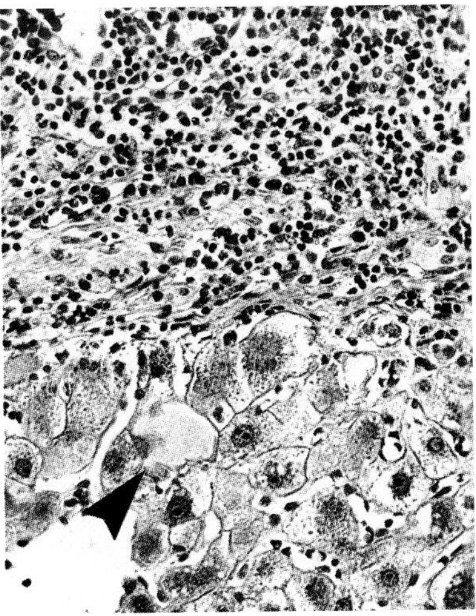

Figure 8.11A Chronic hepatitis B showing piecemeal necrosis, focal necrosis, an apoptotic body, and a ground-glass cell (arrowhead) (hematoxylin and eosin stain; magnification, ×275). Armed Forces Institute of Pathology photograph.

Figure 8.11B Chronic hepatitis B. Numerous ground-glass cells are present (hematoxylin and eosin stain; magnification, ×350). Armed Forces Institute of Pathology photograph.

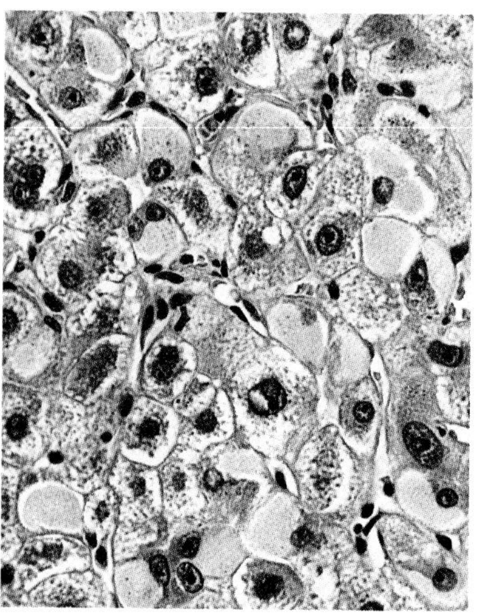

Figure 8.12 Ground-glass cells of chronic hepatitis B are stained positively (black) with aldehyde fuchsin. Magnification, ×250. Armed Forces Institute of Pathology photograph.

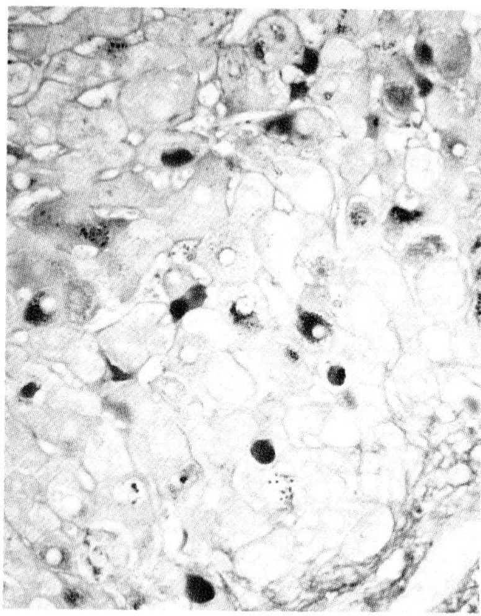

Figure 8.13 HBcAg in hepatic nuclei (as well as the cytoplasm of liver cells) is demonstrated immunohistochemically in a patient with chronic hepatitis B. Magnification, ×630. Armed Forces Institute of Pathology photograph.

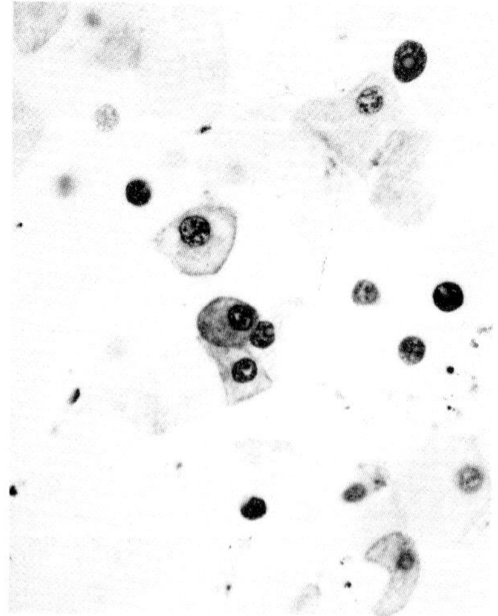

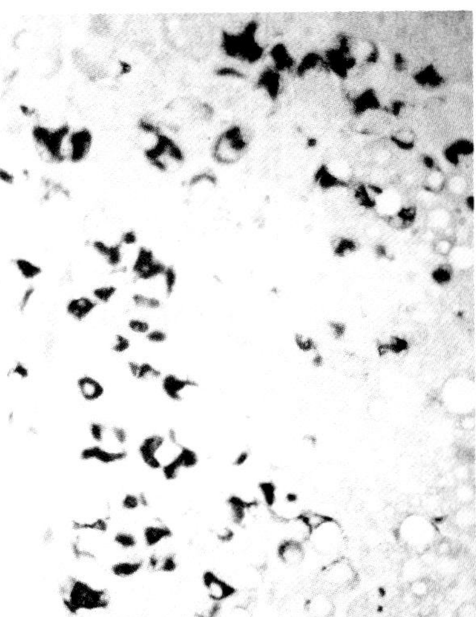

Figure 8.14 HBsAg in cytoplasm of liver cells of a patient with hepatitis B cirrhosis is demonstrated immunohistochemically. Magnification, ×250. Armed Forces Institute of Pathology photograph.

References

1. **Abe, H., P. R. Beninger, N. Ikejiri, H. Setoyama, M. Sata, and K. Tanikawa.** 1982. Light microscopic findings of liver biopsy specimens from patients with hepatitis A and comparison with type B. *Gastroenterology* **82:**938–947.

2. **Alison, M. R., and C. E. Sarraf.** 1994. Liver cell death: patterns and mechanisms. *Gut* **35:**577–581.

3. **Alter, M. J., and S. C. Hadler.** 1993. Delta hepatitis and infection in North America, p. 243–250. *In* S. J. Hadziyannis, J. M. Taylor, and F. Bonino (ed.), *Hepatitis Delta Virus*. Wiley Liss, Inc., New York.

4. **Alter, M. J., S. C. Hadler, F. N. Judson, A. Mares, W. J. Alexander, P. Y. Hu, J. K. Miller, L. A. Moyer, H. A. Fields, D. W. Bradley, and H. S. Margolis.** 1990. Risk factors for acute non-A, non-B hepatitis in the United States and association of hepatitis C virus antibody. *JAMA* **264:**2231–2235.

5. **Alter, M. J., H. S. Margolis, K. Krawczynski, F. N. Judson, A. Mares, W. J. Alexander, P. Y. Hu, J. K. Miller, M. A. Gerber, R. E. Sampliner, E. L. Meeks, and M. J. Beach.** 1992. The natural history of community-acquired hepatitis C in the United States. *N. Engl. J. Med.* **327:**1899–1905.

6. **Anonymous.** 1977. Acute and chronic hepatitis revisited. *Lancet* **ii:**914–919.

7. **Bach, N., S. N. Thung, and F. Schaffner.** 1992. The histological features of hepatitis C. *Hepatology* **15:**567–577.

8. **Baptista, A., L. Bianchi, J. DeGroote, V. J. Desmet, K. G. Ishak, G. Korb, R. N. macSween, H. Pooper, H. Poulsen, P. J. Scheuer, et al.** 1988. The diagnostic significance of periportal hepatic necrosis and inflammation. *Histopathology* **12:**569–579.

9. **Belabbes, E. H., A. Bouguermouh, A. Benatallah, and G. Illoul.** 1985. Epidemic non-A, non-B viral hepatitis in Algeria: strong evidence for its spreading by water. *J. Med. Virol.* **16:**257–263.

10. **Bresee, J. S., E. E. Mast, P. J. Coleman, M. J. Baron, L. B. Schonberger, M. J. Alter, M. M. Jonas, M. W. Yu, P. M. Renzi, and L. C. Schneide.** 1996. Hepatitis C virus infection associated with administration of intravenous immune globulin: a cohort study. *JAMA* **276:**1563–1567.

11. **Broomé, U., A. Scheynius, and R. Hultcrantz.** 1993. Induced expression of heat-shock protein on biliary epithelium in patients with primary sclerosing cholangitis and primary biliary cirrhosis. *Hepatology* **18:**298–303.

12. **Brown, J., S. Dourakis, P. Karayainnis, R. Golden, J. Chiba, H. Ohba, T. Miyamura, and H. C. Thomas.** 1992. Seroprevalence of hepatitis C virus nucleocapsid antibodies with cryptogenic chronic liver disease. *Hepatology* **15:**175–179.

13. **Bryan, J. P., S. A. Tsarev, M. Iqbal, J. Ticehurst, S. Emerson, A. Ahmed, J. Duncan, A. R. Rafiqui, I. A. Malik, R. H. Purcell, and L. J. Legters.** 1994. Epidemic hepatitis E in Pakistan: pattern of serologic response and evidence that antibody to hepatitis E virus protects against disease. *J. Infect. Dis.* **170:**517–521.

14. **Centers for Disease Control.** 1991. Hepatitis B virus. A comprehensive strategy for eliminating transmission in the United States through universal childhood vaccination. Recommendations of the Immunization Practices Advisory Committee (ACIP). *Morbid. Mortal. Weekly Rep.* **40**(RR-13)**:**1–25.

15. **Centers for Disease Control and Prevention.** 1996. Hepatitis A among persons with hemophilia who received clotting factor concentrate—United States, September–December 1995. *Morbid. Mortal. Weekly Rep.* **45:**29–32.

16. **Centers for Disease Control and Prevention.** 1996. Hepatitis Surveillance Report. Centers for Disease Control and Prevention. **56:**1–33.

17. **Centers for Disease Control and Prevention.** 1996. Prevention of hepatitis A through active or passive immunization: recommendations of the Advisory Committee on Immunization Practices (ACIP). *Morbid. Mortal. Weekly Rep.* **45**(RR-15):1–30.

18. **Centers for Disease Control and Prevention.** Unpublished data.

19. **Chu, C. M., and Y. F. Liaw.** 1992. Intrahepatic expression of pre-S1 and pre-S2 antigens in chronic hepatitis B: virus infection in relation to hepatitis B virus replication and hepatitis Delta virus superinfection. *Gut* **33:**1544–1548.

20. **Chu, H.-W., S. Dash, and M. A. Gerber.** 1994. Genomic and replicative hepatitis C virus RNA sequences and histologic activity in chronic hepatitis C. *Hum. Pathol.* **25:**160–163.

21. **Chuttani, H. K., A. S. Sidhu, K. L. Wig, D. N. Gupta, and V. Ramalingaswami.** 1966. Follow-up study of cases from the Delhi epidemic of infectious hepatitis of 1955–6. *Br. Med. J.* **ii:**676–679.

22. **Czaja, A. J., H. A. Carpenter, P. J. Santrach, S. B. Moore, and H. A. Homburger.** 1993. The nature and prognosis of severe cryptogenic chronic active hepatitis. *Gastroenterology* **104:**1755–1761.

23. **Danque, P. O. V., N. Bach, F. Schaffner, M. A. Gerber, and S. N. Thung.** 1993. HLA-DR expression in bile duct damage in hepatitis C. *Mod. Pathol.* **6:**327–332.

24. **Dawson, G. J., K. H. Chau, C. M. Cabal, P. O. Yarbough, G. R. Reyes, and I. K. Mushahwar.** 1992. Solid-phase enzyme-linked immunosorbent assay for hepatitis E virus IgG and IgM antibodies utilizing recombinant antigens and synthetic peptides. *J. Virol. Methods* **38:**175–186.

25. **DiBisceglie, A. M., and J. H. Hoofnagle.** 1991. Serologic interpretation of acute and chronic viral hepatitis. *Semin. Liver Dis.* **11:**73–83.

26. **Everhart, J. E., A. M. Di Bisceglie, L. M. Murray, H. J. Alter, J. J. Melpolder, G. Kuo, and J. H. Hoofnagle.** 1990. Risk for non-A, non-B (type C) hepatitis through sexual or household contact with chronic carriers. *Ann. Intern. Med.* **112:**544–545.

27. **Farci, P., A. Mandas, A. Coiana, M. E. Lai, V. Desmet, P. Van Eyken, Y. Gibo, L. Caruso, S. Scaccabarozzi, and D. Criscuolo.** 1994. Treatment of chronic hepatitis D with interferon alfa-2a. *N. Engl. J. Med.* **330:**88–94.

28. **Favorov, M. O., Y. E. Khudyakov, E. E. Mast, T. L. Yashina, C. N. Shapiro, N. S. Khudyakova, D. Jue, G. G. Onischenko, H. S. Margolis, and H. A. Fields.** 1996. IgM and IgG antibody to hepatitis E virus detected by enzyme immunoassay based on an HEV-specific artificial recombinant mosaic protein. *J. Med. Virol.* **50:**50–58.

29. **Francis, D. P., M. S. Favero, and J. E. Maynard.** 1981. Transmission of hepatitis B virus. *Semin. Liver Dis.* **1:**27–32.

30. **Gerber, M. A., K. Krawczynski, M. J. Alter, et al.** 1992. Histopathology of community acquired chronic hepatitis C. *Mod. Pathol.* **5:**483–486.

31. **Greeve, M., L. Ferrell, M. Kim, C. Combs, J. Roberts, N. Ascher, and T. L. Wright.** 1993. Cirrhosis of undefined pathogenesis: absence of evidence for unknown viruses or autoimmune processes. *Hepatology* **17:**593–598.

32. **Gruber, A., L.-G. Lundberg, and M. Bjorkholm.** 1993. Reactivation of chronic hepatitis C after withdrawal of immunosuppressive therapy. *J. Intern. Med.* **234:**223–225.

33. **Hadler, S. C.** 1991. Global impact of hepatitis A virus infection: changing patterns, p. 14–20. *In* F. B. Hollinger, S. M. Lemon, and H. S. Margolis (ed.), *Viral Hepatitis and Liver Disease.* The Williams & Wilkins Co., Baltimore.

34. **Hiramatsu, N., N. Hayashi, K. Katayama, K. Mochizuki, Y. Kawanishi, A. Kasahara, H. Fusamoto, and T. Kamada.** 1994. Immunohistochemical detection of Fas antigen in liver tissue of patients with chronic hepatitis C. *Hepatology* **19:**1354–1359.

35. **Hoofnagle, J. H., and A. M. DiBisceglie.** 1997. The treatment of chronic viral hepatitis. *N. Engl. J. Med.* **336:**347–356.

36. **Ishak, K. G.** 1976. Light microscopic morphology of viral hepatitis. *Am. J. Clin. Pathol.* **65:**787–827.

37. **Ishak, K. G.** 1976. Viral hepatitis, p. 13. *In* C. H. Binford and D. H. Connor (ed.), *Pathology of Tropical and Extraordinary Diseases*, vol. 1. Armed Forces Institute of Pathology, Washington, D.C.

38. **Ishak, K. G.** 1989. Hepatitis A infection: pathology, p. 15. *In* L. B. Seeff and J. H. Lewis (ed.), *Current Perspectives in Hepatology.* Plenum Medical Book Co., New York.

39. **Ishak, K. G.** 1994. Chronic hepatitis: morphology and nomenclature. *Mod. Pathol.* **7:**690–713.

40. **Kane, M. A., D. W. Bradley, S. M. Shrestha, J. E. Maynard, E. H. Cook, R. P. Mishra, and D. D. Joshi.** 1984. Epidemic non-A, non-B hepatitis in Nepal: recovery of a possible etiologic agent and transmission studies in marmosets. *JAMA* **252:**3140–3145.

41. **Kao, J. H., P. J. Chen, P. M. Yang, M. Y. Lai, J. C. Sheu, T. H. Wang, and D. S. Chen.** 1992. Intrafamilial transmission of hepatitis C virus. The important role of infections between spouses. *J. Infect. Dis.* **166:**900–903.

42. **Khuroo, M. S.** 1980. Study of an epidemic of non-A, non-B hepatitis. Possibility of another human hepatitis virus distinct from post-transfusion non-A, non-B type. *Am. J. Med.* **68:**818–824.

43. **Khuroo, M. S., S. Kamili, M. Y. Dar, R. Moecklii, and S. Jameel.** 1993. Hepatitis E and long-term antibody status. *Lancet* **341:**1355.

44. **Khuroo, M. S., M. Saleem, M. R. Teli, and M. A. Sofi.** 1980. Failure to detect chronic liver disease after epidemic non-A, non-B hepatitis. *Lancet* **ii:**97–98.

45. **Kobayashi, K., E. Hashimoto, and J. Ludwig.** 1993. Liver biopsy features of acute hepatitis C compared with hepatitis A, B, and non-A, non-B, non-C. *Liver* **13:**69–72.

46. **Krawczynski, K., and D. W. Bradley.** 1989. Enterically transmitted non-A, non-B hepatitis: identification of virus associated antigen in experimentally infected cynomologous macaques. *J. Infect. Dis.* **159:**1042–1049.

47. **Kryger, P., and P. Christoffersen.** 1983. Liver histopathology of the hepatitis A virus infection: a comparison with hepatitis type B and non-A, non-B. *J. Clin. Pathol.* **36:**650–654.

48. **Lednar, W. M., S. M. Lemon, J. W. Kirkpatrick, R. R. Redfield, M. L. Fields, and P. W. Kelly.** 1985. Frequency of illness associated with epidemic hepatitis A virus infection in adults. *Am. J. Epidemiol.* **122:**226–233.

49. Lefkowitch, J. H., E. R. Schiff, G. L. Davis, et al. 1993. Pathological diagnosis of chronic hepatitis C: a multicenter comparative study with chronic hepatitis B. *Gastroenterology* **104**:595–603.

50. Lin, H. H., J. H. Kao, H. Y. Hsu, Y. H. Ni, S. H. Yeh, L. H. Hwang, M. H. Chang, S. C. Hwang, P. J. Chen, and D. S. Chen. 1994. Possible role of high-titer maternal viremia in perinatal transmission of hepatitis C virus. *J. Infect. Dis.* **169**:638–641.

51. Lin, H.-H., Y.-F. Liaw, T.-J. Chen, C. M. Chu, and M. J. Huang. 1989. Natural course of patients with chronic type B hepatitis following acute delta virus superinfection. *Liver* **9**:129–134.

52. Linnen, J., J. Wages, Jr., Z. K. Zhang-Yong, K. E. Fry, K. Z. Krawczynski, H. Alter, E. Koonin, M. Gallagher, M. Alter, S. Hadziyannis, P. Karayiannis, K. Fung, Y. Nakatsuji, J. W. Shih, L. Young, M. Piatak, Jr., C. Hoover, J. Fernandez, S. Chen, J. C. Zou, T. Morris, K. C. Hyams, S. Ismay, J. S. Lifson, G. Hess, S. K. Foung, H. Thomas, D. Bradley, H. Margolis, and J. P. Kim. 1996. Molecular cloning and disease association of hepatitis G virus: a transfusion transmissible agent. *Science* **271**:505–508.

53. MacSween, R. N. 1980. Pathology of viral hepatitis and its sequelae. *Clin. Gastroenterol.* **9**:23–45.

54. Margolis, H. S., M. J. Alter, and S. C. Hadler. 1991. Hepatitis B: evolving epidemiology and implications for control. *Semin. Liver Dis.* **11**:84–92.

55. Mast, E. E., and K. Krawczynski. 1996. Hepatitis E: an overview. *Annu. Rev. Med.* **47**:257–266.

56. McCaustland, K. A., S. Bi, M. A. Purdy, and D. W. Bradley. 1991. Application of two RNA extraction methods prior to amplification of hepatitis E virus nucleic acid by the polymerase chain reaction. *J. Virol. Methods* **35**:331–342.

57. McFarlane, I. G. 1993. Hepatitis C and alcoholic liver disease. *Am. J. Gastroenterol.* **88**:982–988.

58. McMahon, B. J., W. L. M. Alward, D. B. Hall, W. L. Heyward, T. R. Bender, D. P. Francis, and J. E. Maynard. 1985. Acute hepatitis B virus infection: relation of age to the clinical expression of disease and subsequent development of the carrier state. *J. Infect. Dis.* **151**:599–603.

59. Mimms, L. T., J. W. Moseley, F. B. Hollinger, R. D. Aach, C. E. Stevens, M. Cunningham, D. V. Vallari, L. H. Barbosa, and G. J. Nemo. 1993. Effect of concurrent acute infection with hepatitis C virus on acute hepatitis B infection. *Br. Med. J.* **307**:1095–1097.

60. Mitsui, T., K. Iwano, K. Masuko, C. Yamazaki, H. Okamoto, F. Tsuda, T. Tanaka, and S. Mishiro. 1992. Hepatitis C virus infection in medical personnel after needlestick accident. *Hepatology* **16**:1109–1114.

61. Morrow, R. H., H. F. Smetana, F. T. Sai, and J. H. Edgcomb. 1968. Unusual features of viral hepatitis in Accra, Ghana. *Ann. Intern. Med.* **68**:1250–1264.

62. Murayama, T., S. Iiono, K. Koike, K. Yasuda, and D. R. Milich. 1993. Serology of acute exacerbation in chronic hepatitis B virus infection. *Gastroenterology* **105**:1141–1151.

63. Nakamura, T., M. Hayama, T. Sakai, M. Hotchi, and E. Tanaka. 1993. Proliferative activity of hepatocytes in chronic viral hepatitis as revealed by immunohistochemistry for proliferating cell nuclear antigen. *Hum. Pathol.* **24**:750–753.

64. Negro, F., D. Pacchioni, A. Mondardini, G. Bussolati, and F. Bonino. 1992. In situ hybridization in viral hepatitis. *Liver* **12:**217–226.

65. Nomoto, M., Y. Uchikosi, N. Kajikazawa, N. Tanaka, and H. Asakura. 1992. Appearance of hepatocyte-like cells in the interlobular bile ducts of human liver in various disease states. *Hepatology* **16:**1199–1205.

66. Oberhammer, F., W. Bursch, R. Tiefenbacher, G. Froschl, M. Pavelka, and T. Purchio. 1993. Apoptosis is induced by transforming growth factor-B1 within hours in regressing liver without significant fragmentation of the DNA. *Hepatology* **18:**1238–1246.

67. Ohto, H., S. Terazawa, N. Sasaki, K. Hino, C. Ishiwata, M. Kako, N. Ujiie, C. Endo, A. Matsui, H. Okamoto, and S. Mishiro. 1994. Transmission of hepatitis C virus from mothers to infants. *N. Engl. J. Med.* **330:**744–750.

68. Okuno, T., A. Sano, T. Deguchi, Y. Katsuma, T. Ogasawara, T. Okanoue, and T. Takinot. 1984. Pathology of acute hepatitis A in humans. Comparison with acute hepatitis B. *Am. J. Clin. Pathol.* **81:**162–169.

69. Osmond, D. H., E. Charlebois, H. W. Sheppard, K. Page, W. Winkelstein, A. R. Moss, and A. Reingold. 1993. Comparison of risk factors for hepatitis C and hepatitis B virus infection in homosexual men. *J. Infect. Dis.* **167:**66–71.

70. Osmond, D. H., N. S. Padian, H. W. Sheppard, S. Glass, S. C. Shiboski, and A. Reingold. 1993. Risk factors for hepatitis C virus seropositivity in heterosexual couples. *JAMA* **269:**361–365.

71. Phillips, M. J., L. M. Blendis, S. Poucell, et al. 1991. Syncytial giant cell hepatitis: sporadic hepatitis with distinctive pathological features, a severe clinical course, and paramyxoviral features. *N. Engl. J. Med.* **324:**455–460.

72. Phillips, M. J., and S. Poucell. 1981. Modern aspects of the morphology of viral hepatitis. *Hum. Pathol.* **12:**1060–1084.

73. Polish, L. B., M. Gallagher, H. A. Fields, and S. C. Hadler. 1993. Delta hepatitis: molecular biology and clinical and epidemiological features. *Clin. Microbiol. Rev.* **6:**211–229.

74. Pontisso, P., M. G. Ruvoletto, G. Fattovich, L. Chemello, A. Gallorini, A. Ruol, and A. Alberti. 1993. Clinical and virological profiles in patients with multiple hepatitis C infections. *Gastroenterology* **105:**1529–1533.

75. Propst, T., A. Propst, O. Dietze, and H. Braunsteiner. 1992. High prevalence of viral infection in adults with homozygous and heterozygous alpha,-antitrypsin deficiency and chronic liver disease. *Ann. Intern. Med.* **117:**641–645.

76. Roberts, J. M., J. W. Searle, and W. G. E. Cooksely. 1993. Histological patterns of prolonged hepatitis C infection. *Gastroenterol. Jpn.* **28:**901–905.

77. Sanchez-Tapias, J. M., J. M. Barrera, J. Costa, M. G. Ercilla, A. Pares, L. Comalrrena, F. Soley, J. Bruix, X. Calvet, M. P. Gil, et al. 1990. Hepatitis C virus infection in patients with nonalcoholic chronic liver disease. *Ann. Intern. Med.* **112:**921–924.

78. Scheuer, P. J. 1991. Classification of chronic viral hepatitis: a need for reassessment. *J. Hepatol.* **13:**372–374.

79. Searle, J., B. V. Harmon, C. J. Bishop, et al. 1987. The significance of cell death by apoptosis in hepatobiliary disease. *J. Gastroenterol. Pathol.* **2:**77.

80. Shapiro, C. N., P. J. Coleman, G. M. McQuillan, M. J. Alter, and H. S. Margolis. 1992. Epidemiology of hepatitis A: seroepidemiology and risk groups. *Vaccine* **10:**S59–S62.

81. **Simons, J. N., T. P. Leary, G. J. Dawson, T. J. Pilot-Matias, A. S. Muerhoff, G. G. Schlauder, S. M. Desai, and I. K. Mushahwar.** 1995. Isolation of novel virus-like sequences associated with human hepatitis. *Nat. Med.* **1:**564–569.

82. **Stechemesser, E., R. Klein, and P. A. Berg.** 1983. Characterization and clinical relevance of liver-pancreas antibodies in autoimmune hepatitis. *Hepatology* **18:**1–9.

83. **Teixeira, M. R., Jr., I. V. D. Weller, and A. Murray.** 1982. The pathology of hepatitis A in man. *Liver* **2:**53–60.

84. **Tsarev, S. A., T. S. Tsareva, S. U. Emerson, A. Z. Kapikian, J. Ticehurst, W. London, and R. H. Purcell.** 1993. ELISA for antibody to hepatitis E virus (HEV) based on complete open-reading frame-2 protein expressed in insect cells: identification of HEV in primates. *J. Infect. Dis.* **168:**369–378.

85. **Vento, S., F. Cainelli, F. Mirandola, et al.** 1996. Fulminant hepatitis on withdrawal of chemotherapy in carriers of hepatitis C. *Lancet* **347:**92–93.

86. **Villa, E., G. Baldini, S. DiStabile, et al.** 1986. Alcohol and hepatitis B virus infection. *Acta Med. Scand. Suppl.* **703:**97.

87. **Vyberg, M.** 1993. The hepatitis-associated bile duct lesion. *Liver* **13:**289–301.

88. **Williams, R., and J. Wendon.** 1994. Indications for orthotopic liver transplantation in fulminant liver failure. *Hepatology* **20:**5S–10S.

chapter 9

Emerging Fungal Infections: Cryptococcosis, Fusariosis, and Penicilliosis Marneffei

Michael M. McNeil, Leo Kaufman, and Francis W. Chandler

Since 1980, much important information has been generated concerning the natural history and outcome of human fungal infections caused by *Cryptococcus neoformans*, *Fusarium* spp., and *Penicillium marneffei*. This has been largely due to the increased frequency of occurrence of these diseases as opportunistic infections in severely immunocompromised patients. Cryptococcal meningitis is the most common life-threatening fungal infection in AIDS patients, occurring in about 6 to 10% of such individuals in North America and in up to 30% in Africa (33). Invasive infection by *Fusarium* spp. has been reported most frequently in severely immunocompromised patients with underlying hematologic malignancies who have received cytotoxic therapy. Penicilliosis marneffei is a recently recognized infection affecting immunocompromised human immunodeficiency virus (HIV)-infected patients who reside in or have visited Southeast Asia.

Michael M. McNeil, Division of Bacterial and Mycotic Diseases, National Center for Infectious Diseases, Centers for Disease Control and Prevention, 1600 Clifton Road, N.E., Mailstop C-09, Atlanta, GA 30333. **Leo Kaufman,** Immunodiagnostic Laboratory, Emerging Bacterial and Mycotic Diseases Branch, National Center for Infectious Diseases, Centers for Disease Control and Prevention, 1600 Clifton Road, N.E., Atlanta, GA 30333. **Francis W. Chandler,** Department of Pathology, Medical College of Georgia, Augusta, GA 30912.

Pathology of Emerging Infections
Edited by C. Robert Horsburgh, Jr., and Ann Marie Nelson
© 1997 American Society for Microbiology, Washington, DC 20005-4171

Epidemiology

Cryptococcosis

C. neoformans is a round or oval yeast that is surrounded by a mucopolysaccharide capsule and that reproduces by budding. The capsule is important for identification of the fungus in tissues and body fluids, in particular in cerebrospinal fluid (CSF), and it has been implicated in host immunosuppression (24). Four serotypes have been identified according to the antigenicity of the capsular mucopolysaccharide. Serotypes A and D have been classified as var. *neoformans*. This variety is found worldwide in soil and bird feces and has been implicated as the cause of most cases of human cryptococcosis. Serotypes B and C (classified as var. *gattii*) cause disease predominantly in tropical regions and have accounted for up to 40% of clinical isolates on the west coast of the United States (24). Of interest, eucalyptus trees (*Eucalyptus camalduensis*), which are common only on the west coast of the United States, have been identified as a natural reservoir for this variety.

Fusariosis

Fusarium spp. are common soil-inhabiting fungi that are distributed worldwide and are known to be plant, animal, and human pathogens. *Fusarium* spp. may affect humans by producing mycotoxicosis (a disease caused by the ingestion of food made toxic by secondary fungal metabolites) or invasive and disseminated disease. Acquisition of invasive infection may result from either inhalation or direct inoculation. Fusariosis is a hyalohyphomycotic infection caused by several *Fusarium* species. The species most often implicated in causing invasive human disease are *F. solani*, *F. oxysporum*, *F. proliferatum*, and *F. moniliforme* (30). These species, once considered pathogenic only for plants, have emerged as serious pathogens in neutropenic patients with underlying malignancies.

F. solani, F. oxysporum, F. proliferatum, and F. moniliforme, once considered pathogenic only for plants, have emerged as serious pathogens in neutropenic patients with underlying malignancies

Pencilliosis marneffei

P. marneffei, the only *Penicillium* species that is dimorphic, was first isolated from a bamboo rat (*Rhizomys sinensis*) in Vietnam in 1956 (4). Subsequently, a laboratory worker acquired the first human *P. marneffei* infection by accidental inoculation which resulted in a localized skin infection (36). The first report of natural human infection with *P. marneffei* was in 1973, in a 61-year-old missionary with Hodgkin's disease who had undergone a splenectomy and had been living in Southeast Asia (12). During the past two decades, there has been a dramatic increase in the number of reported cases; in particular they have been associated with the AIDS epidemic in northern Thailand. In northern Thailand, penicilliosis marneffei is now the third most common AIDS-associated opportunistic infection, behind tuberculosis and cryptococcosis (15).

Diagnosis

Cryptococcosis

Definitive diagnosis of cryptococcal infection requires a positive culture for *C. neoformans*. A positive cryptococcal antigen in the appropriate clinical setting, however, supports a presumptive diagnosis. For cryptococcal meningitis, characteristic CSF findings (leukocyte count, protein, and glucose) may be present. In general, cranial computerized tomographic and magnetic resonance imaging scans are less useful. Direct examination of clinical specimens, i.e., lesional exudate or CSF, by light microscopy often can be diagnostic when encapsulated yeasts are detected. India ink smears of centrifuged spinal fluid show diagnostic encapsulated yeasts in about 50% of meningitis cases. Over 90% of such cases may be recognized by using latex agglutination (LA) tests for cryptococcal antigen (21).

C. neoformans grows well on Sabouraud's agar, on which it produces a white to cream-colored mucoid colony at 25 and 37°C. Niger seed (*Guizotia abyssinica*) agar and L-dopa agar are good primary culture media. Colonies of *C. neoformans* will develop a brown color after 3 to 5 days of incubation at 25°C on niger seed agar and a black color after 24 h on L-dopa agar. Definitive identification can be made by demonstrating growth at 37°C, urease reactivity, and appropriate assimilation patterns by the API 20 kit. If desired, the variety may be determined on canavanine-glycine-bromthymol blue agar. *C. neoformans* var. *gattii* turns the medium blue, whereas var. *neoformans* does not. A commercial DNA probe for identifying *C. neoformans* is also available (Gen-Probe, San Diego, Calif.) (24).

The LA test for cryptococcal antigen is valuable for diagnosing active nonmeningeal and especially meningeal cryptococcosis. The test has a sensitivity of 99% with CSF specimens from culturally proven cases of meningitis. LA titers of 1:8 or higher are considered strong evidence of active infection if care is taken to avoid false positives due to rheumatoid factor or other interfering proteins in sera. The LA test is applicable to CSF, serum, or urine specimens. The antigen titers are not only diagnostic but prognostic. Failure of the titer to decline during therapy suggests inadequate treatment. A commercial enzyme immunoassay (Meridian Diagnostics, Inc., Cincinnati, Ohio) using a polyclonal antibody capture system together with a monoclonal antibody detection system also has proved useful. Unlike the LA test, the enzyme immunoassay does not require any pretreatment of specimens to avoid false-positive reactions (21, 37).

Definitive diagnosis of cryptococcal infection requires a positive culture for C. neoformans. A positive cryptococcal antigen in the appropriate clinical setting, however, supports a presumptive diagnosis

Fusariosis

The diagnosis of fusarial infection depends on the isolation of the fungus from clinical specimens, such as blood or material obtained from cutaneous lesions. In infected patients, there has been a high (60%) rate of isolation of *Fusarium* spp. from the bloodstream. *Fusarium* spp. grow rapidly on Sabouraud's glucose agar. Their growth is often inhibited by cycloheximide. Colonies are cottony to powdery and may be lavender, pink, salmon colored, or greyish white. Microscopically, they show phialidic conidiogenous cells bearing clusters of fusoid, multicelled, curved or canoe-shaped conidia typical of the genus. In addition, all species produce single-celled, pyriform, cylindric to subglobose microconidia from phialidic conidiogenous cells which are held in ball-like masses or in chains at the tip of phialides.

Although all *Fusarium* spp. grow well on Sabouraud's agar, they may not sporulate on this medium. Difficulties in generic identification may occur in the absence of macroconidia. The accurate identification of *Fusarium* species can take 2 to 3 weeks. Potato dextrose or carnation leaf agar is an excellent medium for inducing sporulation, which is necessary for properly identifying these pathogens. The medically important species of *Fusarium* produce specific antigens and may be accurately immunoidentified by exoantigen tests (38). No reliable test for the specific serodiagnosis of fusariosis is currently available.

Penicilliosis Marneffei

Culture isolation of *P. marneffei* alone is inadequate for making a diagnosis, because *Penicillium* spp. are frequent contaminants. The diagnosis is usually established by examination of Wright-stained samples of bone marrow aspirates or touch smears of skin biopsy specimens. The diagnosis of penicilliosis marneffei can be troublesome because its clinical manifestations mimic those of tuberculosis, pneumocystosis, histoplasmosis, and other mycotic infections. The etiologic agent is the only known *Penicillium* species that is dimorphic. At 25°C on Sabouraud's agar, it grows as a mold with a penicillus belonging to the biverticillate series and produces a deep, wine red, water-soluble pigment that diffuses into the medium, whereas at 37°C in vivo or in vitro, it converts to a yeast-like form (fission arthroconidia), displaying ellipsoidal cells measuring 2 to 3 by 2 to 6 μm which multiply by fission rather than budding. The fungus produces two distinct exoantigens, which permits its differentiation from other species of *Penicillium* as well as from other fungi (39). Immunodiffusion tests to detect *P. marneffei* antigens and/or antibodies in human patient sera and an LA test for antigenemia appear to be promising (23, 39).

Pathology

Cryptococcosis

In hematoxylin and eosin (H&E)-stained tissue sections, the pleomorphic yeast-like cells of *C. neoformans* are spherical, oval, or elliptical and eosinophilic or lightly basophilic, have thin walls, and vary in size from 2 to 20 μm but commonly measure 4 to 10 μm in diameter (9). Typical fungal cells are surrounded by optically clear, smoothly contoured spherical zones, or halos, that represent the unstained mucinous capsules (Fig. 9.1). The capsules, which may have a diameter up to five times larger than that of the fungal cells they surround, are readily detected with mucin stains such as Mayer's mucicarmine and Alcian blue. With mucin stains, the capsular material often has a spinous or crenated appearance caused by uneven shrinkage during tissue processing (Fig. 9.2). In active lesions that contain abundant, rapidly proliferating fungal cells, budding is frequent. Single buds

The diagnosis of penicilliosis marneffei can be troublesome because its clinical manifestations mimic those of tuberculosis, pneumocystosis, histoplasmosis, and other mycotic infections

attached by a narrow base are usually seen, but multiple buds and short chains of three to five yeast form cells may also be observed. Germ tubes, pseudohyphae, and true hyphae are rarely produced in tissues (9, 10).

The host reaction to *C. neoformans* is variable and usually depends on the immunologic status of the host, the presence of underlying disease, and whether or not the cryptococci are capsule deficient. In anergic patients, such as those with AIDS, it may be difficult to detect any host reaction at all. In this acellular or paucireactive pattern, the cryptococci multiply profusely, displace normal tissues, and form a "cystic" lesion filled with myriad closely packed fungal cells whose wide mucoid capsules give the lesion a gelatinous, glistening appearance and slimy consistency on gross examination. This appearance is particularly striking in some cases of cryptococcal meningitis, in which compact masses of fungi in the leptomeninges ("soap bubble" appearance at low magnification) displace the underlying brain parenchyma. In healthy, nonimmunocompromised individuals, *C. neoformans* usually elicits a mixed suppurative and granulomatous inflammatory reaction or a purely granulomatous reaction that may contain varying degrees of necrosis. Capsule-deficient cryptococci always elicit a granulomatous inflammatory reaction, with areas of necrosis and suppuration (9, 10, 16). Pleomorphic yeast form cells without conspicuous capsules are present in variable numbers, and many are located within epithelioid histiocytes and multinucleated giant cells (Fig. 9.3).

Chronic infection by *C. neoformans*, similar to that by *Histoplasma capsulatum* var. *capsulatum* and *Coccidioides immitis*, can result in the formation of residual pulmonary granulomas (cryptococcomas). However, unlike residual granulomas caused by the latter two fungi, cryptococcomas rarely calcify (2, 10, 11). They are often found incidentally at autopsy or are suspected of being neoplasms in chest radiographs and then surgically resected. In such lesions, atypical, distorted, and fragmented cells of *C. neoformans* are difficult to detect with H&E but can be readily demonstrated with the Gomori methenamine silver (GMS) stain. Usually, the cryptococci are small (2 to 5 µm in diameter), unevenly stained, and capsule deficient, and it is difficult to culture the fungus from these lesions. In these instances, direct immunofluorescence examination of deparaffinized tissue sections is a valuable diagnostic aid (6, 9, 19) (Fig. 9.4).

Because the cells of *C. neoformans* vary greatly in size and shape and because typical encapsulated forms are not always encountered, cryptococcosis should be considered in the histopathologic differential diagnosis of virtually any yeast form infection. Cryptococci with well-developed capsules are readily visible and can usually be presumptively identified in tissue sections stained with H&E. However, their morphology can be studied to better advantage with the special stains for fungi. When the capsule stains intensely with mucin stains, a definitive diagnosis of cryptococcosis can be made, because *C. neoformans* is the only pathogenic fungus with a mucinous capsule. A histologic diagnosis of cryptococcosis is more difficult to establish when most or all of the cryptococci in a lesion are capsule deficient (9, 16). However, at least some weakly encapsulated cells can almost always be found in such lesions if mucin-stained sections are examined carefully. Capsule-deficient *C. neoformans* can simulate *H. capsulatum* var. *capsulatum* and *Blastomyces dermatitidis* with small tissue forms (so-called microforms), and the potential for confusion with *Sporothrix schenckii*, *Torulopsis glabrata*, *H. capsulatum* var. *duboisii*, blastoconidia of the *Candida* spp., and immature spherules of *C. immitis* also exists (9, 17, 20). If cryptococcosis is not suspected clinically, fresh tissue may not be collected for culture. When fresh tissue is not available, several adjunctive methods can be used to identify cryptococci in fixed tissues.

1. Immunofluorescence. *C. neoformans* can be identified in formalin-fixed, paraffin-embedded tissue sections that contain intact fungal elements by direct immunofluorescence (6, 19, 20). Unfortunately, specific fluorescent-antibody conjugates are not widely available at the present time. The conjugate used at the Centers for Disease Control and Prevention, considered specific for *C. neoformans* when used to test clinical specimens, is directed against capsular polysaccharide antigens. Therefore, capsule-deficient cryptococci are only weakly stained, but at least some immunoreactive cells can almost always be demonstrated in this situation (Fig. 9.4).

2. Transmission electron microscopy. The capsule of *C. neoformans* varies in width but has a characteristic ultrastructural appearance (9). It is separated from the underlying electron-dense cell wall by an electron-lucent zone and is composed of a finely granular matrix that contains radiating filaments and tubules. Most mucicarmine-negative cells of *C. neoformans* seen at the light microscopic level have attenuated capsules that can be readily demonstrated by transmission electron microscopy.

3. Fontana-Masson stain. The Fontana-Masson stain for melanin, as modified by Kwon-Chung et al. (25), stains the cell walls of *C. neoformans* brown or black in tissue sections. A positive reaction highlights silver-reducing substances (melanin-like substances derived from dihydroxyphenylalanine) in the cell walls and does not depend upon the presence of capsular mucopolysaccharide (41). Unfortunately, the reaction is not specific for cryptococci; yeast forms of *S. schenckii* and immature spherules of *C. immitis* sometimes react with this stain.

Occasionally, the cell walls of *Rhinosporidium seeberi* and *B. dermatitidis* are also colored with mucin stains such as Mayer's mucicarmine and Alcian blue (9). However, because these two fungi are nonencapsulated and morphologically distinct, they should not be confused with *C. neoformans*. Mucin stains are not required for their identification in tissue sections.

Fusariosis

In invasive and disseminated fusariosis, gross lesions may resemble abscesses (in nongranulocytopenic patients), infarcts, or granulomas. Histopathologic examination reveals that the lesions are abscesses or nodular infarcts; the latter is a consequence of hyphal vascular invasion and thrombotic occlusion (7). Hyphae are usually abundant in these lesions and are easily delineated with the H&E stain, where they are variably hematoxylinophilic. However, GMS and other special stains for fungi are usually needed to demonstrate hyphal morphology in detail (Fig. 9.5). Erythematous, ulcerated, or necrotic cutaneous nodules often develop during the course of disseminated infection; biopsy and culture are needed to establish the diagnosis (1, 32, 34, 40).

In tissue sections, the *Fusarium* spp. form hyaline, septate hyphae that are 3 to 8 μm wide and that usually branch at right angles (7). Hyphal branches are often constricted at their sites of origin from parent hyphae (Fig. 9.6). Occasionally, varicosities or thick-walled chlamydoconidia up to 20 μm in diameter are found within or at the ends of hyphae. Microconidia or characteristic fusiform, septate macroconidia are rarely formed in tissue exposed to ambient air. Only if the classical, fusiform macroconidia are identified can an unequivocal histopathologic diagnosis of fusariosis be made; otherwise, the presumptive diagnosis should be confirmed by culture or immunofluorescence. The formation of microconidia in tissue can lead to an erroneous pathologic diagnosis of candidiasis or of coexisting yeast form mycoses.

Hyphae of the *Fusarium* spp. are narrower and their septations are much more frequent and prominent than hyphae of the mucoraceous zygomycetes. However, these morphologic features are not entirely reliable for distinguishing hyphae of the *Fusarium* spp. from those of other opportunistic hyaline hyphomycetes, particularly the *Aspergillus* spp. and *Pseudallescheria boydii*. Definitive diagnosis presently requires isolation and identification of the fungus on standard mycologic media or immunofluorescence staining of fungal elements in deparaffinized sections of formalin-fixed tissue (20).

Hyphae of the Fusarium spp. are narrower and their septations are much more frequent and prominent than hyphae of the mucoraceous zygomycetes

Penicilliosis Marneffei

Penicilliosis marneffei is a disseminated fungal infection that involves the mononuclear phagocyte system. *P. marneffei*, the etiologic agent, grows as an intracellular yeast-like fungus in tissue and as a typical species of *Penicillium* on standard mycologic media at 25°C.

Histopathologic examination is the most rapid and reliable means of diagnosis (8, 22). Specific antiglobulins are useful in indirect fluorescent-antibody tests for rapidly identifying *P. marneffei* in tissues (22). In non-AIDS patients, the lymph nodes, liver, lungs, and kidneys are most commonly involved, whereas in AIDS patients, the lymph nodes, skin, bone, and bone marrow are the most frequent organs involved (14). Three inflammatory patterns can be seen in penicilliosis marneffei: granulomatous, suppurative, and anergic or necrotizing (8, 13). The first two patterns are seen in individuals who have intact immunity, and the third occurs in patients with compromised immunity.

In tissue sections, *P. marneffei* is yeast-like and multiplies within macrophages that enlarge to accommodate the fungus (8). The intracellular yeast forms are oval to slightly elongated and 2 to 6 μm in length (Fig. 9.7). When extracellular, the yeast-like cells are sometimes much longer, approaching 12 μm in length, and they often have rounded ends. Some of the elongated fungal cells also may be curved ("sausage" forms). The cells divide at a central septum by fission (schizogony); they do not bud (Fig. 9.8). The central transverse septum usually stains more intensely with GMS and is wider than the external fungal cell wall (28).

Suppurative lesions tend to be more common in pulmonary, cutaneous, and subcutaneous sites. The anergic and necrotizing reactions in immunocompromised individuals usually involve the lungs, skin, and liver. In addition to the histopathology described by Deng et al. (13), the ultrastructural aspects of penicilliosis marneffei have been described (5, 14). In an AIDS patient, a fine-needle aspirate of an enlarged cervical lymph node was used to make the diagnosis of this infection (27).

Because of their similarity in size and shape, the intracellular yeast forms of *H. capsulatum* var. *capsulatum* and *P. marneffei* can be confused (8, 28). However, differences in the division process (budding for *H. capsulatum* and septation for *P. marneffei*) readily separate these two fungal pathogens. The GMS procedure and other special stains for fungi are needed to clearly demonstrate these differences.

Clinical Findings

Cryptococcosis

Healthy people who inhale cryptococcal organisms usually remain asymptomatic or develop a self-limited pneumonitis. Rarely, individuals who are apparently immunologically normal acquire symptomatic and serious cryptococcal disease. However, severely immunocompromised individuals, including those with defects of cell-mediated immunity, such as patients with HIV infection or lymphoma or transplant recipients, are particularly susceptible to opportunistic disseminated infection. The central nervous system is almost invariably involved in disseminated disease, and there often may be accompanying fungemia. Meningitis is found in more than 80% of HIV-associated cryptococcal disease and is most likely to occur in patients with fewer than 200 CD4+ cells per mm^3 (24). The clinical presentation is often indolent and nonspecific, which may significantly delay the diagnosis. However, at the time of diagnosis, headache, fever, and nausea are frequently reported, and nuchal rigidity, focal neurologic deficits, altered mental status, and photophobia are each apparent in 20 to 40% of patients (42). The most common nonmeningeal site of HIV-associated cryptococcal disease is the lungs; however, meningitis is diagnosed in the majority of patients presenting with primary respiratory symptoms (24). The most frequent symptoms include fever, cough, dyspnea, and pleuritic chest pain. Chest radiographic findings include focal and interstitial infiltrates, lymphadenopathy, and pleural effusions, which suggest a broad differential and should always raise concern regarding a coexisting infection (42). Symptomatic prostatic infection is unusual; however, the prostate may serve as an important reservoir from which recurrent dissemination may occur. Lesions observed in mucocutaneous cryptococcosis may be quite variable, and on biopsy, they may yield material diagnostic of disseminated infection. Fungemia is much more common in HIV-infected patients, occurring in 10 to 50% of patients with meningitis, but it appears to have little prognostic significance (24).

Severely immunocompromised individuals, including those with defects of cell-mediated immunity, are particularly susceptible to opportunistic disseminated infection

Fusariosis

Fusarium spp. may occur as throat and conjunctival colonizing microorganisms. They may be the cause of a variety of foreign-body-associated infections (e.g., keratitis in contact lens wearers, peritonitis following chronic ambulatory peritoneal dialysis, and intravenous catheter-associated fungemia). Sites that may be involved in localized *Fusarium* infections include the eyes, nasal sinuses, skin, nails, bones, joints, lungs, and brain. Disseminated fusarial infection was first described in an immunocompromised patient in 1973. Since this report, there has been a significant increase in the incidence of disseminated fusariosis. Disseminated fusarial infections appear to be community acquired, and infections in hospitalized patients are usually a result of colonization prior to hospital admission. Immunosuppression which results from cytotoxic chemotherapy for acute leukemia, in particular severe granulocytopenic immunosuppression, is the predominant risk factor for the infection (30). A frequent clinical presentation is a profoundly granulocytopenic cancer patient with a persistent fever that is unresponsive to broad-spectrum antibiotics. Almost any organ may be affected. Generalized skin lesions are particularly common in patients with disseminated fusariosis and often include erythematous subcutaneous papules, painful erythematous macules and papules, and target lesions (30).

Disseminated fusarial infections appear to be community acquired, and infections in hospitalized patients are usually a result of colonization prior to hospital admission

Pencilliosis Marneffei

The onset of *P. marneffei* infection is often abrupt, with symptoms of persistent fever, chills, painful cough, weakness, and weight loss. There may be generalized lymphadenitis and hepatosplenomegaly. A common presentation is with multiple necrotic skin (lesions often resembling molluscum contagiosum) and subcutaneous abscesses (13, 18). Chest radiographs may reveal localized or patchy infiltrates, abscesses, and cavities in the lungs, but hilar lymph nodes are not calcified.

Treatment

Cryptococcosis

Cryptococcal meningitis is uniformly fatal if left untreated. However, complications may occur even following aggressive antifungal treatment and may include hydrocephalus, dementia, and permanent focal neurologic deficits. Prior to the AIDS epidemic, the standard treatment was amphotericin B in combination with flucytosine. However, this therapy resulted in substantial toxicity in AIDS patients (in particular myelosuppression and gastrointestinal distress associated with flucytosine), which prompted a search for alternative treatments. New triazoles (fluconazole and itraconazole) for the treatment of cryptococcal meningitis have been studied. Fluconazole is well tolerated and orally active and has excellent penetration into body fluids, including CSF. However, two recent randomized trials comparing fluconazole and the standard drug combination suggested that amphotericin B and flucytosine produced better overall results in terms of mortality and time to cure (26, 35). Currently, the best initial therapy for patients with AIDS and acute cryptococcal meningitis appears to be amphotericin B with or without flucytosine for 4 to 8 weeks, using stabilization or disappearance of cryptococcal antigen and normalization of CSF parameters as endpoints (24). Because of the tendency for late relapse in these patients, there is a lifelong requirement for maintenance therapy. Preliminary studies suggest that fluconazole is superior to amphotericin B for this indication (3, 31).

Fusariosis

The most important factors influencing the outcome of fusariosis are the underlying immunologic status of the patient and the extent of the infection (29, 30). Immunocompetent patients with localized infections usually respond to specific antifungal treatment. While optimal antifungal therapy remains to be determined, amphotericin B (the agent demonstrating the most activity in vitro) is the drug of choice for disseminated *Fusarium* infection (29, 30).

Penicilliosis Marneffei

Penicilliosis is usually fatal if left untreated. Treatment with amphotericin B alone or sometimes in combination with flucytosine has been successful in the majority of patients treated to date (13, 18). However, relapse is common once specific antifungal therapy is stopped, suggesting that in the HIV-infected patient, lifelong antifungal therapy should be continued. There have been too few patients treated with either itraconazole or fluconazole for the clinical usefulness of these drugs to be critically assessed.

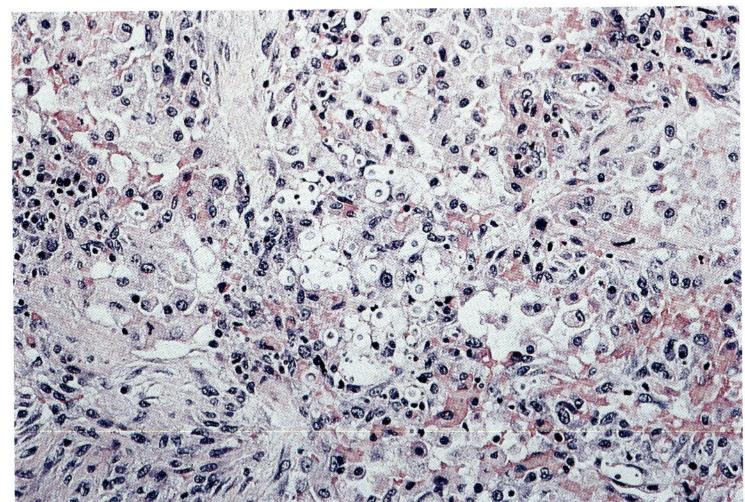

Figure 9.1 Pulmonary cryptococcosis in a patient with AIDS. Pleomorphic yeast-like cells distend the interstitium and are surrounded by wide, unstained (optically clear) capsules (H&E; original magnification, ×100).

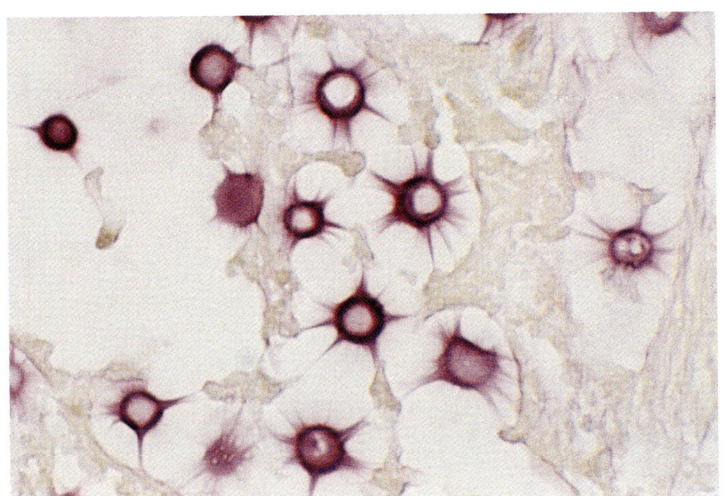

Figure 9.2 Cerebromeningeal cryptococcosis. Numerous yeast-like cells of C. *neoformans* within the leptomeninges elicit little or no inflammation and are surrounded by wide carminophilic capsules that have a crenated or spinous appearance because of uneven shrinkage during tissue processing (Mayer's mucicarmine stain; original magnification, ×500).

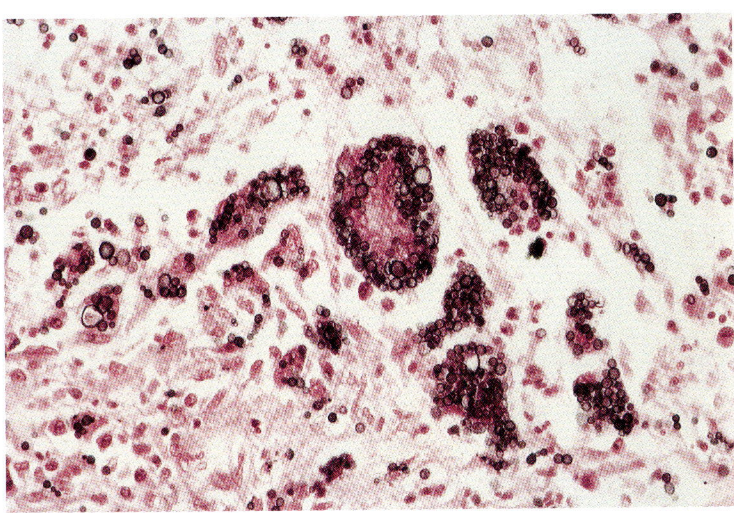

Figure 9.3 Granulomatous pneumonia caused by capsule-deficient cryptococci. Myriad pleomorphic yeast forms are predominantly intracellular and do not have conspicuous capsules. In replicate tissue sections, the attenuated capsules were only weakly reactive or nonreactive with mucin stains (GMS-H&E; original magnification, ×160).

Figure 9.4 Direct immunofluorescence of capsule-deficient cryptococci in a pulmonary granuloma. Attenuated capsules are brightly decorated using a species-specific conjugate against capsular polysaccharide antigens of *C. neoformans*. Immunofluorescence reactivity parallels mucin reactivity but is more sensitive (direct immunofluorescence; original magnification, ×250).

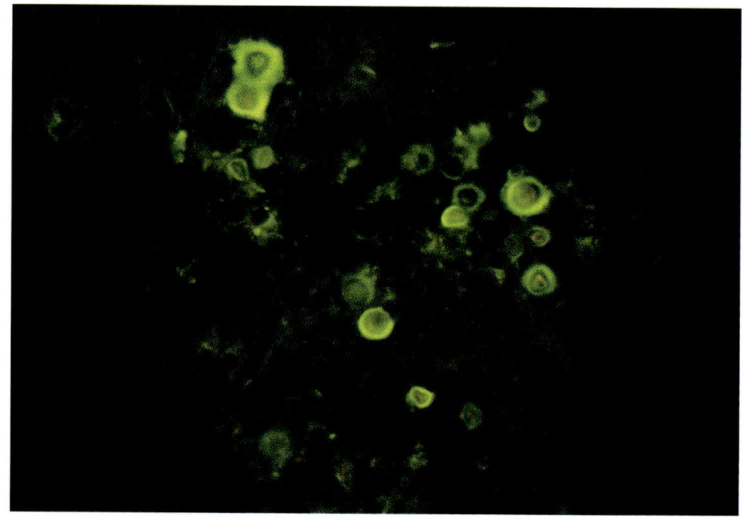

Figure 9.5 Disseminated fusariosis. A nodular infarct contains numerous, elongated, randomly oriented hyphae of a *Fusarium* sp., 3 to 8 μm wide, that resemble those of the *Aspergillus* spp. Some of the hyphae have terminal, spherical to oval, chlamydoconidia-like structures (right center) (GMS-H&E; original magnification, ×100).

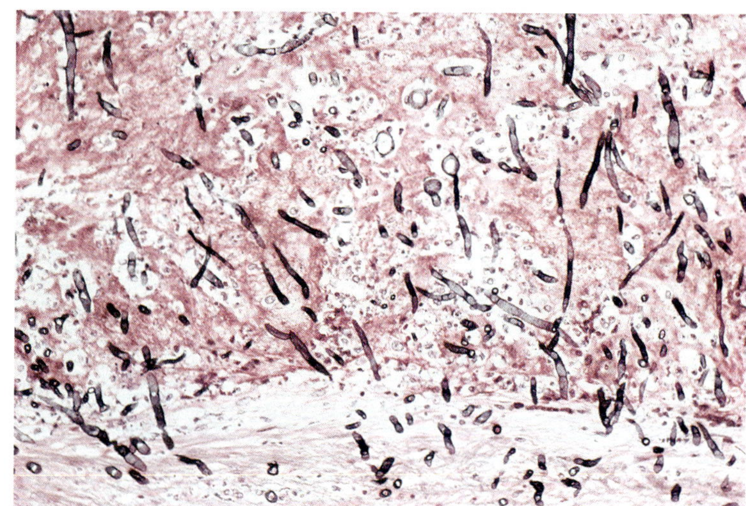

Figure 9.6 Cutaneous fusariosis caused by *F. moniliforme* in a burned patient. The septate hyphae, 3 to 8 μm wide, branch at predominantly right angles. Hyphal branches are often constricted at their origins from parent hyphae (GMS-H&E; original magnification, ×160).

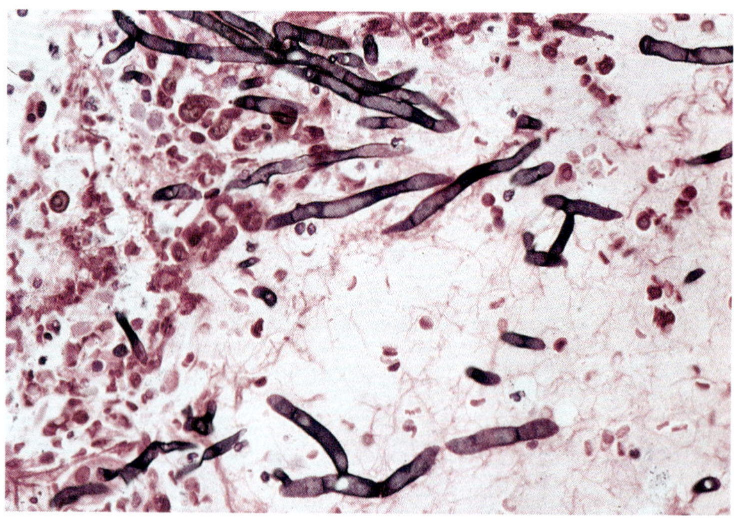

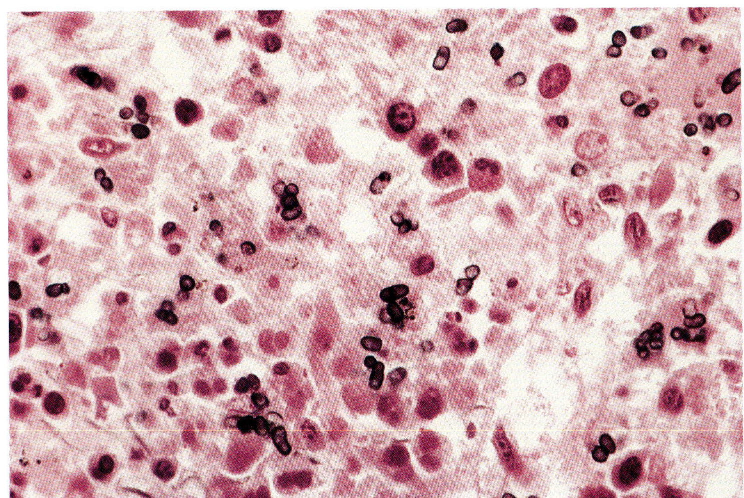

Figure 9.7 Disseminated penicilliosis marneffei. A hepatic granuloma contains individual and clustered, spherical to oval yeast-like forms of *P. marneffei*, 2 to 6 μm in diameter, that resemble the yeast-like cells of *H. capsulatum* var. *capsulatum* (GMS-H&E; original magnification, ×250).

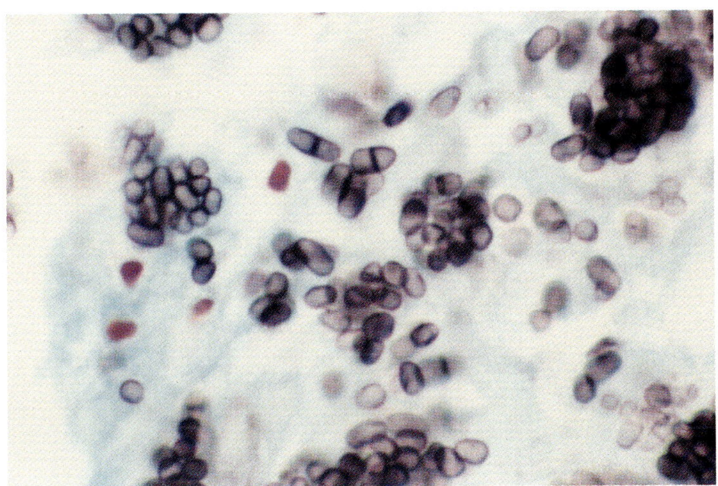

Figure 9.8 Disseminated penicilliosis marneffei. Diagnostic yeast-like cells of *P. marneffei* with single, wide, transverse septa and rounded ends (top center) are located in a hepatic granuloma (GMS; original magnification, ×500).

References

1. **Anaissie, E., H. Kantarjian, J. Ro, R. Hopfer, K. Rolston, V. Fainstein, and G. Bodey.** 1988. The emerging role of *Fusarium* infections in patients with cancer. *Medicine* (Baltimore) **67:**77–83.

2. **Baker, R. D.** 1976. The primary pulmonary lymph node complex of cryptococcosis. *Am. J. Clin. Pathol.* **65:**83–92.

3. **Bozzette, S. A., R. A. Larsen, J. Chiu, M. A. Leal, J. Jacobsen, P. Rothman, P. Robinson, G. Gilbert, J. A. McCutchan, J. Tilles, J. M. Leedom, D. D. Richman, and the California Collaborative Treatment Group.** 1991. A placebo-controlled trial of maintenance therapy with fluconazole after treatment of cryptococcal meningitis in the acquired immunodeficiency syndrome. *N. Engl. J. Med.* **324:**580–584.

4. **Capponi, M., P. Sureau, and G. Segretain.** 1956. Penicillose de *Rhizomys sinensis. Bull. Soc. Pathol. Éxot. Filiales* **49:**418-421.

5. **Chan, Y., and T. C. Chow.** 1990. Ultrastructural observations on *Penicillium marneffei* in natural human infection. *Ultrastruct. Pathol.* **14:**439–452.

6. **Chandler, F. W., W. Kaplan, and L. Ajello.** 1980. *Color Atlas and Text of the Histopathology of Mycotic Diseases,* p. 23–25. Mosby Year Book Medical Publishers, Chicago.

7. **Chandler, F. W., and J. C. Watts.** 1987. *Pathologic Diagnosis of Fungal Infections,* p. 81–84. ASCP Press, Chicago.

8. **Chandler, F. W., and J. C. Watts.** 1987. *Pathologic Diagnosis of Fungal Infections,* p. 209–213. ASCP Press, Chicago.

9. **Chandler, F. W., and J. C. Watts.** 1987. *Pathologic Diagnosis of Fungal Infections,* p. 161–175. ASCP Press, Chicago.

10. **Chandler, F. W., and J. C. Watts.** 1993. Fungal infections, p. 351–428. *In* D. H. Dail and S. P. Hammar (ed.), *Pulmonary Pathology,* 2nd ed. Springer-Verlag, New York.

11. **Cohen, A. A., W. Davis, and S. M. Finegold.** 1965. Chronic pulmonary cryptococcosis. *Am. Rev. Respir. Dis.* **91:**414–423.

12. **DiSalvo, A. F., A. M. Dickling, and L. Ajello.** 1973. Infection caused by *Penicillium marneffei:* a description of the first natural infection in man. *Am. J. Clin. Pathol.* **60:**259–263.

13. **Deng, Z., J. L. Ribas, D. W. Gibson, and D. H. Connor.** 1988. Infections caused by *Penicillium marneffei* in China and Southeast Asia: review of eighteen published cases and report of four more Chinese cases. *Rev. Infect. Dis.* **10:**640–652.

14. **Drouhet, E.** 1993. Penicilliosis due to *Penicillium marneffei:* a new emerging systemic mycosis in AIDS patients travelling or living in southeast Asia. Review of 44 cases reported in HIV infected patients during the last 5 years compared to 44 cases of non AIDS patients reported over 20 years. *J. Mycol. Med.* **4:**195–224.

15. **Dupont, B., D. W. Denning, D. Marriott, A. Sugar, M. A. Viviani, and T. Sirisanthana.** 1994. Mycoses in AIDS patients. *J. Med. Vet. Mycol.* **32:**65–77.

16. **Farmer, S. G., and R. A. Komorowski.** 1973. Histologic response to capsule-deficient *Cryptococcus neoformans. Arch. Pathol.* **96:**383–387.

17. **Gutierrez, F., Y. S. Fu, and H. I. Lurie.** 1975. Cryptococcosis histologically resembling histoplasmosis: a light and electron microscopical study. *Arch. Pathol.* **99:**347–352.

18. **Hilmarsdottir, I., J. L. Meynard, O. Rogeaux, G. Guermonprez, A. Datry, C. Katlama, G. Brucker, A. Coutellier, M. Danis, and M. Gentilini.** 1993. Disseminated *Penicillium marneffei* infection associated with human immunodeficiency virus: a report of two cases and a review of 35 published cases. *J. Acquired Immun. Defic. Syndr.* **6:**466–471.

19. **Kaplan, W., and D. E. Kraft.** 1969. Demonstration of pathogenic fungi in formalin-fixed tissues by immunofluorescence. *Am. J. Clin. Pathol.* **52:**420–432.

20. **Kaufman, L.** 1992. Immunohistologic diagnosis of systemic mycoses: an update. *Eur. J. Epidemiol.* **8:**377–382.

21. **Kaufman, L., and E. Reiss.** 1985. Serodiagnosis of fungal diseases, p. 924–944. *In* E. H. Lennette, A. Balows, W. J. Hausler, Jr., and H. J. Shadomy (ed.), *Manual of Clinical Microbiology*, 4th ed. American Society for Microbiology, Washington, D.C.

22. **Kaufman, L., P. G. Standard, S. A. Anderson, M. Jalbert, and B. L. Swisher.** 1995. Development of specific fluorescent-antibody test for tissue form of *Penicillium marneffei. J. Clin. Microbiol.* **33:**2136–2138.

23. **Kaufman, L., P. G. Standard, M. Jalbert, P. Kantipong, K. Limpakarnjanarat, and T. D. Mastro.** 1996. Diagnostic antigenemia tests for Pencilliosis marneffei. *J. Clin. Microbiol.* **34:**2503–2505.

24. **Kwon-Chung, K. J., and J. E. Bennett.** 1992. *Medical Mycology.* Lea and Feibiger, Philadelphia.

25. **Kwon-Chung, K. J., W. B. Hill, and J. E. Bennett.** 1981. New, special stain for histopathological diagnosis of cryptococcosis. *J. Clin. Microbiol.* **13:**383–387.

26. **Larsen, R. A., M. A. Leal, and L. S. Chan.** 1990. Fluconazole compared with amphotericin B plus flucytosine for cryptococcal meningitis in AIDS. A randomized trial. *Ann. Intern. Med.* **113:**183–187.

27. **Ma, K., M. Tsui, and D. N. C. Tsang.** 1991. Fine needle aspiration diagnosis of *Penicillium marneffei* infection. *Acta Cytol.* **35:**557–559.

28. **McGinnis, M. R.** 1994. *Penicillium marneffei*, dimorphic fungus of increasing importance. *Clin. Microbiol. Newsl.* **4:**29–31.

29. **Merz, W. G., J. E. Karp, M. Hoagland, M. Jett-Goheen, J. M. Junkins, and A. F. Hood.** 1988. Diagnosis and successful treatment of fusariosis in the compromised host. *J. Infect. Dis.* **158:**1046–1055.

30. **Nelson, P. E., M. C. Dignani, and E. J. Anaissie.** 1994. Taxonomy, biology, and clinical aspects of *Fusarium* species. *Clin. Microbiol. Rev.* **7:**479–504.

31. **Powderly, W. G., M. S. Saag, G. A. Cloud, P. Robinson, R. D. Meyer, J. M. Jacobson, J. R. Graybill, A. M. Sugar, V. J. McAuliffe, S. E. Follansbee, C. U. Tuazon, J. J. Stern, J. Feinberg, R. Hafner, W. E. Dismukes, The NIAID AIDS Clinical Trials Group, and The NIAID Mycoses Study Group.** 1992. A controlled trial of fluconazole or amphotericin B to prevent relapse of cryptococcal menigitis in patients with the acquired immunodeficiency syndrome. *N. Engl. J. Med.* **326:**793–798.

32. **Rabodonirina, M., M. A. Piens, M. F. Monier, E. Gueho, D. Fiere, and M. Mojon.** 1994. *Fusarium* infections in immunocompromised patients; case reports and literature review. *Eur. J. Clin. Microbiol. Infect. Dis.* **13:**152–161.

33. **Richard, M. D., and D. W. Warnock.** 1993. *Fungal Infection: Diagnosis and Management.* Blackwell Scientific Publications, Boston.

34. **Richardson, S. E., R. M. Bannatyne, R. C. Summerbell, J. Milliken, R. Gold, and S. S. Weitzman.** 1988. Disseminated fusarial infection in the immunocompromised host. *Rev. Infect. Dis.* **10:**1171–1181.

35. **Saag, M. S., W. G. Powderly, G. A. Cloud, P. Robinson, M. H. Grieco, P. K. Sharkey, S. E. Thompson, A. M. Sugar, C. U. Tuazon, J. F. Fisher, N. Hyslop, J. M. Jacobson, R. Hafner, W. E. Dismukes, The NIAID Mycoses Study Group, and the AIDS Clinical Trials Group.** 1992. Comparison of amphotericin B with fluconazole in the treatment of AIDS-associated cryptococcal meningitis. *N. Engl. J. Med.* **326:**83–89.

36. **Segretain, G.** 1959. *Penicillium marneffei:* n. sp., agent d'une mycose du système réticulo-endothelial. *Mycopathol. Mycol. Appl.* **11:**327–353.

37. **Sekhon, A. S., A. K. Garg, L. Kaufman, G. S. Kobayashi, Z. Hamir, M. Jalbert, and N. Moledina.** 1993. Evaluation of a commercial enzyme immunoassay for the detection of cryptococcal antigen. *Mycoses* **36:**31–34.

38. **Sekhon, A. S., L. Kaufman, N. Moledina, R. C. Summerbell, A. A. Padhye, E. A. Ambrosie, and T. Panter.** 1995. An exoantigen test for the rapid identification of medically significant *Fusarium* species. *J. Med. Vet. Mycol.* **33:**287–289.

39. **Sekhon, A. S., J. S. K. Li, and A. K. Garg.** 1982. Penicilliosis marneffei: serological and exoantigen studies. *Mycopathologia* **77:**51–57.

40. **Venditti, M., A. Micozzi, G. Gentile, L. Polonelli, G. Morace, P. Bianco, P. Avvisati, G. Papa, and P. Martino.** 1988. Invasive *Fusarium solani* infections in patients with acute leukemia. *Rev. Infect. Dis.* **10:**653–660.

41. **Wheeler, M. H., and A. A. Bell.** 1987. Melanins and their importance in pathogenic fungi. *Curr. Top. Med. Mycol.* **2:**338–387.

42. **White, M. H., and D. Armstrong.** 1994. Cryptococcosis. *Infect. Dis. Clin. North Am.* **8:**383–398.

chapter 10

Streptococcal Disease

Monica M. Farley and Ronald Neafie

n the past decade, several streptococcal infections have emerged (or reemerged) as important clinical problems. These include invasive group A streptococcal (GAS) disease, acute rheumatic fever (ARF), and drug-resistant pneumococcal infections. The reasons for the recent reemergence of severe manifestations of invasive GAS disease and outbreaks of ARF are unclear. One potential explanation is the circulation of rheumatogenic strains or particularly virulent strains producing exotoxins, capsules, and cross-reactive M protein epitopes. Alternatively, the presence of a large susceptible population lacking preexisting humoral immunity may be partially responsible for the resurgence.

Epidemiology

Increased reports of serious manifestations of invasive GAS infections have been noted since the mid-1980s (2, 6, 21, 30). Cases of rapidly fatal pneumonia, toxic shock syndrome, and necrotizing fasciitis (the "flesh-eating"

Monica M. Farley, Atlanta VA Medical Center and Division of Infectious Diseases, Emory University School of Medicine, 69 Butler Street, S.E., Atlanta, GA 30303. **Ronald Neafie,** Parasitic Disease Pathology Branch, Geographic Pathology Division, Armed Forces Institute of Pathology, Washington, DC 20306-6000.

Pathology of Emerging Infections
Edited by C. Robert Horsburgh, Jr., and Ann Marie Nelson
© 1997 American Society for Microbiology, Washington, DC 20005-4171

The incidence of invasive disease is highest in the young and the elderly

infection) have stimulated renewed interest in GAS. More than half the cases of invasive GAS infection occur in individuals between 10 and 65 years of age, with a mean age of 40.8 years. However, the incidence of invasive disease is highest in the young and the elderly. The overall annual incidence is 5 cases per 100,000 population. Among individuals <10 years of age, the incidence is 8.1/100,000; in individuals 10 to 65 years of age, it is 3.4/100,000; and in those over 65 years of age, it is 13.3/100,000. The overall mortality is 21%, with many of the deaths occurring in elderly patients. Certain underlying or concurrent conditions may increase the risk of invasive GAS infections. Approximately 39% of children with invasive GAS infection had concurrent varicella infections. Skin disorders, chronic heart and lung disease, diabetes, and malignancy are common underlying conditions noted in adults with invasive GAS disease.

Despite a dramatic and sustained decline in the incidence of ARF earlier in this century, an increase in the number of reports has been noted in recent years (7, 27, 28). A number of outbreaks of ARF have occurred in the United States in the last decade, despite a lack of change in the prevalence of pharyngitis. In contrast to epidemiologic characteristics of ARF in the pre-World War II era, recent cases have most often affected suburban or rural white populations that are well above the poverty line. However, the epidemiologic association with crowding, which can occur in settings such as households with large families and military camps, remains. School-aged children are affected most commonly, but recent outbreaks have involved a significant number of adults.

A recent study of invasive pneumococcal disease in Atlanta, Ga., demonstrated the striking emergence of significant levels of antibiotic resistance in the community (10). Five hundred twenty-seven cases of invasive pneumococcal disease occurred over a 10-month period in 1994; the mean age of patients was 35.3 years (range, 2 days to 94 years). Fifty-five percent were African-American, 44% were white, and 1% were Asian or other racial or ethnic groups. The annual incidence of invasive pneumococcal disease was 30 cases per 100,000 population (18 cases per 100,000 for whites and 58 cases per 100,000 for African-Americans). The prevalence of antimicrobial resistance is shown in Table 10.1.

Drug resistance was found in isolates from both children and adults; penicillin resistance in isolates from children less than 6 years of age was 27% compared with 24% in isolates from all others. Isolates from young children were more likely to be cefotaxime resistant or multiple drug resistant. A higher proportion of whites were infected with penicillin-resistant or multidrug-resistant isolates (32 and 30%, respectively) than African-Americans (19 and 20%, respectively). White children under 6 years of age were at the highest risk of being infected with a resistant isolate: 41% of the isolates had some level of resistance to penicillin, 22% had some resistance to cefotaxime, and 47% had some resistance to multiple antibiotics. Several studies have identified the following risk factors for the development and transmission of resistant pneumococci: intensive antimicrobial use, confined and/or crowded conditions, and large numbers of children in close person-to-person contact, such as in day care centers (1, 4, 10, 16).

Table 10.1 Pneumococcal antimicrobial resistance—Atlanta, 1994

Antimicrobial agent and resistance	% Nonsusceptible
Penicillin	
Intermediate	18
High level	7
Total	25
Cefotaxime	
Intermediate	5
High level	4
Total	9
TMP/SMX[a]	
Intermediate	18
High level	7
Total	26
Multi-drug resistance[b]	25

[a] TMP/SMX, trimethoprim-sulfamethoxazole.
[b] Resistance to two or more drugs.

Clinical Manifestations

The clinical manifestations of invasive GAS infection may vary from a relatively mild bacteremia to severe, life- or limb-threatening disease. Specific syndromes include sepsis and bacteremia, necrotizing fasciitis and myositis, and streptococcal toxic shock syndrome (STSS) (23). An abbreviated STSS case definition is shown in Table 10.2.

Necrotizing fasciitis and STSS may occur concurrently and are the most serious manifestations of invasive GAS infection. Skin and soft tissues are the primary focus of infection in the majority of patients; respiratory infections and bacteremia from an unknown source are the next most common infections (6, 21). Severe pain that is out of proportion to the initial skin and soft tissue findings has been cited as a predictor of necrotizing fasciitis. Fever and hypotension are common findings. Laboratory abnormalities may include leukocytosis, thrombocytopenia, disseminated intravascular coagu-

Table 10.2 STSS case definition (abbreviated)

Definite case = 1A + 2A + 2B
1. Isolation of group A streptococci
    A. From normally sterile site
    B. From nonsterile site
2. Clinical signs of severity
    A. Hypotension: systolic BP[a] of ≤90 mm Hg in adults or <5th percentile for age in children
    B. ≥2 of the following
        1. Renal impairment
        2. Coagulopathy
        3. Liver involvement
        4. Acute respiratory distress syndrome
        5. Generalized rash
        6. Soft-tissue necrosis or gangrene

[a] BP, blood pressure.

lation, and hypoalbuminemia. Creatine phosphokinase (CPK) is often elevated with necrotizing fasciitis. In contrast to the findings with staphylococcal TSS, blood cultures are usually positive in STSS. However, pharyngeal cultures are rarely positive. Necrotizing fasciitis is rare in children. The mortality ranges between 30 and 60% among patients with STSS and/or necrotizing fasciitis, with most deaths occurring in adults.

The revised Jones criteria for the diagnosis of ARF are shown in Table 10.3 (20). In recent ARF outbreaks, arthritis was reported in 47 to 100% of cases, while carditis was noted in 30 to 72% of cases. Only one-quarter to one-third of patients reported symptoms of pharyngitis significant enough to seek medical care preceding the onset of ARF. In one study, only 12% of children received antibiotic treatment for pharyngitis. The majority of patients with ARF have measurable streptococcal antibodies. However, very few have GAS recoverable from throat cultures.

Bacterial Characteristics

M protein serotypes 1, 3, and 12 are most commonly associated with serious invasive GAS infections, but a wide variety of M types have been isolated (23, 25). Streptococcal pyrogenic exotoxin A expression has also been associated with serious GAS disease. Streptococcal pyrogenic exotoxin A has been shown to be a superantigen and a potent inducer of tumor necrosis factor. A mucoid phenotype that reflects the presence of a hyaluronic capsule is more common in invasive disease than in uncomplicated infections (21 versus 3%). GAS protease production has been associated with necrotizing fasciitis. A number of M protein serotypes have been associated with ARF (rheumatogenic strains), including types 1, 3, 5, 6, and 18. Rheumatogenic serotypes may contain epitopes shared with human tissues (24). Up to half of GAS isolates associated with ARF demonstrate the mucoid phenotype.

Penicillin resistance in pneumococci results from the synthesis of high-molecular-weight penicillin-binding proteins (PBPs) with reduced binding affinity for penicillin G (26). High-level resistance is associated with multiple abnormal PBPs. Penicillin resistance is acquired through genetic recom-

Table 10.3 Revised Jones criteria for diagnosis of acute rheumatic fever[a]

Major manifestations	Minor manifestations[b]
Polyarthritis	Clinical:
Carditis	Arthralgias
Arthritis	Fever
Chorea	Laboratory:
Subcutaneous nodules	Elevated acute phase reactants
Erythema marginatum	Erythrocyte sedimentation rate
	C-Reactive Protein
	Prolonged PR interval on EKG

[a] If supported by evidence of preceding streptococcal infection, the presence of two major or one major and two minor manifestations indicates a high probability of acute rheumatic fever.

[b] Plus supporting evidence of preceding streptococcal infection: throat culture or rapid streptococcal antigen test, increased or rising streptococcal antibodies.

bination with genes encoding PBPs from penicillin-resistant commensal bacteria and through horizontal transfer to other pneumococci. Cephalosporin and penicillin resistance may involve different PBPs (11). Both single-step and incremental acquisition of cephalosporin resistance have been demonstrated. The mechanisms for acquisition of other resistance genes (e.g., Tm/Sulfa, Tcn, and Ery) are less well understood.

Oxacillin disk testing (1 mg/ml) is a reliable qualitative screening test for penicillin and cephalosporin resistance. The method is highly sensitive but less specific for pneumococcal resistance. The E-test strip, which contains an antibiotic concentration gradient, provides quantitative data, and its relative simplicity and low cost make it particularly suitable for clinical laboratories. Minimal inhibitory concentrations (MICs) can best be assessed by broth dilution using Mueller-Hinton broth supplemented with lysed horse blood.

The following susceptibility standards for penicillin have been adopted (15a):

- Sensitive = <0.12 µg/ml
- Intermediate = 0.12–1.2 µg/ml
- High-level resistance = ≥2 µg/ml

Six pneumococcal serotypes (14, 6B, 9V, 23F, 19A, and 6A) account for over 85% of isolates resistant to penicillin, cefotaxime, or multiple drugs (10). Serotype 23F is significantly associated with cefotaxime resistance and high-level resistance to both cefotaxime and penicillin; among 15 isolates with high-level penicillin and cefotaxime resistance in the Atlanta study, 13 were serotype 23F, one was 6A, and one was 6B.

Pathophysiology

GAS infection of the deep tissues, also called necrotizing fasciitis, is an uncommon, acute necrotizing process that involves the fascia and subcutaneous tissue (29). It was first described in 1924 by Meleney (12) who called the condition "streptococcal gangrene." Although necrotizing fasciitis was first ascribed exclusively to group A beta-hemolytic streptococci, recent reports have shown that a variety of bacteria can cause it (3, 5). This disease, also referred to as "flesh-eating" bacterial infection, should probably be considered a clinical entity and not a specific bacterial infection.

Regardless of the etiologic agent, the histopathologic features of necrotizing fasciitis are very similar. The epidermis may be spared or involved. The epidermis may become necrotic and infiltrated with neutrophils; bullae may form. The upper dermis may be involved by edema, necrosis, and inflammation. Subepidermal vesicles and blister formation can be prominent features. Vascular ectasia may be prominent throughout the dermis, and vessels may be dilated and stuffed with erythrocytes. The deep dermis and panniculus are infiltrated with inflammatory cells, and there is a massive necrotizing process.

Lesions show intense edema, granulation tissue, hemorrhage, and frank abscess formation. There is inflammation of the septae with necrosis and

Although necrotizing fasciitis was first ascribed exclusively to group A beta-hemolytic streptococci, recent reports have shown that a variety of bacteria can cause it

acute inflammation extending into the fat lobule. Intravascular thrombosis is frequently present. The inflammation and necrosis occasionally extend into adjacent muscle. An exaggerated superantigen-mediated immune response is likely to contribute to the severity of GAS disease (13).

The causative bacterium can frequently be found in hematoxylin and eosin-stained sections of the lesion, although they may not be uniformly distributed. Special stains, including the Brown-Hopps Gram, Brown-Brenn Gram, Giemsa, and Gomori methenamine silver, are frequently necessary to properly demonstrate the etiologic agent. *Streptococcus pyogenes* occurs as spherical or ovoid cells 0.6 to 1.0 µm in diameter. They form pairs and short to moderate chains. They are gram-positive facultative anaerobes.

Streptococcus pneumoniae lives harmlessly in the upper respiratory tract of humans. However, *S. pneumoniae* causes 60% of all culturally proven cases of acute pneumonias in the United States (19). In children, it is the leading cause of acute bacteremia, otitis media, sinusitis, and bacterial meningitis (15). It also causes a variety of other uncommon infectious diseases, such as tubo-ovarian abscess (9). Regardless of the organ involved, *S. pneumoniae* causes a purulent exudate.

S. pneumoniae is the most common cause of lobar pneumonia and a lesser cause of bronchopneumonia. On the basis of the duration of the reaction, lobar pneumonia can be divided into four histologic phases:

- Phase I is marked by multiplication of the diplococcus and prominent edema that enables the bacteria to spread between alveoli. Neutrophils migrate into the alveoli.
- Phase II is characterized by early consolidation. The involved lobe has a redness caused primarily by marked hyperemia. The alveolar fluid is replaced by numerous neutrophils, fine strands of fibrin, and some erythrocytes. Pneumococci are abundant.
- Phase III is that of gray hepatization, a gradual transformation. The fluid portion of the exudate has been removed and replaced by abundant fibrin. Mononuclear cells increasingly become a component of the exudate. The pneumococci decrease in number and are found predominantly within mononuclear cells.
- Phase IV is the stage of resolution, as the exudate softens and the fibrin undergoes lysis. There are large numbers of macrophages that engulf neutrophils and debris. The diplococci are gone. In most instances, full anatomic and functional restitution is to be expected.

S. pneumoniae are oval or spherical, coccal-like forms 0.5 to 1.25 µm in diameter that occur typically in pairs and sometimes singly or in short chains. The distal end of each pair tends to be pointed or lance shaped. They are gram-positive facultative anaerobes.

Treatment

GAS are highly susceptible to penicillin, and high-dose penicillin G remains an effective treatment for uncomplicated invasive GAS infections. However, the treatment recommendations vary somewhat for more severe

> *The causative bacterium can frequently be found in hematoxylin and eosin-stained sections of the lesion, although they may not be uniformly distributed*

invasive disease, particularly STSS and necrotizing fasciitis. A phenomenon known as the "Eagle effect" results in reduced efficacy of penicillin in eradicating streptococci from tissue sites if the organisms are present in very high concentrations (22). The effect may be due to a slow rate of replication (most organisms in stationary phase) and diminished expression of penicillin-binding proteins. Clindamycin has been shown to be superior to penicillin in a mouse model of myositis. In theory, clindamycin may decrease production of M proteins and potentially harmful exotoxins. Most experts recommend the combination of penicillin and clindamycin for treatment of STSS and necrotizing fasciitis. The use of intravenous immunoglobulin infusion as adjuvant therapy for severe GAS infections is currently under investigation.

The optimal therapy for infections with drug-resistant pneumococci is not well defined. Studies have suggested that cephalosporins or high-dose penicillin may be effective in patients with nonmeningeal bacteremic infections if the MIC of penicillin is 2 μg/ml or less (8, 18). In the setting of suspected pneumococcal meningitis or other life-threatening pneumococcal infection, the use of both an extended-spectrum cephalosporin and vancomycin should be strongly considered until results of susceptibility testing are available (17). For the treatment of less serious infections, the addition of vancomycin is currently not routinely recommended.

Prevention

With the continuing spread of drug-resistant strains of pneumococci, treatment options for invasive disease will become more limited and prevention measures will become more critical. The prevention of infections with invasive drug-resistant pneumococci will require strategies to encourage judicious antibiotic use and to optimize immunization with the 23-valent pneumococcal vaccine in targeted populations. Pneumococcal conjugate vaccines hold promise for the prevention of invasive disease in children under 2 years of age and are currently under evaluation (14).

Figure 10.1 Severe group A streptococcal cellulitis of the lower extremity.

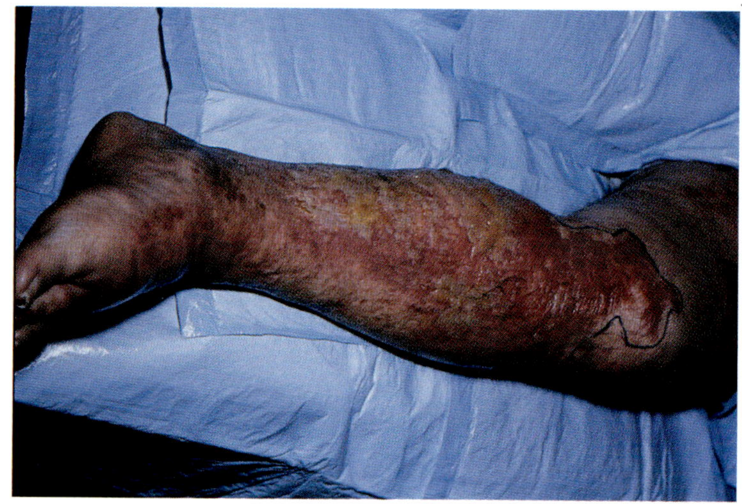

Figure 10.2 Bullous lesion in patient with GAS necrotizing faciitis. Courtesy of Dr. Larry Slack, Vanderbilt University.

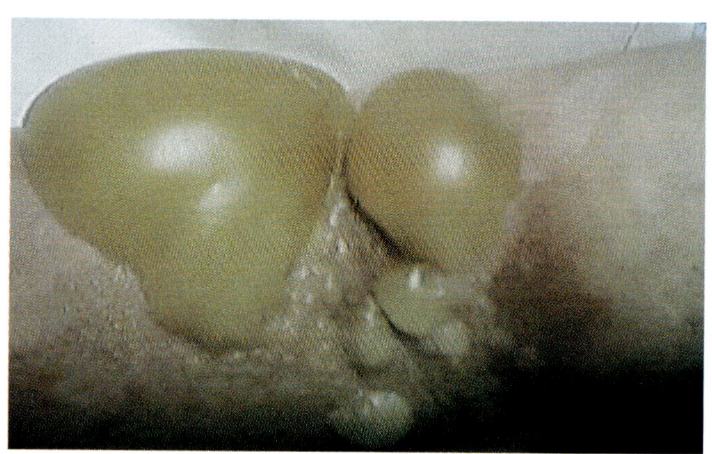

Figure 10.3 E-test method of pneumococcal sensitivity testing showing intermediate resistance to penicillin G (MIC, 0.5 µg/ml).

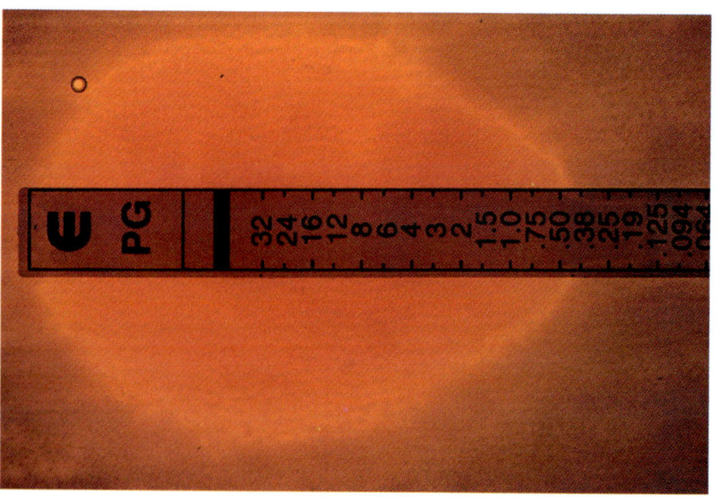

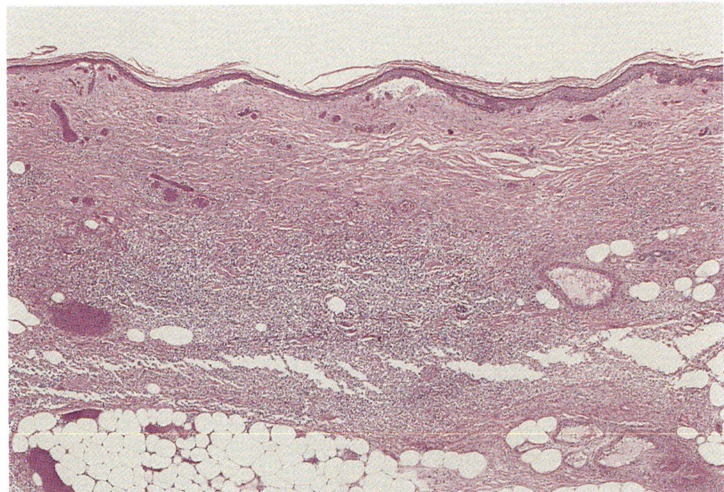

Figure 10.4 Necrotizing fasciitis in the skin and subcutis of the left lower leg in a 64-year-old man from California. A predominantly neutrophilic infiltrate is concentrated in the lower dermis and panniculus (hematoxylin and eosin; original magnification, ×10).

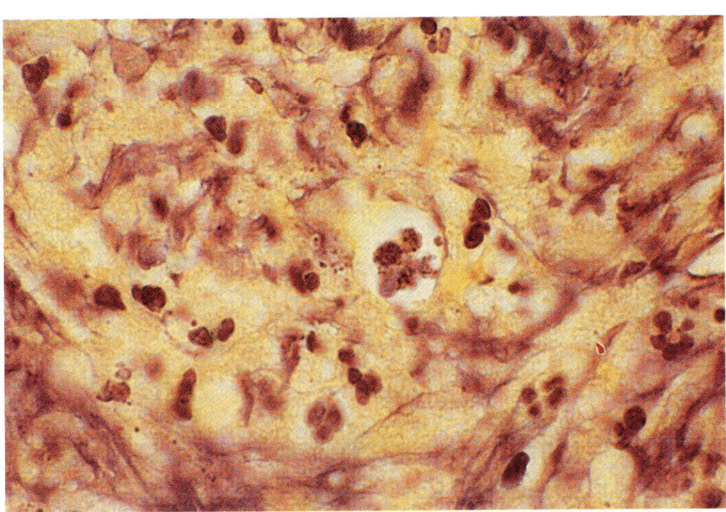

Figure 10.5 Necrotizing fasciitis in the skin and subcutis of the left thigh in a 31-year-old patient. Intracellular gram-positive cocci are centered in areas of necrosis. A group A beta-hemolytic streptococcus was cultured (B&H; original magnification, ×330).

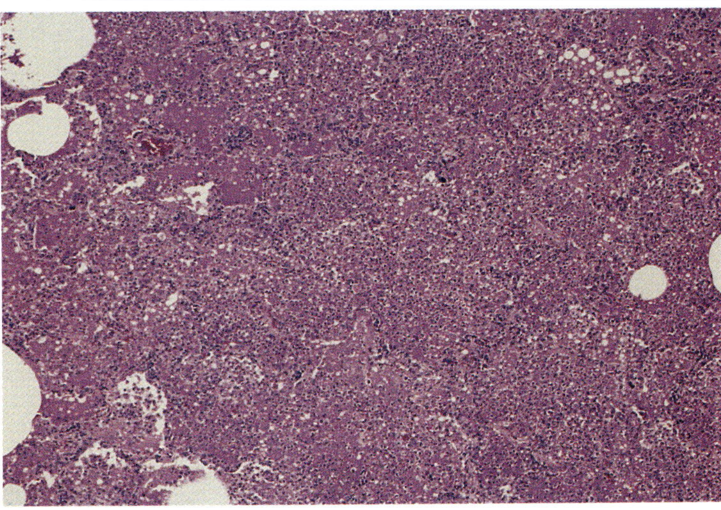

Figure 10.6A *S. pneumoniae* from the lung of a 48-year-old Zairian who died of pneumococcal pneumonia. The lung is consolidated, and there are large numbers of neutrophils and small numbers of histiocytes within the alveoli (hematoxylin and eosin; original magnification, ×25).

Figure 10.6B   Same patient as in Fig. 10.6A. Large numbers of gram-positive diplococci are within the exudate. The diplococci are lancet shaped and 1 to 3 μm long (B&H; original magnification, ×330).

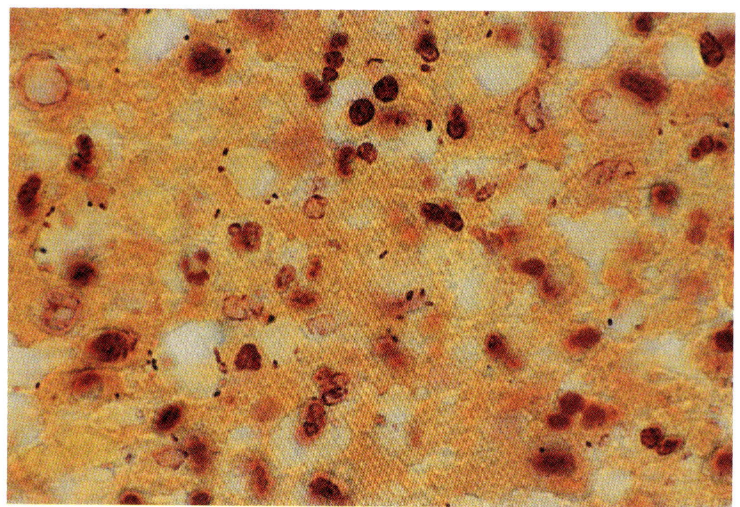

References

1. **Breiman, R. F., J. C. Butler, F. C. Tenover, J. A. Elliott, and R. R. Facklam.** 1994. Emergence of drug-resistant pneumococcal infection in the United States. *JAMA* **271:**1831–1835.

2. **Bronze, M. S., and J. B. Dale.** 1996. The reemergence of serious group A streptococcal infection and acute rheumatic fever. *Am. J. Med. Sci.* **311:**41–54.

3. **Brook, I., and E. H. Frazier.** 1995. Clinical and microbiological features of necrotizing fasciitis. *J. Clin. Microbiol.* **33:**2382–2387.

4. **Centers for Disease Control.** 1994. Drug resistant *Streptococcus pneumoniae*—Kentucky and Tennessee, 1993. *Morbid. Mortal. Weekly Rep.* **43:**23–31.

5. **Choudhri, S. H., R. Brownstone, F. Hashem, C. M. Magro, and A. N. Crowson.** 1995. A case of necrotizing fasciitis due to *Streptococcus pneumoniae. Br. J. Derm.* **133:**128–131.

6. **Demers, B., A. E. Simor, H. Vellend, P. M. Schlievert, S. Bryne, F. Jamieson, S. Walmsley, and D. E. Low.** 1993. Severe invasive group A streptococcal infections in Ontario, Canada: 1987–1991. *Clin. Infect. Dis.* **16:**792–800.

7. **Ferguson, G. W., J. M. Shultz, and A. L. Bisno.** 1991. Epidemiology of acute rheumatic fever in a multiethnic, multiracial urban community: the Miami-Dade County experience. *J. Infect. Dis.* **164:**720–725.

8. **Friedland, I. R., M. Med, and G. H. McCracken, Jr.** 1994. Management of infections caused by antibiotic-resistant *Streptococcus pneumoniae. N. Engl. J. Med.* **331:**377–382.

9. **Hadfield, T. L., R. C. Neafie, and L. O. Lanoie.** 1990. Tubo-ovarian abscess caused by Streptococcus pneumoniae. *Hum. Pathol.* **21:**188–189.

10. **Hofmann, J., M. S. Cetron, M. M. Farley, W. S. Baughman, R. R. Facklam, J. A. Elliott, K. A. Deaver, and R. F. Breiman**. 1995. The prevalence of drug-resistant *Streptococcus pneumoniae* in Atlanta. *N. Engl. J. Med.* **333:**481–486.

11. **Klugman, K. P., I. R. Friedland, and J. S. Bradley.** 1995. Bactericidal activity against cephalosporin-resistant *Streptococcus pneumoniae* in cerebrospinal fluid of children with acute bacterial meningitis. *Antimicrob. Agents Chemother.* **39:**1988–1992.

12. **Meleney, F. L.** 1924. Hemolytic streptococcus gangrene. *Arch. Surg.* **9:**317–364.

13. **Michie, C., A. Scott, J. Cheesborough, P. Beverley, and G. Pascal.** 1994. Streptococcal toxic shock-like syndrome: evidence of superantigen activity and its effects on T lymphocyte subsets in vivo. *Clin. Exp. Immunol.* **98:**140–144.

14. **Munford, R. S., and T. V. Murphy.** 1994. Antimicrobial resistance in *Streptococcus pneumoniae*: can immunization prevent its spread? *J. Invest. Med.* **42:**613–621.

15. **Musher, D. M.** 1992. Infections caused by Streptococcus pneumoniae: clinical spectrum, pathogenesis, immunity, and treatment. *Clin. Infect. Dis.* **14:**801.

15a. **National Committee for Clinical Laboratory Standards.** 1994. *Performance Standards for Antimicrobial Susceptibility Testing.* Fifth informational supplement, M100-S5. National Committee for Clinical Laboratory Standards, Villanova, Pa.

16. **Pallares, R., J. Linares, M. Vadillo, C. Cabellos, F. Manresa, P. F. Viladrich, R. Martin, and F. Gudiol.** 1995. Resistance to penicillin and cephalosporin and mortality from severe pneumococcal pneumonia in Barcelona, Spain. *N. Engl. J. Med.* **333:**474–480.

17. **Paris, M. M., S. M. Hickey, M. I. Uscher, S. Shelton, K. D. Olsen, and G. H. McCracken.** 1994. Effect of dexamethasone on therapy of experimental penicillin- and cephalosporin-resistant pneumococcal meningitis. *Antimicrob. Agents Chemother.* **38:**1320–1324.

18. **Paris, M. M., O. Ramilo, and G. H. McCracken.** 1995. Management of meningitis caused by penicillin-resistant *Streptococcus pneumoniae*. *Antimicrob. Agents Chemother.* **39:**2171–2175.

19. **Simon, H. B.** 1983. Gram positive cocci, p. 1E. *In* E. Rubenstein and D. D. Federman (ed.), *Scientific American Medicine.* Scientific American, Inc., New York.

20. **Special Writing Group of the Committee on Rheumatic Fever, Endocarditis, and Kawasaki Disease of the Council on Cardiovascular Disease in the Young of the American Heart Association.** 1992. Guidelines for the diagnosis of rheumatic fever. *JAMA* **268:**2969–2973.

21. **Stevens, D. L.** 1992. Invasive group A streptococcus infections. *Clin. Infect. Dis.* **14:**2–13.

22. **Stevens, D. L., A. E. Gibbons, R. Bergstrom, and V. Winn.** 1988. The eagle effect revisited: efficacy of clindamycin, erythromycin, and penicillin in the treatment of streptococcal myositis. *J. Infect. Dis.* **158:**23–28.

23. **Stevens, D. L., M. H. Tanner, J. Winship, R. Swarts, K. M. Ries, P. M. Schlievert, and E. Kaplan.** 1989. Severe group A streptococcal infections associated with a toxic shock-like syndrome and scarlet fever toxin A. *N. Engl. J. Med.* **321:**1–8.

24. **Stollerman, G. H.** 1993. Variation in group A streptococci and the prevalence of rheumatic fever: a half-century vigil. *Ann. Intern. Med.* **118:**467–469.

25. **Talkington, D. F., B. Schwartz, C. M. Black, J. K. Todd, J. Elliott, R. F. Breiman, and R. R. Facklam.** 1993. Association of phenotypic and genotypic characteristics of invasive *Streptococcus pyogenes* isolates with clinical components of streptococcal toxic shock syndrome. *Infect. Immun.* **61:**3369–3374.

26. **Tomasz, A., and R. Munoz.** 1995. Beta-lactam antibiotic resistance in gram-positive bacterial pathogens of the upper respiratory tract: a brief overview of mechanisms. *Microb. Drug Resist.* **1(2):**103–108.

27. **Veasy, L. G., S. E. Wiedmeier, G. S. Orsmond, H. D. Ruttenberg, M. M. Boucek, S. J. Roth, V. F. Tait, J. A. Thompson, J. A. Daly, and E. L. Kaplan.** 1987. Resurgence of acute rheumatic fever in the intermountain area of the United States. *N. Engl. J. Med.* **316:**421–427.

28. **Wallace, M. R., P. D. Garst, T. J. Papadimos, and E. C. Oldfield III.** 1989. The return of acute rheumatic fever in young adults. *JAMA* **262:**2557–2561.

29. **Wilkerson, R., W. Paull, and F. V. Coville.** 1987. Necrotizing fasciitis: review of the literature and case report. *Clin. Ortho.* **216:**187–192.

30. **The Working Group on Severe Streptococcal Infections.** 1993. The Working Group on Severe Streptococcal Infections. *JAMA* **269:**390–391.

chapter 11

Bartonella Infections

Molly Eaton and Ann Marie Nelson

Bartonellae are small gram-negative rods that belong to the alpha-2 subgroup of the class *Proteobacteria* most closely related to *Brucella abortus*. Three species are now identified as important causes of disease in humans: *Bartonella bacilliformis*, *Bartonella quintana*, and *Bartonella henselae* (7, 29). The two original infections ascribed to the bartonellae (formerly rochalimae) attracted minimal attention because of limited geographic distribution (*B. bacilliformis*) or limited mortality (*B. quintana*).

In the early 1900s, *B. bacilliformis* was recognized as the cause of Oroyo fever and verruga peruana, two phases of the same illness. Oroyo fever derives its name from the epidemic of 1870 that killed 7,000 railroad workers on the Lima-Oroyo line (4). Verruga peruana, characterized by eruptive skin lesions, was described in ancient times; pre-Columbian artifacts indicate that the disease was present in the mountains of Peru and the coastal province of Manabi, Ecuador, at least 1,000 years prior to the arrival of Europeans (2, 38). Bartonellosis is sometimes referred to as Carrion's disease, in honor of the medical student Daniel Carrion, who died of Oroyo fever af-

Molly Eaton, Division of Infectious Diseases, Emory University School of Medicine, 69 Butler Street, S.E., Atlanta, GA 30303. **Ann Marie Nelson,** Division of AIDS Pathology, Department of Infectious and Parasitic Disease Pathology, Armed Forces Institute of Pathology, Washington, DC 20306-6000.

Pathology of Emerging Infections
Edited by C. Robert Horsburgh, Jr., and Ann Marie Nelson
© 1997 American Society for Microbiology, Washington, DC 20005-4171

ter inoculating himself with organisms from a verruga lesion. Decades later, Noguchi produced the eruptive lesion in monkeys with organisms cultured from a patient with Oroyo fever (4, 38). Thus, modern science was able to prove the belief held by native Peruvians that the two diseases were different phases of the same process.

Trench fever, a louse-borne febrile illness caused by *B. quintana*, was epidemic in both World Wars. In World War I, as many as a million soldiers contracted the "five-day fever," Wolhynia (42). Since the infection was nonfatal and rarely occurred outside of these epidemics, it was of little interest.

Although the French physician Debré recognized patients with cat scratch disease (CSD) in 1931, he did not formally report his findings until 1950 (14). By the mid-1950s, CSD was recognized as a relatively common cause of regional lymphadenitis, especially affecting children. As early as 1889, Parinaud described an infectious conjunctivitis that he thought was transmitted from animals to humans (30). Verhoeff described filamentous organisms within these oculoglandular lesions that he thought were an unusual mycotic infection (47). The cause of both of these diseases remained elusive until 1983, when Wear and colleagues at the Armed Forces Institute of Pathology (AFIP) detected pleomorphic bacilli in lymph nodes from patients with CSD by using the Warthin-Starry method of silver impregnation (51). Two years later, the same group demonstrated CSD bacilli in lesions of patients with Parinaud's oculoglandular syndrome (50). In 1988, English et al. cultured an organism later named *Afipia felis* (6) from lymph nodes of 10 patients with CSD (18). *A. felis* causes some cases of CSD, but subsequent studies (culture, serology, and polymerase chain reaction [PCR]) indicated that *B. henselae* is the most common etiologic agent (15, 34, 45).

Also in 1983, Stoler and colleagues first described a patient with AIDS who developed multiple subcutaneous nodules (41). These pseudoneoplastic vascular proliferations were infiltrated by small bacillary forms seen only with Warthin-Starry techniques. It was another 5 years before others began to recognize this syndrome, bacillary angiomatosis (BA). Although organisms were easily seen in tissues, usual microbiologic techniques were unsuccessful in growing the bacteria. Novel techniques for unculturable pathogens identified the organisms as belonging to the genus *Rochalimaea* (36) and later were used for their reclassification into the genus *Bartonella* (7). Imaginative culture techniques led to successful isolation of the organisms from blood, skin lesions, and solid organs of patients with BA (20, 39, 44, 52).

The recognition of organisms from the genus *Bartonella* as the cause of CSD and BA stimulated increased interest in the genus. These organisms have since been found to cause other syndromes, including fever of unknown etiology and culture-negative endocarditis, especially in the homeless (17, 35, 40). The full spectrum of disease(s) caused by bartonellae may not yet be elucidated.

Bacteriology

The organisms now classified as the genus *Bartonella* of the alpha-2 subdivision of the *Proteobacteria* were combined from a divergent group of infectious agents (7). In the 1900s, Barton identified small bacilli in erythrocytes of pa-

> *A. felis causes some cases of CSD, but studies have indicated that B. henselae is the most common etiologic agent*

tients with Oroyo fever (38). This organism, *B. bacilliformis*, considered an obligate intracellular parasite, was classified in the order *Rickettsiales*, family *Bartonellaceae*. *B. quintana* (originally *Rochalimaea quintana*, order *Rickettsiales*, family *Rickettsiaceae*) was cultured on acellular media from patients in Mexico City with trench fever in the 1960s and could therefore no longer be considered an obligate intracellular parasite (48). Gram-negative, argyrophilic bacteria from lymph nodes of patients with CSD were identified in 1983 by Wear et al. (51) and were later cultured by English and Wear and colleagues in 1988 (18). *Rochalimaea henselae* was first cultured from patients with bacteremia in 1990 and from patients with BA and peliosis hepatis in 1991 by Slater et al. and Welch et al. in Oklahoma (39, 52); it was cultured from patients with CSD by Lucey's laboratory in Texas in 1990 (49).

BA was emerging as a complication of human immunodeficiency virus (HIV) infection during this same period (3, 11, 19). Histologic identification of argyrophilic organisms similar to the CSD bacillus and the recognition that these reactive vascular proliferations resembled the little known verruga peruana led to a series of molecular and microbiologic studies that united these seemingly diverse diseases. Attempts to culture the organisms of BA were initially unsuccessful, but phylogenetic DNA analysis of the 16S rRNA gene sequences revealed that the organisms were more closely related to members of the order *Proteobacteria* than members of the order *Rickettsiales* (29). Relman demonstrated homology with *R. quintana*, leading to the name *R. henselae*. PCR techniques using primers and probes specific for *Rochalimaea* spp. have been used to detect rochalimal DNA in tissues of patients with BA and CSD, and material from skin test antigens has been used to diagnose CSD (15, 31, 36). Subsequent studies showed >98% RNA homology with *B. bacilliformis* and led to the reclassification of these organisms into the genus *Bartonella* (7). Species of *Afipia* are unique but are closely related by a unique fatty acid, 11-methyloctadec-12-enoic acid, found on gas chromatography (49).

Bartonella species can now be cultured, although with difficulty. Enriched erythrocyte media (brain heart infusion or tryptic soy broth and agar with rabbit or sheep blood) or chocolate agar are recommended with incubation at 35 to 37°C in 5% CO_2. Growth requires 7 to 30 days (or more) and is often missed in blood culture systems unless the laboratory is alerted to keep the cultures and to perform stains and/or subcultures at appropriate intervals. Lysis centrifugation appears to be the most sensitive method of detecting these organisms. Initial colonies on agar are embedded in the media and are cauliflower-like; with subsequent passages, the colonies become raised and transparent. There may be morphologic heterogeneity in the same culture (9, 39 ,44, 52). The organisms are slightly curved, pleomorphic gram-negative rods measuring 0.5 to 0.6 by 1.0 to 2.0 µm. They exhibit ratchety motility. *B. bacilliformis* has multiple polar flagella. Biochemical reactions with oxidase, urease, and catalase are negative in all species. Goat sera or other systems such as PCR and gas-liquid chromatography are used to identify the bacteria (37). Diagnosis of BA is still made by biopsy in most cases, although culture and indirect fluorescent-antibody tests (IFA) may be confirmatory.

Lysis centrifugation appears to be the most sensitive method of detecting Bartonella spp.

Epidemiology and Clinical Manifestations of Bartonellosis

The acute phase of bartonellosis, Oroyo fever, is characterized by the sudden onset of fever, chills, myalgia, and hemolysis, which can be profound

Bartonellosis, or Carrion's disease, is found only in the river valleys of Peru, Ecuador, and Colombia, on both slopes of the Andes Mountains between 800 and 2,500 meters. This area corresponds to the habitat of the phlebotomine sandfly vector that transmits the *Bartonella* bacteria. The incubation period between the nocturnal bite of the sandfly and onset of symptoms may range from 7 to 100 days (2, 4, 16, 53). The acute phase of illness, Oroyo fever, is characterized by the sudden onset of fever, chills, myalgia, and hemolysis, which can be profound. The bacteria invade virtually all peripheral erythrocytes, resulting in macrocytic anemia (mild in survivors and severe in fatal cases). Reticulocyte counts can reach 50%. Case-fatality rates of untreated cases range from 40 to 90%, with most patients dying of infectious complications such as salmonellosis or malaria. Asymptomatic infection is common (16, 53).

From one to several months after the acute phase subsides, the verrucous phase, known as verruga peruana, develops. Skin lesions begin as subcutaneous nodules and rapidly enlarge; clinically they resemble pyogenic granuloma, although they bleed much more easily. This eruptive phase may last 4 to 6 months and is often recurrent. Eruptions may be miliary or nodular. Miliary lesions are small and occur in crops, usually on extensor surfaces. Nodular lesions are larger and fewer in number, may bleed profusely, and may be deeper in the subcutaneous tissue and quite painful (4, 16, 53). During this phase, the patient is otherwise asymptomatic. Without antibiotic treatment, the lesions regress over several months, leaving a scar.

Pathophysiology of Bartonellosis

The organism enters the blood during the bite of the sandfly, and the bacteria adhere to the erythrocytes and enter through a vacuole. They replicate within the vacuole, causing an alteration of the cytoskeleton with increased erythrocyte fragility and hemolytic anemia (often severe) (5, 38). In fatal cases of Oroyo fever, autopsy reveals extreme pallor and/or jaundice of the viscera, hepatosplenomegaly, and hyperplasia of the bone marrow. Organisms are found on erythrocytes and in reticuloendothelial cells. The infected cells are markedly enlarged and packed with organisms. There is erythrophagocytosis in the Kupffer cells, centrilobular necrosis of the liver, and significant hemosiderosis of both the liver and the spleen. Thrombosis and infarction are common (4, 16).

Histologically, the verruga peruana presents as a granulomatous reaction with an associated vascular proliferation that causes an elevation of the epidermis (4, 5, 16). In larger lesions, an epidermal collarette surrounds the superficial portion, where there is also edema and necrosis. In the deeper parts of the lesion, one sees increased cellularity, with a predominance of neutrophils and endothelial cells. Macrophages, mast cells, and plasma cells are also present. Endothelial swelling and neutrophilic vasculitis are common.

In ulcerated lesions there is an increase in the acute inflammatory component. Organisms are easily seen by silver impregnation methods. Electron microscopy of verruga peruana shows organisms in various stages of the life cycle within the stroma of the lesion and in neutrophils but not in endothelial cells or macrophages (5).

Epidemiology and Clinical Manifestations of Trench Fever and *Bartonella* Bacteremia and Endocarditis

Trench fever is an acute febrile disease resembling typhus. It is caused by louse-borne transmission of B. *quintana* and was epidemic in Europe during World War I and II (33, 35, 42). There have also been reported outbreaks in Africa and Mexico. Although it is seldom recognized outside of epidemics, it probably does persist in populations with chronic louse infestation. B. *quintana* infections causing some cases of BA have been documented in HIV-seropositive patients. There are several recent reports of febrile illnesses associated with blood cultures that are positive for B. *quintana* in homeless persons in the United States and France (see below) (17, 35, 40).

The clinical illness begins after an incubation phase of 4 to 35 days (average, 22 days) and may have an insidious or abrupt onset which can vary from a mild flu-like illness to a more severe systemic disease. The typical episode presents with acute onset of fever with chills, headache, malaise, conjunctivitis, eye pain, myalgia, arthralgia, and bone pain (especially in the shins). These symptoms last 4 to 6 days and subside spontaneously but may recur multiple times over weeks to years. Some patients have a short-lived maculopapular rash. Fever patterns are variable, ranging from a single febrile episode to continuous fevers to recurrent quartan or quintan fevers (33, 54). B. *quintana* can be isolated from blood of these patients (48).

Since 1990, several patients with fever and blood cultures positive for *Bartonella* species, but no other skin or visceral manifestations of BA or CSD, have been reported (17, 39, 40, 44). Fever, malaise, fatigue, anorexia, and weight loss begin insidiously and often persist for weeks to months before a diagnosis can be made. Bacteremia has not been seen exclusively in immunocompromised patients. Ten homeless men from Seattle, Wash., with this syndrome and B. *quintana* bacteremia, with the same clinical picture as trench fever, were reported (40). In addition to B. *quintana*, B. *henselae* and *Bartonella elizabethae* also cause bacteremia and endocarditis (1).

The typical episode of trench fever presents with acute onset of fever with chills, headache, malaise, conjunctivitis, eye pain, myalgia, arthralgia, and bone pain

Pathophysiology of Trench Fever and *Bartonella* Bacteremia and Endocarditis

Little is known about the pathophysiology of trench fever. Endocarditis may involve either aortic or mitral valves. Despite antibiotics, most of these patients have required valve replacement.

Epidemiology and Clinical Manifestations of CSD

CSD usually presents as a benign, subacute to chronic, regional lymphadenitis. Although some cases may be caused by *A. felis* (6), the majority of cases are caused by inoculation of *B. henselae* through cat exposure (1, 8, 43, 46). Estimates of incidence range from 3.3 to 9.3 per 100,000 in ambulatory populations. Incidence is seasonal, peaking between September and January. Children are most commonly affected, with 54 to 87% of cases occurring in patients 18 years old or younger (8). Males are affected slightly more often than females. CSD has been reported from all states in the United States, as well as in Europe and Japan. Cats are clearly the vector in this zoonosis. Cat exposure is found in over 90% of patients with CSD (8), and bacteremia with *B. henselae* and antibodies to *Bartonella* spp. have been found in many cats, including those associated with cases of CSD and BA (1, 45, 46). Vector cats are usually less than 1 year old. A cat scratch is most often associated with transmission, but other salivary exposures, such as cat bite or licking of a preexisting skin break, may also lead to disease (8).

Patients with CSD present with tender lymphadenopathy, usually affecting only one node or group of nodes. The incubation period following inoculation averages 2 weeks (range, 7 to 50 days). Axillary nodes are most commonly involved, followed by cervical, groin, and preauricular nodes. Nodes suppurate in 15 to 30% of cases. Within 10 days of the inoculation, 60 to 93% of patients develop a 3- to 5-mm macule at the site. The lesion may go unnoticed, as it is nontender and nonpruritic. It usually becomes papular over time (1).

Systemic symptoms occur in the majority of patients but are usually mild, with malaise, generalized myalgia, fatigue, and anorexia. Only about one-third of patients have fever greater than 38.3°C. Symptoms usually spontaneously improve over 2 to 4 months. About 2 to 4% of patients may have severe CSD (26), characterized by either more severe or prolonged systemic symptoms (fever lasting more than 2 weeks, weight loss, more prolonged fatigue) or extranodal manifestations, including neuroretinitis, encephalopathy, hepatosplenomegaly, hemolytic anemia, thrombocytopenic purpura, erythema nodosa, oculoglandular syndrome with parotitis, and atypical pneumonia. Patients over 21 years old are more likely to develop severe CSD. Although spontaneous resolution occurs even with severe CSD, the course is more prolonged, occasionally lasting as long as 1 to 2 years (26).

Clinical diagnosis of CSD previously required at least three of the following four criteria: (i) regional lymphadenopathy without alternative explanation, (ii) history of cat exposure, often with a characteristic papule at the inoculation site, (iii) histopathology of lymph node or other tissue consistent with CSD, and (iv) positive CSD skin test.

The CSD skin test was made by slowly heating material from nodes of patients with biopsy-proven CSD; it could be problematic in the era of AIDS. The new IFA for bartonella-specific antibody is sensitive and specific for the diagnosis of CSD. Preliminary studies found *Bartonella* antibody (IFA titers of >64) in 84 to 88% of patients with suspected CSD, while background

> *A cat scratch is most often associated with transmission of CSD, but other salivary exposures, such as cat bite or licking of a preexisting skin break, may also lead to disease*

seroprevalence was only 4 to 6% (34). A recently published study of samples submitted from patients suspected of having CSD found *B. henselae* antibody in 95% of those who had cat scratch, papule formation, and regional adenopathy (13). In the future, the typical clinical scenario combined with positive IFA serology should be adequate for diagnosis of CSD, obviating the need for expensive and scarring lymph node biopsies.

Pathophysiology of CSD

The histopathologic presentation of CSD covers a full range, from anergy (BA, peliosis) to hypergy (8, 28, 49). Skin, lymph node, conjunctiva, and internal organs such as the liver, spleen, and bone all demonstrate a similar host response to bacterial invasion. In the immunocompetent host, the bacteria proliferate in the walls of capillaries and in the lining macrophages of adjacent lymphatics. From there, the organisms spread throughout the vascular arborization; vessel walls become thickened or expanded, and the lumina becomes occluded. Local anoxia and/or bacterial products produce karyorrhexis; these early lesions are often near the subcapsular sinuses. Neutrophils and macrophages invade the areas of necrosis, with abscess formation occurring, often near germinal centers. Macrophages commonly, and neutrophils rarely, phagocytize the bacteria. Macrophages ring the area of necrosis and eventually become epithelioid cells. Depending upon the initial vasculitis, lesions may be round (targeting one vessel) or serpentine (following vessel channels), hence producing round or stellate granulomas. Bacilli are numerous in early lesions (up through karyorrhexis) and few in abscesses or suppurating granulomas. In the hypergic patient, one or two bacteria may be captured by macrophages lining lymphatics or captured by dendritic cells. A massive macrophage response to the bacterial antigen surrounds the few bacilli. Neutrophils invade the centers of these round granulomas. Noninvolved areas of the node often show reactive changes with follicular and paracortical hyperplasia (8, 28).

Biopsies of skin at the inoculation site typically show acanthosis, a lymphohistiocytic perivasculitis, and a small central zone of dermal necrosis; there may or may not be ulceration. The necrotic areas are surrounded by a larger zone of acellular necrobiosis, which in turn is ringed by epithelioid macrophages and lymphocytes. Eosinophils and neutrophils are prominent in early lesions; argyrophilic bacteria are in macrophages and areas of necrosis (27). Lesions of the conjunctiva have focal to diffuse necrosis of the substantia propria, mixed inflammatory infiltrates with karyorrhexis, and a peculiar arteritis. The presence of ulceration, exudates, and granulomas is variable (50). Granulomatous hepatitis has been reported in immunocompetent patients with CSD; lesions are similar to those in the lymph node (24).

Silver impregnation methods, such as the Warthin-Starry technique, are required to demonstrate bacteria in tissue. The method of fixing tissue makes a significant difference in the interpretation of special stains; B-5 or other mercury-containing fixatives as well as some of the new alcohol-based fixatives interfere with the Warthin-Starry silver impregnation method. A

> *Skin, lymph node, conjunctiva, and internal organs such as the liver, spleen, and bone all demonstrate a similar host response to bacterial invasion in CSD*

proper Warthin-Starry stain has a golden yellow background and stains the nuclear chromatin black. For an etiologic diagnosis of the bacteria in tissue, Wear (49) uses the following criteria: the presence of (i) branching, filamentous, silvered bacilli in collagen fibers in any stage of the lesion; (ii) Y-shaped branching bacteria (Chinese figures), intra- or extracellular in viable tissue or the area of necrosis; and (iii) single bacilli in macrophages, if present, and in the same lesion on at least two consecutive sections. Areas most likely to yield a positive diagnosis are vascular proliferation with only karyorrhexis, necrotic vessels, some polymorphonuclear leukocytes and macrophages (look in walls of necrotic vessels), round or stellate granulomas with homogeneous caseation necrosis (look for ghosted vessels), pure abscesses (bacteria are in macrophages or collagen remnants in center of lesion), suppurative granuloma (usually only one to two bacilli in center of lesion but could be anywhere), and solid granuloma with a few neutrophils in center (look in dendritic cell processes between neutrophils). Prolonged incubation, altered pH, and other factors may cause precipitation, which can be confused with organisms. Control slides from known cases of early CSD are recommended, especially in those laboratories that perform this technique on an irregular basis.

Epidemiology and Clinical Manifestations of BA

BA was first reported in 1983 (41) and was not further described until 1987 (11). Cases are characterized by skin lesions and constitutional symptoms and often by extracutaneous involvement. BA occurs primarily in patients with AIDS, but it has also been reported in patients with immunosuppression following organ transplantation and in a few immunocompetent patients. Traumatic exposure to a cat, most often a kitten, either through a scratch or bite, is strongly associated with BA (1). *Bartonella* organisms have been cultured or found by PCR techniques in the blood, claws, and fleas of cats owned by patients with BA (1). However, one-third of patients with BA report no cat exposure (43). *Bartonella* species are also indigenous to the soil and may enter injured epidermal or mucosal surfaces via inoculating injuries, such as punctures by splinters, thorns, or porcupine quills; paper cuts; or direct transfer from soil or tropical plants. Other unknown mechanisms may account for some infections. Immune suppression is an important risk factor for disease. Although BA has not been included in the list of AIDS-defining opportunistic infections, most HIV-infected patients with BA have had CD4+ cells of less than 200 cells per mm^3 (43).

After initial multiplication at the portal of entry (skin, conjunctiva, or other injured mucosal surfaces), we believe that these microorganisms go to draining regional lymph nodes and then to the liver, spleen, and other viscera, where they grow before occasionally sending multiple satellite colonies to random target areas of skin or mucosae. It should be assumed that all infections are systemic. Cutaneous involvement is the most common presentation of BA (10, 19, 21). The appearance of skin lesions can be variable; they can be cutaneous or subcutaneous, single or multiple, dome shaped or acuminate, and red, purple, or skin colored. The differential diagnosis of le-

BA occurs primarily in patients with AIDS, but it has also been reported in patients with immunosuppression following organ transplantation

sions includes pyogenic granuloma, hemangioma, and Kaposi's sarcoma (3, 11, 23). Mucosal surfaces and the retina may also be involved. Affected patients are often systemically ill. Fever, chills, malaise, headache, and anorexia usually accompany the skin lesions.

Visceral involvement is common (1, 19–21, 32); lesions have been reported in cardiac, respiratory, gastrointestinal, musculoskeletal, reticuloendothelial, soft tissue, and central nervous systems. Bone lesions are found in 35% of cases, often underlying an adjacent skin lesion. Lymph nodes can be enlarged, producing the clinical picture of CSD. Several different clinicopathologic findings in the liver and spleen, including abscesses, necrotizing granulomas, necrotizing splenitis, and peliosis hepatis or splenis, have been described (32). Peliosis is commonly associated with nausea, vomiting, diarrhea, abdominal distention, fever, pancytopenia, and hepatosplenomegaly. Central nervous system involvement may present with behavioral changes or focal neurologic defects. Systemic symptoms and skin lesions often, but not invariably, accompany visceral lesions.

Pathophysiology of Bacillary Angiomatosis

In immunocompetent individuals, bartonella infections will produce the classical features of CSD, with well-formed granulomas, stellate necrosis, and few argyrophilic bacilli. In immunodeficient patients (e.g., HIV infection and/or AIDS), they induce a modified response characterized by aborted or poorly formed granulomas or miliary seeding with no protective granulomas (22). Histomorphologic features are closely related to the degree of integrity of the host immune system, to the organ or tissue involved, and to the stage of evolution of the lesions from onset of infection.

Histomorphologic features of BA are closely related to the degree of integrity of the host immune system, to the organ or tissue involved, and to the stage of evolution of the lesions from onset of infection

The bacteria grow in a collagen matrix around blood vessels, with a resulting vascular proliferation. The lesions have an angiomatoid appearance mimicking a benign (vascular) tumor; small capillaries often ring ectatic vessels (23). This type of vascular proliferation is also seen in the lymph nodes (7%) and conjunctivae (>50%) of immunocompetent patients (3, 21, 49). *B. henselae* and *B. quintana* have been shown to enhance vascular proliferation and migration in cell culture of human umbilical vein endothelial cells (12), suggesting that these neovascular manifestations are produced by an angiogenic factor produced by the bacteria.

Angritt (unpublished data) describes three main histologic stages. (i) Early granulomatoid (rarely biopsied) lesions show epithelioid and foamy macrophages, karyorrhexis, and necrobiosis of collagen. (ii) Intermediate angiomatoid lesions are the most frequently biopsied; diagnostic features include a lobular vascular proliferation with ectasia and protuberant endothelial cells and a collagen network with necrobiosis and overlying granular masses. The superficial portions often have stromal edema; deeper regions are cellular. In papular or nodular lesions the overlying epidermis is thin, often with a collarette; ulceration with acute inflammation and bleeding may occur at this stage. (iii) Resolving lesions (rarely biopsied) are hyalinized and have fibroconnective rather than vascular proliferation.

Mucosal lesions often resemble those seen in skin and subcutaneous tissues. Gastrointestinal lesions are rare in the medical literature, but they are probably more common than thought. In those cases studied at the AFIP, there has been mucosal ulceration with typical necroepithelioid angiomatosis and bacterial clusters. Parenchymal lesions of the liver, spleen, and lung present as abortive granulomas, fibrosis (similar to that seen in the skin), and bacillary peliosis. Histologically, these are large blood-filled spaces surrounded by a myxoid network of collagen with mixed inflammatory cells and karyorrhectic debris in the interstitium. Macrophages may be large with foamy cytoplasm and phagocytized cellular debris. Neutrophils may be less common in peliosis than in other lesions (22, 52).

Bacteria are abundant in early and intermediate stages in the necrobiotic areas, between collagen fibers, in the walls of vessels, or surrounding the peliotic spaces. The tiny filamentous bacteria appear as granular "clouds" or clusters, which appear as tangled masses with the silver impregnation. The bacteria stain red on Brown-Hopps (B&H)-stained sections, blue with Giemsa stain, black with Warthin-Starry and Wenger-Angritt stains, blue-grey on hematoxylin and eosin (H&E), and blue on the methylene blue counterstain of the Ziehl-Neelsen method. The Wenger-Angritt method (developed by Angritt and Wenger at the AFIP) is easier to perform than the Warthin-Starry method and can be used with B5- or mercurial-fixed tissues. Bacteria are not seen with the Gomori methenamine silver stain and are only rarely seen with the Steiner stain.

BA has both clinical and histologic characteristics which resemble those of Kaposi's sarcoma or pyogenic granuloma (10, 23). Careful histologic examination readily differentiates BA from these other lesions. The vascular proliferation is composed of round rather than spindled cells; hyaline globules, siderophages, and extravasation of erythrocytes are absent. The degree of necrosis and karyorrhexis is also greater in BA than in pyogenic granuloma. The granular clusters of bacteria are not seen in either Kaposi's sarcoma or pyogenic granuloma; identification of argyrophilic organisms is diagnostic.

B. henselae is by far the most common organism implicated in CSD, and *B. henselae* and *B. quintana* have both been found in patients with BA (1, 20). Identification is made by using multiple techniques, including culture, PCR, and evaluation of tissue for the eubacterial 16S rRNA. At this point, it is not possible to differentiate clinical disease due to *B. henselae* from that due to *B. quintana*.

Treatment of *Bartonella* Infections

In vitro susceptibility tests of *Bartonella* spp. are not standardized, but they have shown consistent patterns of susceptibility to third-generation cephalosporins, tetracyclines, macrolides, and rifampin (15). Some have also shown susceptibility to trimethoprim-sulfamethoxazole and aminoglycosides. The organisms are resistant to first- and second-generation cephalosporins, oxacillin, and clindamycin by laboratory as well as clinical criteria. For *B. bacilliformis*, tetracyclines or chloramphenicol is the recom-

> *BA has both clinical and histologic characteristics which resemble those of Kaposi's sarcoma or pyogenic granuloma; careful histologic examination readily differentiates BA from these other lesions*

mended therapy, with the latter also effective against the frequent salmonella coinfection. Trench fever mimics epidemic typhus and is therefore usually treated with tetracycline.

The role of antibiotics in CSD remains unclear (25). There are multiple reports in the literature of failed treatment with antibiotics to which *B. henselae* shows in vitro susceptibility (15). There are no controlled trials. Because CSD is usually not a serious illness and resolves spontaneously, antibiotics are often not prescribed. However, for the 1 to 2% of patients with serious CSD, quinolones, third-generation cephalosporins, or aminoglycosides have been tried with mixed reported results.

Treatment of BA, bacillary peliosis, and *Bartonella* bacteremias has been more successful. Erythromycin is the drug of choice, and doxycycline is used for patients who cannot tolerate erythromycin (1). Clinical response is usually rapid, with clearing of skin lesions and resolution of fevers. The optimal duration of treatment is not known. The initial course should be 2 to 4 weeks, with the longer duration in patients who are immunocompromised. Relapses are very common, especially in persistently immunocompromised patients. Patients with AIDS often require lifelong suppressive therapy with erythromycin or doxycycline. Patients with endocarditis may require more prolonged courses of antibiotics, often with valve replacement.

Figure 11.1 BA. Angiomatous nodules of finger and scrotum. (Courtesy of Jane Koehler and Jordan Tappero [19].)

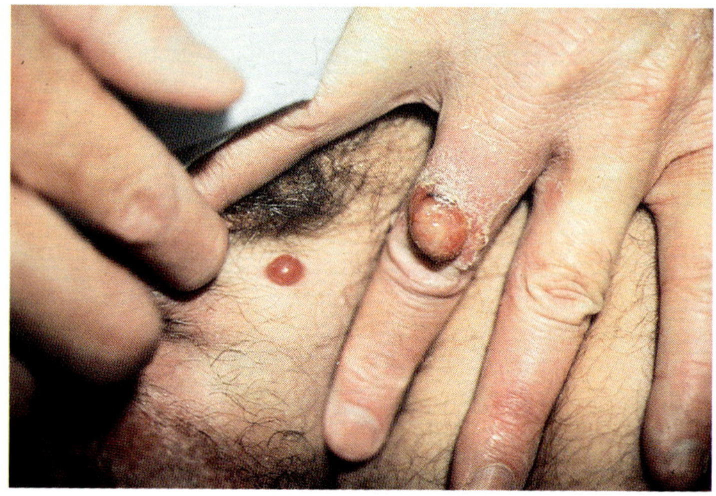

Figure 11.2 BA. Multiple tender vascular oozing lesions overlying the right thigh. (Courtesy of Jane Koehler and Jordan Tappero [20].)

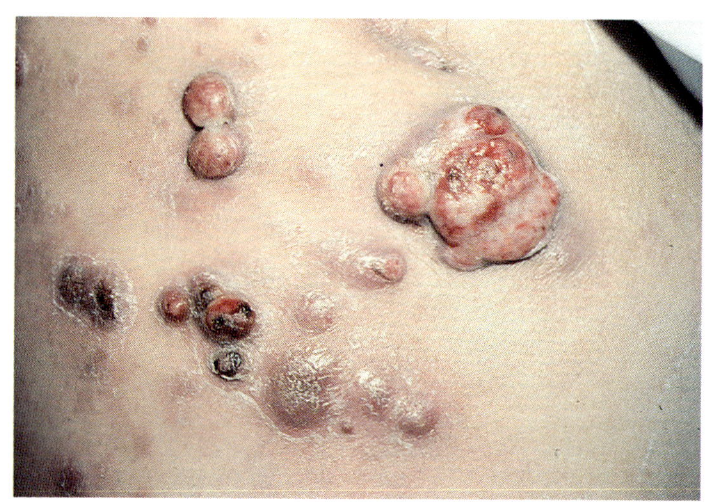

Figure 11.3 BA. Papular lesion of left lower extremity with collarette of hyperkeratotic skin and serous crust. (Courtesy of Jane Koehler and Jordan Tappero [20].)

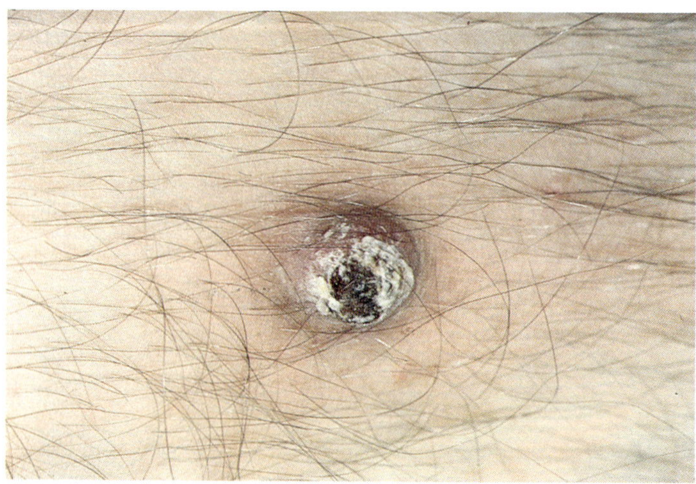

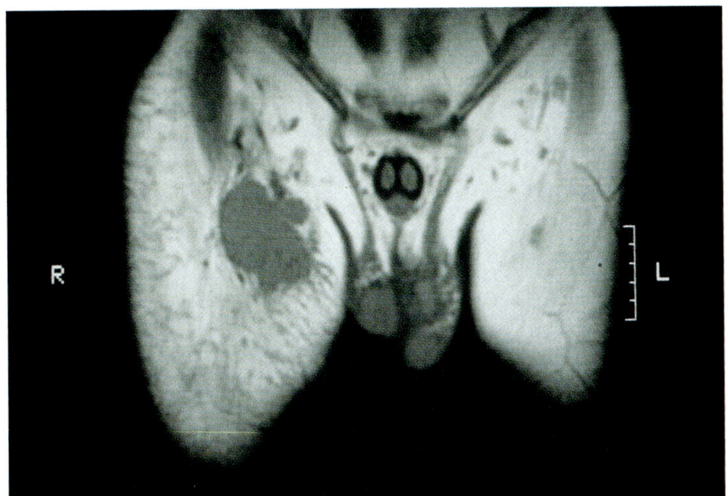

Figure 11.4 BA. Magnetic resonance imaging showing highly vascular soft tissue mass in right thigh underlying the skin lesions shown in Fig. 11.2. (Courtesy of Jane Koehler and Jordan Tappero [20].)

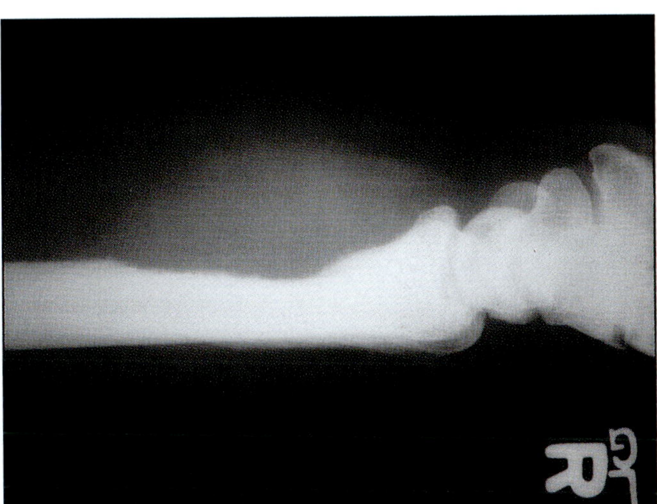

Figure 11.5 BA. Bony defect underlying right wrist mass. (Courtesy of Jane Koehler and Jordan Tappero [19].)

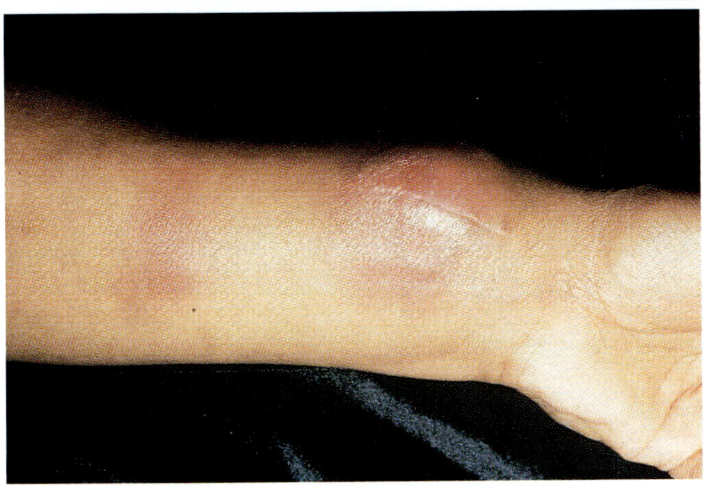

Figure 11.6 BA. Painful right wrist mass over bony defect shown in Fig. 11.5. (Courtesy of Jane Koehler and Jordan Tappero [19].)

Figure 11.7 BA. Photomicrograph of skin showing elevated lesion with epidermal collarette and superficial necrosis (H&E; original magnification, ×2.5).

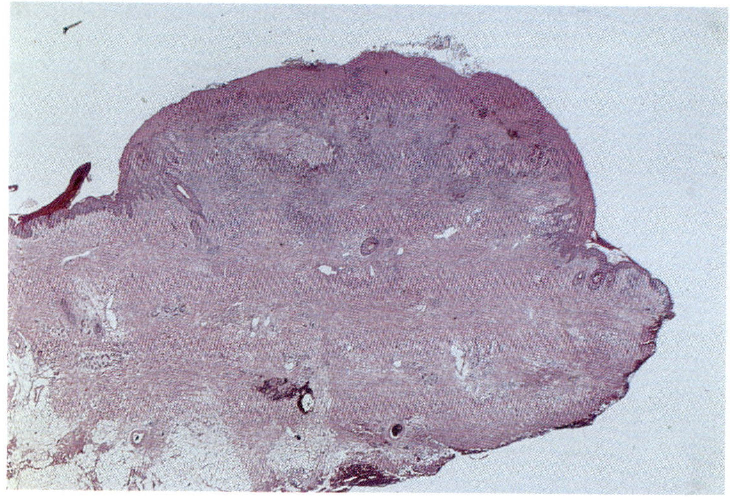

Figure 11.8 BA. High-power magnification of the same case as that shown in Fig. 11.7, showing vascular proliferation (angiomatoid) with epithelioid cells. Blue-purple granular "clouds" along collagen represent clusters of bacteria (H&E; original magnification, ×100).

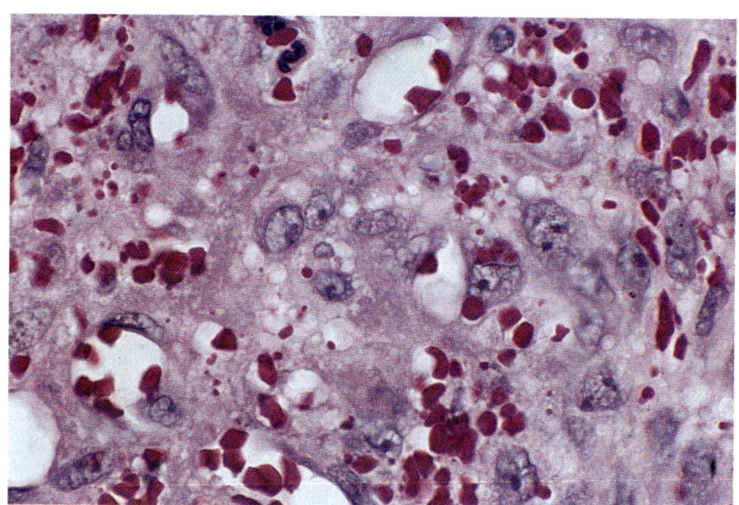

Figure 11.9 BA. Silver impregnation on same case as in Fig. 11.7 and 11.8, which shows masses of tangled argyrophilic bacilli along collagen and adjacent to dilated vessels (Warthin-Starry; original magnification, ×330).

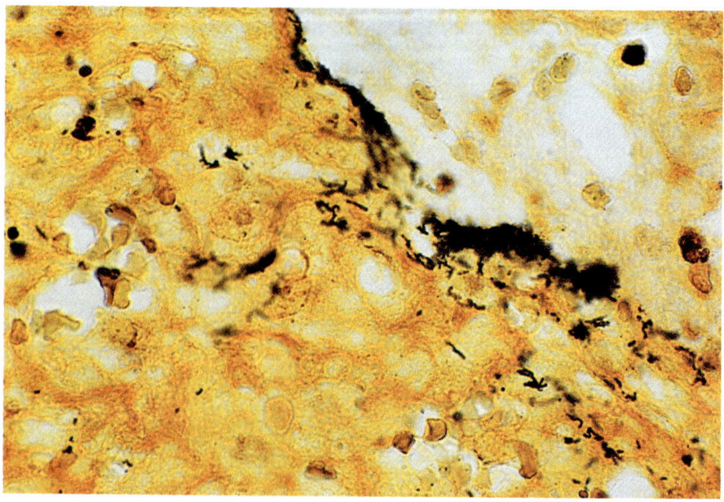

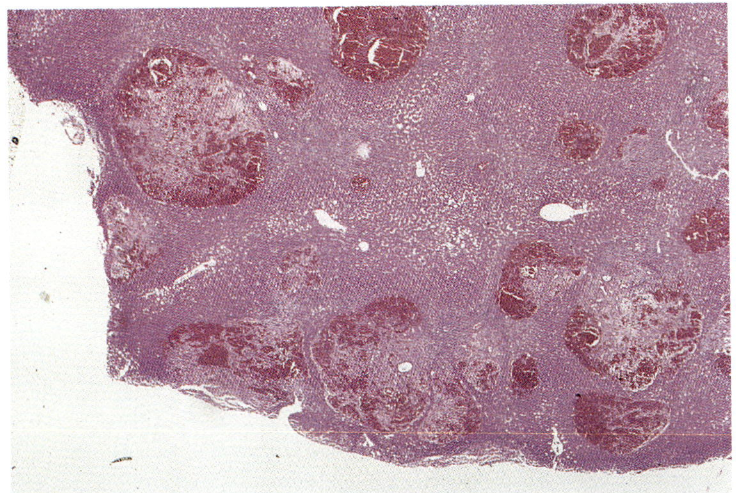

Figure 11.10   Peliosis hepatis. Liver showing multiple blood-filled spaces and poorly formed granulomas (H&E; original magnification, ×10).

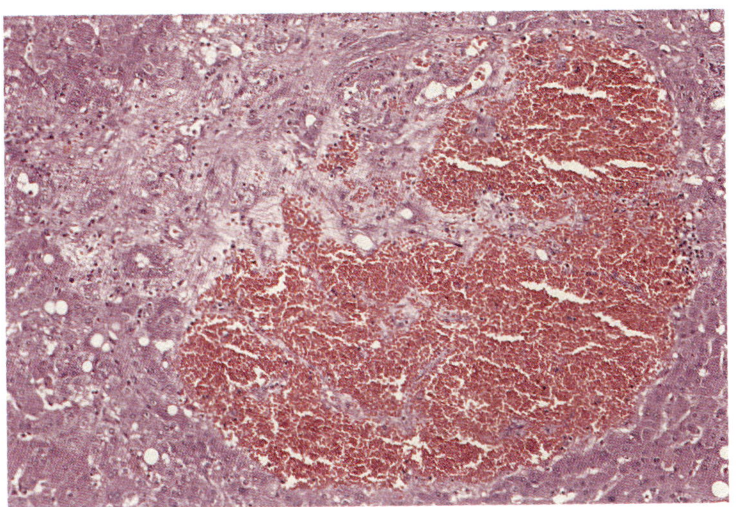

Figure 11.11   Peliosis hepatis. The figure shows the same case as that in Fig. 11.10; a single, large blood-filled space with adjacent granuloma is seen (H&E; original magnification, ×50).

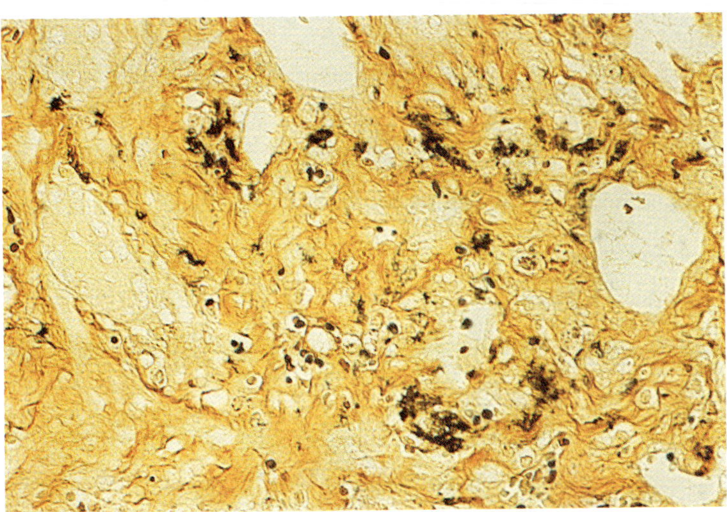

Figure 11.12   Peliosis hepatis, same case as that in Fig. 11.10 and 11.11. Tangles of argyrophilic bacilli tracking along collagen can been seen (Warthin-Starry; original magnification, ×400).

References

1. **Adal, K. A., C. J. Cockerell, and W. A. Petri, Jr.** 1994. Cat scratch disease, bacillary angiomatosis, and other infections due to *Rochalimaea*. *N. Engl. J. Med.* **330:**1509–1515.

2. **Alexander, B.** 1995. A review of bartonellosis in Ecuador and Colombia. *Am. J. Trop. Med. Hyg.* **52:**354–359.

3. **Angritt, P., S. M. Turr, K. J. Smith, C. S. Park, F. P. Hobin, and C. Myrie-Williams.** 1988. Epithelioid angiomatosis in HIV infection: neoplasm or cat-scratch disease? *Lancet* **i:**996.

4. **Ash, J. E., and S. Spitz.** 1945. Oroyo Fever/Verruga Peruana, bartonellosis, p. 25–29. *In* J. E. Ash and S. Spitz (ed.), *Pathology of Tropical Diseases: An Atlas.* Armed Forces Institute of Pathology, Washington, D.C.

5. **Bhutto, A. M., S. Nonaka, Y. Hishiguchi, and E. A. Gomez.** 1994. Histopathologic and electron microscopic features of skin lesions in a patient with bartonellosis (verruga peruana). *J. Dermatol.* **21:**178–184.

6. **Brenner, D. J., D. G. Hollis, C. W. Moss, C. K. English, G. S. Hall, J. Vincent, J. Radosevic, K. A. Birkness, W. F. Bibb, F. D. Quinn, B. Swaminathan, R. E. Weaver, M. W. Reeves, S. P. O'Connor, P. S. Hayes, F. C. Tenover, A. G. Steigerwalt, B. A. Perkins, M. I. Daneshvar, B. C. Hill, J. A. Washington, T. C. Woods, S. B. Hunter, T. L. Hadfield, G. W. Ajello, A. F. Kaufmann, D. J. Wear, and J. D. Wenger.** 1991. Proposal of *Afipia* gen. nov., with *Afipia felis* sp. nov. (formerly the cat scratch disease bacillus), *Afipia clevelandensis* sp. nov. (formerly the Cleveland Clinic Foundation strain), *Afipia broomeae* sp. nov., and three unnamed genospecies. *J. Clin. Microbiol.* **29:**2450–2460.

7. **Brenner, D. J., S. P. O'Connor, H. H. Winkler, and A. G. Steigerwalt.** 1993. Proposals to unify the genera *Bartonella* and *Rochalimaea*, with descriptions of *Bartonella quintana* comb. nov., *Bartonella vinsonii* comb. nov., *Bartonella henselae* comb. nov., and *Bartonella elizabethae* comb. nov., and to remove the family *Bartonellaceae* from the order *Rickettsiales*. *Int. J. Syst. Bacteriol.* **43:**777–786.

8. **Carithers, H. A.** 1985. Cat-scratch disease. An overview based on a study of 1200 patients. *Am. J. Dis. Child.* **139:**1124–1133.

9. **Cockerell, C. J., and E. J. Bottone.** 1995. *Bartonella* infections—evolution from the esoteric. *Am. J. Clin. Pathol.* **104:**487–490.

10. **Cockerell, C. J., and P. E. LeBoit.** 1990. Bacillary angiomatosis: a newly characterized, pseudoneoplastic, infectious, cutaneous vascular disorder. *J. Am. Acad. Dermatol.* **22:**501–512.

11. **Cockerell, C. J., G. F. Webster, M. A. Whitlow, and A. E. Friedman-Kien.** 1987. Epithelioid angiomatosis: a distinct vascular disorder in patients with the acquired immunodeficiency syndrome or AIDS-related complex. *Lancet* **ii:**654–656.

12. **Conley, T., L. Slater, and K. Hamilton.** 1994. *Rochalimaea* species stimulate human endothelial cell proliferation and migration in vitro. *J. Lab. Clin.* **124:**521–528.

13. **Dalton, M. J., L. E. Robinson, J. Cooper, R. L. Regnery, J. G. Olson, and J. E. Childs.** 1995. Use of *Bartonella* antigens for serologic diagnosis of cat-scratch disease at a national referral center. *Arch. Intern. Med.* **155:**1670–1676.

14. **Debré, R., M. Lamy, M. L. Jammet, L. Costil, and P. Mozziconacci.** 1950. La maladie des griffes de chat. *Bull. Mém. Soc. Méd. Paris* **66:**76.

15. **Dolan, M. J., M. T. Wong, R. L. Regnery, J. H. Jorgensen, M. Garcia, J. Peters, and D. Drehner.** 1993. Syndrome of *Rochalimaea henselae* adenitis suggesting cat scratch disease. *Ann. Intern. Med.* **118:**331–336.

16. **Dooly, J. R.** 1976. Bartonellosis, p. 190–193. *In* C. H. Binford and D. H. Connor (ed.), *Pathology of Tropical and Extraordinary Disease: An Atlas.* Armed Forces Institute of Pathology, Washington, D.C.

17. **Drancourt, M., J. L. Mainardi, P. Brouqui, F. Vandenesch, A. Carta, F. Lehnert, J. Etienne, F. Goldstein, J. Acar, and D. Raoult.** 1995. *Bartonella (Rochalimaea) quintana* endocarditis in three homeless men. *N. Engl. J. Med.* **332:**419–423.

18. **English, C. K., D. J. Wear, A. M. Margileth, C. R. Lissner, and G. P. Walsh.** 1988. Cat-scratch disease: isolation and culture of the bacterial agent. *JAMA* **259:**1347–1352.

19. **Koehler, J. E., P. E. LeBoit, B. M. Egbert, and T. G. Berger.** 1988. Cutaneous vascular lesions and disseminated cat-scratch disease in patients with the acquired immunodeficiency syndrome (AIDS) and AIDS-related complex. *Ann. Intern. Med.* **109:**449–455.

20. **Koehler, J. E., F. D. Quinn, T. G. Berger, P. E. LeBoit, and J. W. Tappero.** 1992. Isolation of *Rochalimaea* species from cutaneous and osseous lesions of bacillary angiomatosis. *N. Engl. J. Med.* **327:**1625–1631.

21. **LeBoit, P. E.** 1990. The expanding spectrum of a new disease, bacillary angiomatosis. *Arch. Dermatol.* **126:**808–811.

22. **LeBoit, P. E.** 1995. Bacillary angiomatosis. *Mod. Pathol.* **8:**218–222.

23. **LeBoit, P. E., T. G. Berger, B. M. Egbert, J. H. Beckstead, T. S. B. Yen, and M. H. Stoler.** 1989. Bacillary angiomatosis: the histopathology and differential diagnosis of a pseudoneoplastic infection in patients with human immunodeficiency virus disease. *Am. J. Surg. Pathol.* **13:**909–920.

24. **Lenoir, A. A., G. A. Storch, K. DeSchryver-Kecskemeti, G. D. Shackelford, R. J. Rothbaum, D. J. Wear, and J. L. Rosenblum.** 1988. Granulomatous hepatitis associated with cat scratch disease. *Lancet* **i:**1132–1136.

25. **Margileth, A. M.** 1992. Antibiotic therapy for cat-scratch disease: clinical study of therapeutic outcome in 268 patients and a review of the literature. *Pediatr. Infect. Dis. J.* **11:**474–478.

26. **Margileth, A. M., D. J. Wear, and C. K. English.** 1987. Systemic cat scratch disease: report of 23 patients with prolonged or recurrent severe bacterial infection. *J. Infect. Dis.* **155:**390–402.

27. **Margileth, A. M., D. J. Wear, T. L. Hadfield, C. J. Schlagel, G. T. Spigel, and J. E. Muhlbauer.** 1984. Cat-scratch disease: bacteria in skin at the primary site of inoculation. *JAMA* **252:**928–931.

28. **Miller-Catchpole, R., D. Variakojis, J. W. Vardiman, J. M. Loew, and J. Carter.** 1986. Cat scratch disease: identification of bacteria in seven cases of lymphadenitis. *Am. J. Surg. Pathol.* **10:**276–281.

29. **O'Connor, S. P., M. Dorsch, A. G. Steigerwalt, D. J. Brenner, and E. Stackebrandt.** 1991. 16S rRNA sequences of *Bartonella bacilliformis* and cat scratch disease bacillus reveal phylogenetic relationships with the alpha-2 subgroup of the class *Proteobacteria. J. Clin. Microbiol.* **29:**2144–2150.

30. **Parinaud, H.** 1889. Conjonctivité infectieuse paraissant transmisé à l'homme par les animaux. *Rec. Opthamol.* **11:**176–180.

31. **Perkins, B. A., B. Swaminathan, and L. A. Jackson.** 1992. Case 22-1992. Pathogenesis of cat scratch disease. *N. Engl. J. Med.* **327:**1599–1600.

32. **Perkocha, L. A., S. M. Geaghan, T. S. B. Yen, S. L. Nishimura, S. P. Chan, R. Garcia-Kennedy, G. Honda, A. C. Stoloff, H. Z. Klein, R. L. Goldman, S. Van Meter, L. D. Ferrel, and P. E. LeBoit.** 1990. Clinical and pathological features of bacillary peliosis hepatis in association with human immunodeficiency virus infection. *N. Engl. J. Med.* **323:**1581–1586.

33. **Pinkerton, H., and A. J. Strano.** 1976. Rickettsial disease: trench fever, p. 99. In C. H. Binford and D. H. Connor (ed.), *Pathology of Tropical and Extraordinary Disease: An Atlas,* vol. 1. Armed Forces Institute of Pathology, Washington, D.C.

34. **Regnery, R. L., J. G. Olson, B. A. Perkins, and W. Bibb.** 1992. Serological response to *Rochalimaea henselae* antigen in suspected cat-scratch disease. *Lancet* **339:**1443–1445.

35. **Relman, D. A.** 1995. Has trench fever returned? *N. Engl. J. Med.* **332:**463–464.

36. **Relman, D. A., J. S. Loutit, T. M. Schmidt, S. Falkow, and L. S. Tompkins.** 1990. The agent of bacillary angiomatosis—an approach to identification of uncultured pathogens. *N. Engl. J. Med.* **323:**1573–1580.

37. **Roux, V., and D. Raoult.** 1995. Inter- and intraspecies identification of *Bartonella* (*Rochalimaea*) species. *J. Clin. Microbiol.* **33:**1573–1579.

38. **Schultz, M. G.** 1968. A history of bartonellosis (Carrion's disease). *Am. J. Trop. Med. Hyg.* **17:**503–515.

39. **Slater, L. N., D. F. Welch, D. Hensel, and D. W. Coody.** 1990. A newly recognized fastidious gram-negative pathogen as a cause of fever and bacteremia. *N. Engl. J. Med.* **323:**1587–1593.

40. **Spach, D. H., A. S. Kanter, M. J. Dougherty, A. M. Larson, M. B. Coyle, D. J. Brenner, B. Swaminathan, G. M. Matar, D. F. Welch, R. K. Root, and W. E. Stamm.** 1995. *Bartonella* (*Rochalimaea*) *quintana* bacteremia in inner-city patients with chronic alcoholism. *N. Engl. J. Med.* **332:**424–428.

41. **Stoler, M. H., T. A. Bonfiglio, R. T. Steigbigel, and M. Pereira.** 1983. An atypical subcutaneous infection associated with acquired immune deficiency syndrome. *Am. J. Clin. Pathol.* **80:**714–718.

42. **Swift, H. F.** 1920. Trench fever. *Arch. Intern. Med.* **26:**76–98.

43. **Tappero, J. W., J. Mohle-Boetani, J. E. Koehler, B. Swaminathan, T. G. Berger, P. E. LeBoit, L. L. Smith, J. D. Wenger, R. W. Pinner, C. A. Kemper, et al.** 1993. The epidemiology of bacillary angiomatosis and bacillary peliosis. *JAMA* **269:**770–775.

44. **Tierno, P. M., Jr., K. Inglima, and M. T. Parisi.** 1995. Detection of Bartonella henselae bacteremia using BacT/Alert blood culture system. *Am. J. Clin. Pathol.* **104:**530–536.

45. **Tompkins, D. C., and R. T. Steigbigel.** 1993. *Rochalimaea's* role in cat scratch disease and bacillary angiomatosis. *Ann. Intern. Med.* **118:**388–389.

46. **Ueno, H., Y. Muramatsu, B. B. Chomel, T. Hohdatsu, H. Koyama, and C. Morita.** 1995. Seroepidemiological survey of *Bartonella* (*Rochalimaea*) *henselae* in domestic cats in Japan. *Microbiol. Immunol.* **39:**339–341.

47. **Verhoff, F. H.** 1913. Parinaud's conjunctivitis; a mycotic disease due to a hitherto undescribed filamentous organism. *Arch. Opthalmol.* **17:**345–351.

48. **Vinson, J. W.** 1966. In vitro cultivation of the rickettsial agent of trench fever. *Bull. W. H. O.* **35:**155–164.

49. **Wear, D. J.** 1994. Cat scratch disease and bacillary angiomatosis, p. 29–36. *In* A. M. Marty and A. M. Nelson (ed.), *Advances in Diagnostic Pathology of Infectious Diseases*. Armed Forces Institute of Pathology, Washington, D.C.

50. **Wear, D. J., R. H. Malaty, L. F. Zimmerman, T. L. Hadfield, and A. M. Margileth.** 1985. Cat scratch disease bacilli in the conjunctivae of patients with Parinaud's oculoglandular syndrome. *Ophthalmology* **92:**1282–1287.

51. **Wear, D. J., A. M. Margileth, T. L. Hadfield, G. W. Fischer, C. J. Schlagel, and F. M. King.** 1983. Cat scratch disease: a bacterial infection. *Science* **221:**1403–1404.

52. **Welch, D. F., D. A. Pickett, L. N. Slater, A. G. Steigerwalt, and D. J. Brenner.** 1992. *Rochalimaea henselae*, sp. nov., a cause of septicemia, bacillary angiomatosis, and parenchymal bacillary peliosis. *J. Clin. Microbiol.* **30:**275–280.

53. **Wignall, F. S.** 1991. Bartonellosis, p. 426–429. *In* G. T. Strickland (ed.), *Hunter's Tropical Medicine*, 7th ed. The W. B. Saunders Co., Philadelphia.

54. **Wisseman, C. L., Jr.** 1991. Trench fever, p. 285–286. *In* G. T. Strickland (ed.), *Hunter's Tropical Medicine*, 7th ed. The W. B. Saunders Co., Philadelphia.

chapter 12

Helicobacter pylori

Benjamin D. Gold and Aileen Marty

Mucosal ulceration in the gastric mucosa occurs when the mucosal "defensive factors," such as mucus, the bicarbonate and ion layers, lamina propria blood flow, free radical scavengers, and prostaglandins and phospholipids, are overwhelmed by "aggressive factors," such as excessive acid, drugs (nonsteroidal anti-inflammatory agents), and alcohol. For decades, the concept of "too much acid equals peptic ulceration" has been taught in and among medical circles and has been widely accepted in the lay community (17, 35). However, the discovery of a novel, spiral-shaped bacterium associated with gastroduodenal inflammation in 1983 changed this dogma (47).

Gastroduodenal inflammation and mucosal ulceration had been previously classified as type A ulcers, which are usually associated with pernicious anemia, and type B ulcers, which are associated with a variety of disorders. Peptic ulceration of the gastroduodenal mucosa can now be classified as primary or secondary (17, 60, 65). In most cases, primary peptic ulceration in adults and children occurs as a result of *Helicobacter pylori* colonization of the

Benjamin D. Gold, Division of Pediatric Gastroenterology and Nutrition, Department of Pediatrics, Emory University School of Medicine, 2040 Ridgewood Drive, N.E., Atlanta, GA 30322. **Aileen Marty,** Infectious Disease Pathology Branch, Geographic Pathology Division, Department of Infectious and Parasitic Disease Pathology, Armed Forces Institute of Pathology, Washington, DC 20306-6000.

Pathology of Emerging Infections
Edited by C. Robert Horsburgh, Jr., and Ann Marie Nelson
© 1997 American Society for Microbiology, Washington, DC 20005-4171

gastric mucosa (18). Secondary peptic ulceration occurs as a result of diseases that are usually more systemic in nature (17, 37, 75). Secondary ulcers can occur because of "systemic" stress, associated with major head trauma, burns, or other major systemic illnesses that result in elevation of circulating catecholamines and adrenal corticosteroids. Secondary ulcers can also occur in conditions where there is excessive acid production, e.g., gastrinomas associated with excessive gastrin secretion in conditions such as Zollinger-Ellison syndrome. In addition, ingestion of exogenous agents such as nonsteroidal anti-inflammatory agents, aspirin, or alcohol can result in gastric mucosal ulceration. Finally, illnesses such as Crohn's disease or sickle-cell disease are associated with secondary ulcers of the gastrointestinal mucosa (17, 35, 65).

Although the "discovery" of *H. pylori* was believed to have occurred in 1983, evidence of gram-negative organisms in the stomachs of patients at autopsy has appeared in the literature since the late 19th century (1, 47, 49, 63). However, the interpretation has been that these unidentified organisms were incidental and had nothing to do with inflammation. More reports describing gram-negative organisms in the stomachs of various mammalian species appeared over the next few decades (46, 56). In 1975, Steer and Colin-Jones demonstrated, again, gram-negative organisms in the stomachs of humans with mucosal inflammation (70). These investigators came very close to culturing the organisms but grew *Pseudomonas* species, which were subsequently believed to be oral pathogens. The landmark discovery of Marshall and Warren, from Perth, Australia, was published in the *Lancet* in 1983 (47, 49). These researchers described the association of gastric colonization by a novel gram-negative, spiral-shaped organism, with gastroduodenal inflammation. Furthermore, Marshall isolated a primary culture of this organism from gastric biopsies (49). Finally, in 1989, further molecular (16S RNA) and biochemical (unique cellular fatty acids) analyses of these gastric organisms were performed, and a separate novel genus was created for this organism, which is now properly referred to as *H. pylori* (24, 77).

Microbiology of *H. pylori*

H. pylori is a gram-negative organism that resides under microaerobic conditions (38). It has two primary morphological shapes, bacillary ("curved" and "spiral" are morphological descriptions that have been used) and coccoid (38, 66). However, the biological relevance of each morphological form is not clearly understood. This organism is highly motile with multiple unipolar flagella (30, 42). It is oxidase, catalase, and urease producing; its urease enzyme is used to metabolize the urea present in the gastric mucus, creating a neutral microenvironment in which it lives and replicates at the apical surface of gastric epithelial cells (24, 77).

At least 11 other species of *Helicobacter* have now been identified (72, 73). *H. fennelliae* and *H. cinaedi* are both human pathogens that reside in the lower gastrointestinal tract and cause diarrheal disease in immunocompromised patients, particularly those with human immunodeficiency virus in-

> *Evidence of gram-negative organisms in the stomachs of patients at autopsy has appeared in the literature since the late 19th century*

fection and/or AIDS. However, most of the other *Helicobacter* spp. are animal pathogens. In particular, much attention has been given to *Helicobacter felis*, an organism that infects domestic and some wild cats and that causes chronic gastritis in the feline stomach (40). Researchers have been using *H. felis* in a mouse model of chronic and acute gastritis for the development of vaccine constructs against gastric *Helicobacter* infection (8). Another *Helicobacter* sp. of great interest is the newly discovered *H. hepaticus*, which infects certain strains of mice (e.g., SCID, AJCr) and has satisfied Koch's postulates as a causative agent of hepatocellular carcinoma in these murine strains (22). *Gastrospirillum hominis*, or *Helicobacter heilmannii*, has been observed by histologic staining of gastric biopsies obtained during upper endoscopy performed on patients with chronic active gastritis (26). However, primary culture of these organisms has not been successfully performed, and the clinical relevance of these gastric spirochetes remains unclear.

> *The newly discovered H. hepaticus, which infects certain strains of mice and has satisfied Koch's postulates as a causative agent of hepatocellular carcinoma in these murine strains, is also of great interest*

Epidemiology of *H. pylori* Infection in Humans

The epidemiology of *H. pylori* infection in humans is quite interesting, particularly in relations to the gastroduodenal disease associated with gastric colonization by the organisms (34, 52). Unfortunately, the literature is amply endowed with studies of the prevalence of *H. pylori* infection, yet is notably lacking in studies of the incidence of this infection (57). To determine incidence of a particular infection, one needs both (i) the number of newly diagnosed infections in the population and (ii) the proportion of new infections that typically remain undiagnosed. Thus, a target population can be surveyed for disease diagnosis, new cases can be counted, and the total case load can be estimated (57). However, most epidemiological studies of *H. pylori* infection have been performed with adults, who likely were infected for decades before diagnosis (16). In addition, acute *H. pylori* infection is not known to be present with specific diagnostic symptoms. Furthermore, studies of pediatric populations, in which *H. pylori* infection is acquired, are lacking (54). Therefore, true incidence cannot be directly determined and has been extrapolated from prevalence data.

The few studies that have been carried out prospectively to determine acquisition of infection in uninfected subjects or treated patients provide some insight into the incidence of *H. pylori* infection (57, 79). The incidence of *H. pylori* infection in industrialized countries has been estimated to be ~0.5% of the susceptible population per year. This incidence has been decreasing; thus, infected adults are more likely to have been infected in childhood (79). The incidence of *H. pylori* infection continues to be high in developing countries; it is estimated to be between 3 and 10% per year (52). Furthermore, throughout the world, incidence of *H. pylori* infection appears to be higher in children than adults (8).

The route of transmission of *H. pylori* is postulated to be fecal-oral or oral-oral. Several studies have identified *H. pylori* DNA in the dental plaque and saliva of adults and children by using polymerase chain reaction techniques

(2, 31, 52). The mouth may be either a reservoir for this infection or an initial site of colonization prior to seeding the stomach and colonizing the gastric epithelia (51). The fecal-oral route of transmission has been definitively characterized in ferrets (38). Ferrets are naturally colonized by their own species of *Helicobacter, H. mustelae,* and are infected some time after weaning. Gastric colonization of ferret stomachs by *H. mustelae* results in pathology similar to that seen in humans infected with *H. pylori*. Ferrets get chronic gastritis and duodenal and gastric ulcers and develop gastric carcinoma as the end result of long-term *H. mustelae* infection.

H. pylori primarily infects children, and there are many risk factors for acquiring the infection at an early age (69). The risk factors that have been described are familial overcrowding, country of origin in which *H. pylori* is endemic, poor socioeconomic circumstances, and being of certain ethnicities. In particular, in the United States, the prevalence rates among African-Americans and Hispanics are similar to those of people residing in developing countries (54, 69, 83).

Clinical Characteristics and Pathogenesis of *H. pylori* Infection

The first link between *H. pylori* infection and gastroduodenal disease was the observation that this bacterium is consistently associated with chronic superficial gastritis (49). There is abundant evidence demonstrating that this organism satisfies Koch's postulates as a human gastric pathogen associated with gastroduodenal inflammation (48). In addition to its association with chronic superficial gastritis, *H. pylori* has been associated with chronic active gastritis and with primary duodenal ulcers in >90% of infected adults and children (4, 11, 32, 61). It is now estimated that the lifetime risk for developing peptic ulcer disease is >10% in *H. pylori*-infected individuals (55, 81). Furthermore, the recurrence rate of duodenal ulcers is markedly reduced following successful treatment of *H. pylori* infection, which provides additional evidence delineating its etiologic role (13, 25). *H. pylori* infection is less commonly associated with gastric ulcers, and its association with Barrett's esophagus and nonulcer dyspepsia is still controversial (20, 67, 68). Of particular interest is the association of *H. pylori* infection, particularly if acquired in early childhood, with the development of gastric cancer (83). Multiple studies have demonstrated that concurrent or previous *H. pylori* infection is associated with a 2.7- to 12-fold-increased risk of developing gastric cancer. Moreover, in regions of the world with high rates of gastric cancer, the prevalence of *H. pylori* infection is also high, and infection tends to be acquired early in life (12, 21, 43, 71). In addition to the link between *H. pylori* infection and gastric cancer, this organism is also thought to play a role in the development of low-grade B-cell lymphomas of the gastric mucosa-associated lymphoid tissue (MALT) type (5, 58).

The interrelationship between bacterial virulence properties and the host immune response which then results in mucosal disease is still not clearly

> *There is abundant evidence demonstrating that H. pylori satisfies Koch's postulates as a human gastric pathogen associated with gastroduodenal inflammation*

characterized. Many bacterial virulence factors for *H. pylori* have been described, and the genetic bases for many of these have been elucidated (6, 19, 59, 74, 85). Specifically, urease (*ureA*, *ureB*, and *ureC* genes) is produced in large quantities by all *H. pylori* isolates, as well as the other gastric *Helicobacter* spp. identified (66, 73). *H. pylori* is highly motile and utilizes its flagella (*flaA* and *flaB* genes) to navigate through the thick, viscous gastric mucus to reach the apical surface of the gastric epithelial cells where it adheres, replicates, and occupies its biological niche (30, 42). Recently, attention has been given to the vacuolating cytotoxin produced by at least half of the *H. pylori* strains isolated. This cytotoxin was first characterized by Cover and Blaser and produces vacuoles in the cytoplasm of eukaryotic cells in vitro (10). The gene (*vacA*) for this vacuolating cytotoxin, an 87-kDa protein, has at least two alleles and is quite variably expressed among *H. pylori* isolates (36, 84). In addition to cytotoxin activity, *H. pylori* strains also differ in a high-molecular-weight protein, designated CagA, which ranges from 105 to 140 kDa in size (10). About 60% of *H. pylori* isolates produce this protein, and its presence strongly correlates with the expression of the vacuolating cytotoxin activity. The *cagA* gene is absent from those strains lacking the CagA protein product (54).

A vigorous local and systemic host immune response after gastric colonization by *H. pylori* organisms is observed. A monocyte and macrophage response can be seen in the gastric mucosa of infected children, with both polymorphonuclear cells and plasma cells also present in the inflammatory infiltrate (23). T cells do not seem to play a major role in the inflammation associated with *H. pylori* infection, but elevated levels of interleukin-1 (IL-1), IL-2, IL-6, and IL-8, as well as tumor necrosis factor alpha, are detectable in the gastric epithelia of infected individuals (15, 66, 76, 85). Circulating immunoglobulin G (IgG) antibodies in *H. pylori*-infected individuals are easily detectable, and many diagnostic assays have been developed on the basis of these circulating IgG antibodies (7). The answer to why, despite this vigorous immune response to *H. pylori* infection, no spontaneous clearance of this organism has been described and why, although reinfection rates are low, individuals in areas of endemicity can be reinfected after successful treatment of their gastric *H. pylori* infection still eludes researchers in this field.

Methods for Detection of *H. pylori* Infection

At present, the "gold standard" for the diagnosis of active *H. pylori* infection is upper endoscopy and esophagogastroduodenoscopy with gastric biopsies (7, 29). However, there are numerous, fairly accurate detection assays that recently have become commercialized and available for clinical use (28). Methods for detection of *H. pylori* infection can therefore be divided into two primary categories: (i) those that are invasive and (ii) those that are noninvasive. The invasive methods used to detect *H. pylori* infection require endoscopy and gastric biopsies. The optimal number of biopsies and the anatomic location within the stomach necessary for the best yield are

At present, the "gold standard" for the diagnosis of active H. pylori infection is upper endoscopy and esophagogastroduodenoscopy with gastric biopsies

still quite controversial. At minimum, a gastric biopsy is needed both for pathologic review of the inflammatory infiltrate and for histologic identification of *H. pylori* organisms. Although the Steiner stain or a modified silver stain (Warthin-Starry) is considered the best method for the identification of *H. pylori* organisms, a trained pathologist can readily see the curved, spiral organisms on a Giemsa stain of the gastric biopsy sections (45, 55).

In addition, there are commercially available rapid tests used in the endoscopy suite that involve placement of a gastric biopsy into a kit (CLO test) that detects the urease production of the organisms (62). Since primary culture of *H. pylori* organisms from gastric biopsy is 100% specific but is far less sensitive and is also time-consuming and labor-intensive to perform, very few laboratories in the country offer this service. Polymerase chain reaction techniques in capable hands are exquisitely sensitive but can be fraught with false positives, resulting from, e.g., contaminated forceps or endoscopy equipment (80). Finally, because *H. pylori* colonization of the stomach of infected individuals can be patchy in its distribution, biopsy sampling errors can occur. Therefore, if histologic evidence of gastric inflammation is apparent but there is no evidence of *H. pylori* organisms, a high level of suspicion, and in some cases even empirical anti-*H. pylori* therapy, could be warranted.

Noninvasive methods should be used with much caution in the diagnosis of the infection, particularly if they and only they are being used to determine whether therapy should be initiated

There are several noninvasive methods for the detection of *H. pylori* infection and they have been touted as being "near perfection" in their sensitivity, specificity, and positive and negative predictive values (7, 64). However, these tests should be used with much caution in the diagnosis of the infection, particularly if they and only they are being used to determine whether therapy should be initiated. The most promising noninvasive method is based on urease enzyme production of *H. pylori* organisms; it involves the administration of a ^{13}C- or ^{14}C-labeled urea meal and subsequent testing of expired breath samples over a 2-h period (45, 78). This test is semiquantitative, in that it measures the approximate bacterial load in the entire stomach, and of all the noninvasive tests, it may be the best predictor of treatment success. Commercially available serological assays, which are primarily based on levels of IgG antibody against *H. pylori* antigens, are too numerous to count, but all have reasonable accuracy in detecting the presence of *H. pylori* infection. However, caution must be used when depending on these assays for patient management, particularly when deciding on therapy (14, 65). The assays may be limited in their accuracy when they are used in populations different from those in which the assays were developed (e.g., a developing country such as Peru compared with the United States). In addition, most commercially available assays have been standardized and validated (against esophagogastroduodenoscopy with biopsy) in adult populations; therefore, they may have cutoff values different from what might be appropriate for their use in children. Finally, the IgG response to *H. pylori* infection persists for at least 3 months and even >1 year in the face of successful antimicrobial treatment of the infection; thus, the use of serology for posttreatment monitoring may be limited (28, 33). Therefore, selection of the appropriate test should be individualized to the particular patient, which depends on the clinical situation.

Pathology

Gross Findings

Thickened gastric folds indicate inflammation, and this inflammation is most often a result of *H. pylori*. Lobulated, markedly thickened folds have a very high correlation with *H. pylori* and with neoplasms (41). Endoscopically, the changes of nonspecific gastritis or a peptic ulcer mimic those of MALT lymphoma.

Thickened gastric folds indicate inflammation, and this inflammation is most often a result of H. pylori

Histology

H. pylori colonizes only the gastric epithelium. However, it will localize to the gastric epithelium outside of the stomach, such as in gastric metaplasia in the duodenum, Barrett's esophagus, and gastric heterotopia in a Meckel's diverticulum, rectum, or other site. (Gastric heterotopia differs from gastric surface metaplasia by the presence of underlying parietal and chief cells.) We have not yet determined the precise nature of the eukaryotic cell receptor or the *H. pylori* adhesin, but we do know that the gastric epithelial cell receptor contains a glycoconjugate and may be related to the Lewis B blood group antigen (6).

Inflammatory lesions are initially acute and later chronic. Acute gastritis involves the entire stomach. Biopsies show surface epithelial degeneration, which leads to mucin depletion and compensatory foveolar hyperplasia. In adult biopsies, there is then mucosal infiltration by neutrophils, with little or no chronic inflammatory cells. Neutrophils sometimes aggregate around the narrow isthmus of gastric pits. Strains of *H. pylori* that are positive for cytotoxin-associated protein (*cagA*) cause gastric epithelial cells to produce the powerful neutrophil attractant IL-8. Except in human volunteer studies and following accidental infection in endoscopy personnel, these lesions only rarely contain *H. pylori*.

The principal histological features of acute *H. pylori* gastritis, i.e., surface epithelial degeneration and neutrophil infiltration, are also the most sensitive indicators of the activity of infection in the chronic phase. Features of chronic gastritis caused by *H. pylori* usually include the following.

- Plasma cell and T-cell infiltrates that are especially prominent in the lamina propria of the mucosa between gastric pits
- Reactive lymphoid hyperplasia of the stomach. This is very common in both adults and children with *H. pylori* infection. Lymphoid follicles are present in nearly all cases of *H. pylori* infection (particularly in children) if at least 10 biopsy sections are reviewed. The high prevalence of lymphoid hyperplasia perhaps reflects that *H. pylori* is a major determinant of the development of gastric lymphoid tissue (MALT) (15).
- "Active components" (neutrophil infiltration) that are present in both the lamina propria and the epithelium. Bacterial *cagA* protein stimulates cytokines, including production of IL-8 by epithelial cells leading to this infiltration.
- Epithelial degeneration, which usually varies with the density of *H. pylori* and with the number of *H. pylori* organisms attached to epithelial cells. The gastric mucosa reverts to normal following antibiotic therapy.

In 1973, Strickland and Mackay recognized two major categories of chronic gastritis with atrophy: type A (autoimmune type), which mainly affects the body mucosa in patients who have hypo- or achlorhydria, high gastrin levels, and anti-parietal cell antibodies; and type B, which is characterized by predominantly antral involvement without parietal cell antibodies. In chronic type B antral gastritis, patients have full thickness infiltration by chronic inflammatory cells and glandular atrophy (71). Glass and Pitchumoni (cited in reference 71) added a third category, AB gastritis, in which patchy involvement by gastritis and multifocal atrophy in both the antrum and the corpus are seen. AB gastritis is atrophic gastritis with or without intestinal metaplasia. These biopsies have glandular atrophy and intestinal metaplasia in the antral and/or corpus mucosa.

H. pylori does not attach to areas of intestinal metaplasia, but countless *H. pylori* organisms may carpet the adjacent normal gastric epithelium. The numbers of *H. pylori* decrease as the gastric mucosa develops intestinal metaplasia or becomes atrophic. The atrophy could result from direct bacterial effects, i.e., from cellular destruction by cytotoxins, ammonia products, proteases, or antibodies reacting to cross-reactive antigens. The prevalence of atrophy in chronically infected persons increases with the age of the patient. As the numbers of *H. pylori* organisms decrease, the numbers of inflammatory cells in the underlying lamina propria decrease. In end-stage chronic gastritis, there are usually very few inflammatory cells. AB gastritis with intestinal metaplasia carries an increased risk of ulceration and carcinoma. The newer, but not widely adopted, Sydney system for grading and classifying gastritis is based on the intensity of the chronic inflammation, neutrophil activity, glandular atrophy, intestinal metaplasia, and *H. pylori* density.

Peptic ulcers are defects in the integrity of the mucosa of the proximal digestive tract which by definition are at least 0.5 cm in diameter and penetrate through the muscularis mucosae (34). The majority of gastric ulcers worldwide are related to *H. pylori* infection. Far less common than gastric ulcers are duodenal ulcers; the majority of patients with these are older, have *H. pylori* in the gastric corpus as well as the antrum, and have decreased acid output and atrophic gastritis of the corpus with loss of specialized cells (68). Duodenal ulcer disease is characterized by a patchy chronic inflammation with villus blunting, neutrophil infiltration of the epithelium, and gastric metaplasia. *H. pylori* in the stomach predominantly colonizes the gastric antrum, and patients have a large acid output, no atrophic signs of the corpus mucosa, and gastric metaplasia in the duodenal bulb. In the duodenum, *H. pylori* is present in areas of gastric metaplasia.

Low-grade B-cell lymphomas, known as MALT lymphomas (CD20+), that arise from lymphoid aggregates in the lamina propria are seen in association with *H. pylori* disease. Early MALT lymphomas may completely regress after eradication of *H. pylori*. *H. pylori* has also been associated with high-grade B-cell lymphomas that are CD30+. These have a diffuse distribution. In addition, *H. pylori* has been associated with well-differentiated, "intestinal type" gastric adenocarcinoma (29, 43). There is evidence suggesting that toxigenic strains of *H. pylori*, in particular strains with the cytotoxin-associated gene *cagA* (12), are specifically associated with gastric cancer. The tumors display irregular tubular glands formed by atypical epithelial cells with several mitotic figures, but *H. pylori* is not seen in the tumor. In biopsies of diffuse-type adenocarcinoma, there is a lack of cellular cohesiveness and diffuse infiltration of the gastric wall; again, *H. pylori* does not attach to areas with severe atrophy, intestinal metaplasia, or cancer. Biopsies from patients with more than one of these tumors display histologic features of both lymphoma and gastric adenocarcinoma.

Treatment and Prevention of *H. pylori* Infection

The recurrence of duodenal ulcers can be dramatically reduced and prevented by a single course of antimicrobial therapy directed at the eradication of *H. pylori* organisms infecting the gastric mucosa (25). Because of the economic impact of peptic ulcer disease (e.g., treatment costs, morbidity, and mortality) as well as the prevalence of *H. pylori* worldwide, a Consensus Development Conference of the National Institutes of Health recommended that all patients with ulcers who are also infected by *H. pylori* receive antimicrobial therapy (55). There is a notable lack of consensus on which patients should receive therapy when infected by *H. pylori* and manifesting other gastroduodenal disease (e.g., gastritis) (67). Reports of reinfection rates in the literature vary, but cross-infection may occur and can be quite high in families with small children.

The recurrence of duodenal ulcers can be dramatically reduced and prevented by a single course of antimicrobial therapy directed at the eradication of H. pylori organisms infecting the gastric mucosa

   H. pylori is a difficult organism to treat, and success of therapy requires the concurrent administration of two or more antimicrobial drugs (3, 13, 27, 50, 82). In treatment trials, the success of therapy usually has been arbitrarily defined as the absence of detectable organisms, as shown by tissue sampling or carbon-labeled urea breath tests, one month or more after treatment has been discontinued. Most treatment trials have also been performed with adults, and there is a notable lack of information on treating *H. pylori*-infected children (44). None of the drug regimens currently used to treat *H. pylori* eradicates the organism successfully 100% of the time, and some regimens are associated with a relatively high frequency of side effects (82). In addition, *H. pylori* is resistant to only a few antimicrobial agents (e.g., vancomycin and nalidixic acid), but it can readily become resistant to metronidazole and, to a lesser extent, clarithromycin. Therefore, the success of the therapeutic regimen depends highly upon patient compliance, the resistance that may develop in *H. pylori* strains colonizing the infected individual, and adverse reactions.

   Therefore, as recommended by the National Institutes of Health Consensus Committee for adults, the combination of a bismuth compound (two 262-mg tablets four times daily), tetracycline (500 mg four times daily), and metronidazole (1.0 to 1.5 g/day) can be quite efficacious. Although studies are still necessary, the combination of a bismuth compound, amoxicillin, and metronidazole is recommended for therapy in children (65). The recommended duration of therapy is quite controversial. However, the average therapeutic regimen is 2 weeks. Many alternative therapies, which vary in the number of antimicrobial agents, their duration, and the manner in which they are delivered, have been reported, but further clinical trials are necessary.

The most promising treatment and possible prevention of *H. pylori* infection and its significant gastroduodenal disease sequelae lie in the development of an efficacious vaccine (8, 39). Development of a vaccine against *H. pylori* infection was first initiated by the demonstration that *H. felis* proteins could protect mice from infection by *H. pylori* (14). Several important steps are critical for the development of an appropriate vaccine, and many laboratories throughout the world are therefore working to (i) characterize and identify appropriate antigens; (ii) identify and develop appropriate and biologically relevant animal models to test the safety, efficacy, and immunogenicity of the vaccine candidate; (iii) characterize the type of host immunity required to confer protection against *H. pylori* infection; and (iv) appropriately choose a vaccine delivery system to stimulate the necessary immunity at the right anatomic site. Recent work in this area by Michetti et al. has demonstrated a mouse model of superficial gastric ulcers following infection by *H. felis* that are prevented by the administration of a recombinant urease oral vaccine, with *Escherichia coli* heat-labile toxin given as adjuvant (53). More recently, Corthésy-Theulaz et al. have demonstrated that not only are oral vaccines using the *H. pylori* urease protein as antigen and cholera toxin as adjuvant efficacious in the prevention of *H. felis* colonization of the murine stomach, but these oral vaccines can also be used to successfully treat active infection, with the resolution of the mucosal inflammation (9).

Therefore, although a great deal of information on the understanding of gastroduodenal disease associated with gastric colonization by *H. pylori* has emerged since its "discovery" in Perth, Australia, in 1983, many critical questions still remain unanswered. Future research addressing the environmental reservoir(s) and the organism's narrow host range and highly specific tissue tropism will be critical to add to our present understanding. Furthermore, prospective studies of the natural history of this pathogen after its initial acquisition are necessary to understand the evolution of the host immune/inflammatory response and the progression to malignancy. Finally, the molecular basis for the bacterial virulence factors, either already identified or yet to be characterized, particularly in relation to vaccine development, will be important for eventual clinical trials with novel vaccine constructs aimed at both the treatment and widespread prevention of this common human infection.

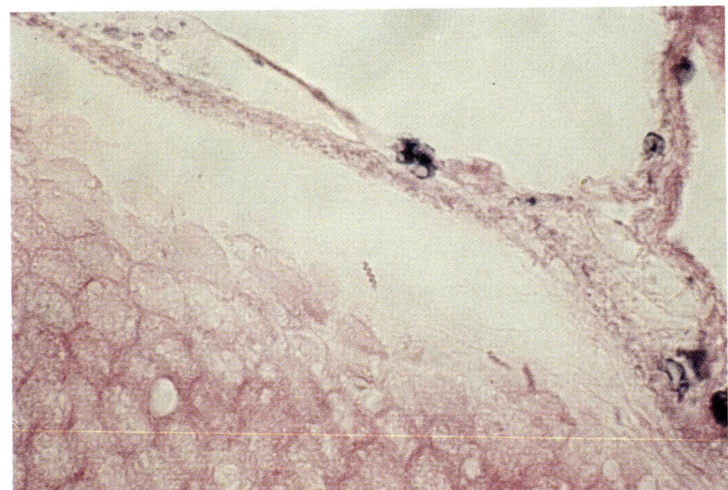

Figure 12.1 *H. heilmannii* (hematoxylin and eosin; original magnification, ×330).

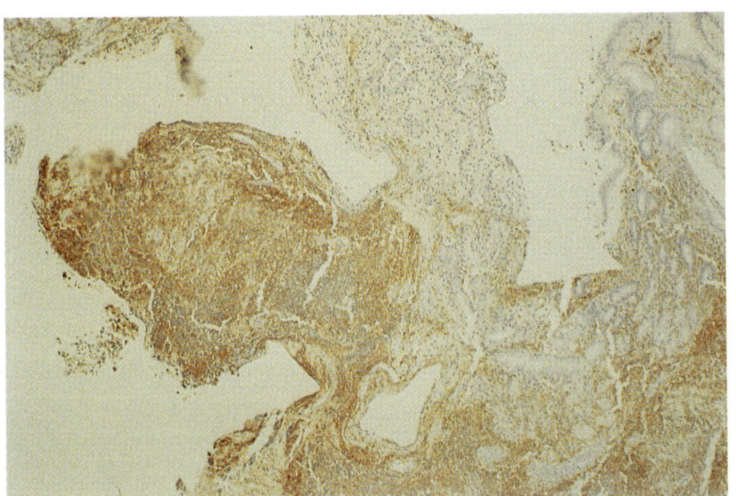

Figure 12.2 Gastric biopsy of a patient with a MALT lymphoma demonstrating monoclonality (L-26 [immunohistochemical stain for B-cell lymphocytes]; original magnification, ×50).

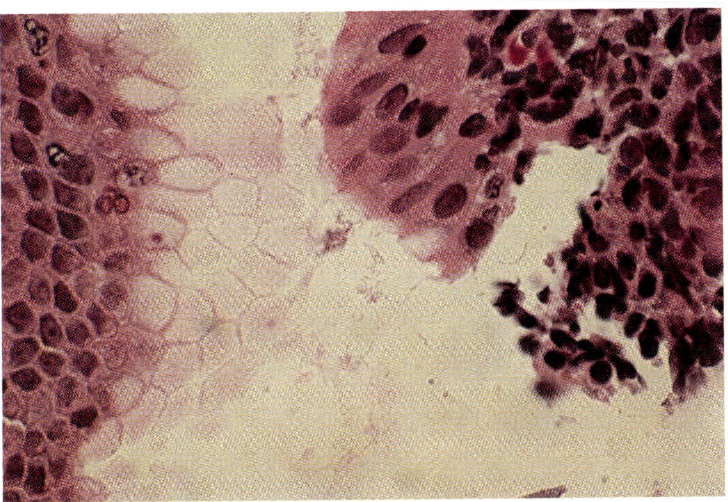

Figure 12.3 Higher magnification of gastric biopsy shown in Fig. 12.2 in an area with normal gastric glands infected with *H. pylori* (hematoxylin and eosin; original magnification, ×250).

Figure 12.4 Gastric biopsy of patient with gastric adenocarcinoma who had *H. pylori* in the adjacent normal gastric epithelium (hematoxylin and eosin; original magnification, ×25).

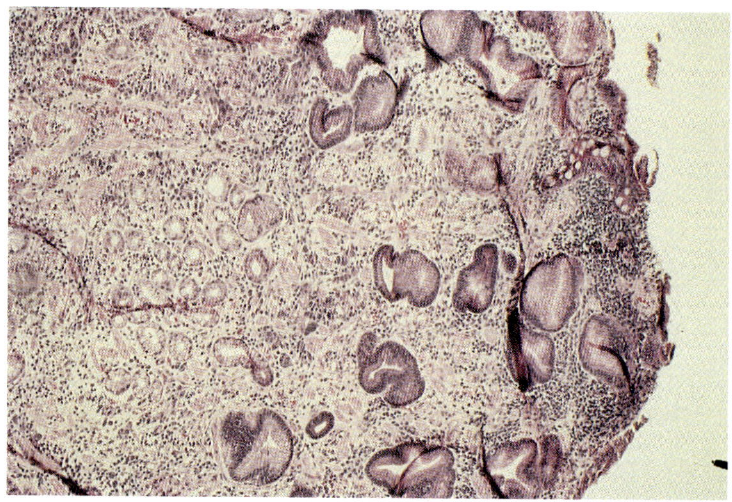

Figure 12.5 Gastric biopsy of patient with gastric adenocarcinoma in an area with normal glands demonstrating *H. pylori* (monoclonal antibody stain for *H. pylori*; original magnification, ×100).

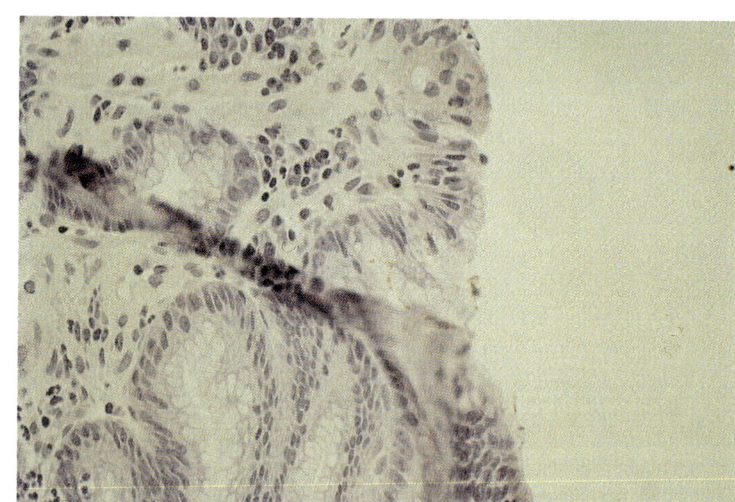

Figure 12.6 Wenger-Angrit stain of *H. pylori*. Original magnification, ×400.

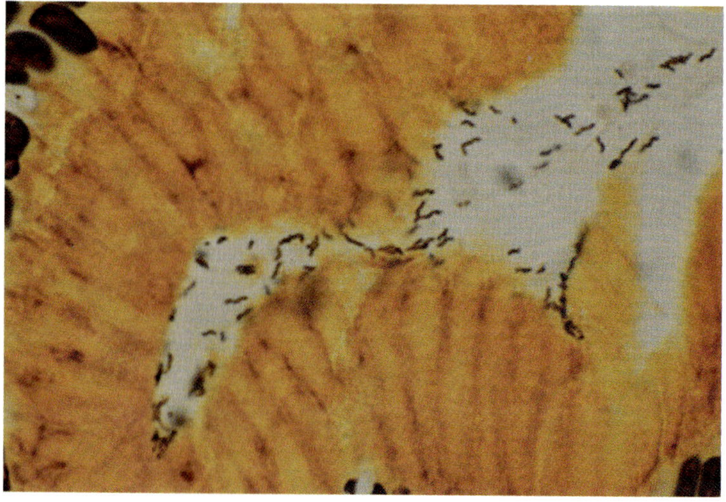

References

1. **Balfour, A.** 1906. A haemogregarine of mammals and some notes on trypanosomiasis in the Anglo-Egyptian Sudan. *J. Trop. Med.* **9:**81–92.

2. **Banatvala, N., C. R. Lopez, R. J. Owen, A. Hurtado, Y. Asai, G. Davies, J. Hardies, and R. Feldman.** 1994. Use of the polymerase chain reaction to detect *Helicobacter pylori* in the dental plaque of healthy and symptomatic volunteers. *Microbiol. Ecol. Health Dis.* **7:**1–8.

3. **Bayerdorffer, E., S. Miehlke, G. A. Mannes, A. Sommer, N. Hochter, J. Weingart, W. Heldwein, H. Klann, T. Simon, and W. Schmidt.** 1995. Double-blind trial of omeprazole and amoxicillin to cure *Helicobacter pylori* infection in patients with duodenal ulcer. *Gastroenterology* **108:**1412–1417.

4. **Blaser, M. J.** 1992. Hypotheses on the pathogenesis and natural history of *Helicobacter pylori* induced inflammation. *Gastroenterology* **102:**720–727.

5. **Blecker, U., T. W. McKeithan, and B. S. Kirschner.** 1995. Resolution of *Helicobacter pylori*-associated gastric lymphoma disease in a child. *Gastroenterology* **109:**973–977.

6. **Borén, T., P. Flak, K. A. Roth, G. Larson, and S. Normark.** 1993. Attachment of *H. pylori* to human gastric epithelium mediated by blood group antigens. *Science* **262:**1892–1895.

7. **Brown, K. E., and D. A. Peura.** 1993. Diagnosis of *Helicobacter pylori* infection. *Gastroenterol. Clin. North Am.* **22:**105–115.

8. **Chen, M. H., A. Lee, S. Hazell, P. J. Hu, and Y. Y. Li.** 1993. Immunization against gastric infection with *Helicobacter* species—first step in the prophylaxis against gastric cancer. *Int. J. Microbiol. Virol. Parasitol. Infect. Dis.* **280:**155–165.

9. **Corthésy-Theulaz, I., N. Porta, M. Glauser, E. Saraga, A. C. Vaney, R. Haas, J. P. Kraehenbuhl, A. L. Blum, and P. Michetti.** 1995. Oral immunization with *Helicobacter pylori* urease B subunit as a treatment against *Helicobacter* infection in mice. *Gastroenterology* **109:**115–121.

10. **Cover, T. L., and M. J. Blaser.** 1992. Purification and characterization of the vacuolating toxin from *Helicobacter pylori*. *J. Biol. Chem.* **267:**10570–10575.

11. **Cover, T. L., and M. J. Blaser.** 1992. *Helicobacter pylori* and gastroduodenal disease. *Annu. Rev. Med.* **43:**135–145.

12. **Crabtree, J. E., J. I. Wyatt, G. M. Sobala, G. Miller, D. S. Tompkins, J. N. Primrose, and A. G. Morgan.** 1993. Systemic and mucosal humoral responses to *Helicobacter pylori* in gastric cancer. *Gut* **34:**1339–1343.

13. **Cutler, A. F., and T. T. Schubert.** 1993. Long term *Helicobacter pylori* recurrence after successful eradication with triple therapy. *Am. J. Gastroenterol.* **88:**1359–1361.

14. **Czinn, S. J., and J. G. Nedrud.** 1991. Oral immunization against *Helicobacter pylori*. *Infect. Immun.* **59:**2359–2363.

15. **Dixon, M. F.** 1995. Histologic responses to *Helicobacter pylori* infection: gastritis, atrophy, and preneoplasia. *Bailliere's Clin. Gastroenterol.* **9:**467–485.

16. **Drumm, B.** 1993. *Helicobacter pylori* and the pediatric patient. *Gastroenterol. Clin. North Am.* **22:**169–182.

17. **Drumm, B., S. Gormally, and P. M. Sherman.** 1996. Gastritis and peptic ulcer disease, p. 506–527. *In* A. W. Walker, P. R. Durie, J. R. Hamilton, J. A. Walker-Smith, and J. B. Watkins (ed.), *Pediatric Gastrointestinal Disease: Pathophysiology, Diagnosis, Management*, 2nd ed., vol. 1. Mosby-Year Book, Inc., St. Louis.

18. **Drumm, B., P. Sherman, E. Cutz, and M. Karmali.** 1987. Association of *Campylobacter pylori* on the gastric mucosa with antral gastritis in children. *N. Engl. J. Med.* **316:**1557–1561.

19. **Fauchere, J. L., A. Rosenau, and F. Bonneville.** 1989. Virulence factors of *Campylobacter pylori. Gastroenterol. Clin. Biol.* **13:**59–64.

20. **Ferreres, J.-C., F. Fernandez, A. R. Vives, I. Gonzalez-Rodilla, I. Ursua, R. Ramos, and J. F. Val-Bernal.** 1991. *Helicobacter pylori* in Barrett's esophagus. *Histol. Histopathol.* **6:**403–408.

21. **Forman, D., D. G. Newel, F. Fullerton, J. W. Yarnell, A. R. Stacey, M. Wald, and F. Sitas.** 1991. Association between infection with *Helicobacter pylori* and risk of gastric cancer: evidence from a prospective investigation. *Br. Med. J.* **302:**1302–1305.

22. **Fox, J. G., F. E. Dewhirst, J. G. Tully, B. J. Paster, L. Yan, N. S. Taylor, M. J. Collins, Jr., P. L. Gorelick, and J. M. Ward.** 1994. *Helicobacter hepaticus* sp. nov., a microaerophilic bacterium isolated from livers and intestinal mucosal scrapings from mice. *J. Clin. Microbiol.* **32:**1238–1245.

23. **Genta, R. M., H. W. Hamner, and D. Y. Graham.** 1993. Gastric lymphoid follicles in Helicobacter pylori infection: frequency, distribution, and response to triple therapy. *Hum. Pathol.* **24:**577–583.

24. **Goodwin, C. S., J. A. Armstrong, T. Chilvers, M. Peters, M. D. Collins, L. Sly, W. McConnell, and W. E. S. Harper.** 1989. Transfer of *Campylobacter pylori* and *Campylobacter mustelae* to *Helicobacter* gen. nov. as *Helicobacter pylori* comb. nov. and *Helicobacter mustelae* comb. nov., respectively. *Int. J. Syst. Bacteriol.* **39:**397–405.

25. **Graham, D. Y., G. M. Lew, D. G. Evans, D. J. Evans, Z. A. Saeed, and H. M. Malatay.** 1992. Effect of treatment of *Helicobacter pylori* infection on the long term recurrence of gastric or duodenal ulcer: a randomized, controlled study. *Ann. Intern. Med.* **116:**705–708.

26. **Heilmann, K. L., and F. Borchard.** 1991. Gastritis due to spiral shaped bacteria other than *Helicobacter pylori*: clinical, histological, and ultrastructural findings. *Gut* **32:**137–140.

27. **Hentschel, E., G. Brandstätter, B. Dragosics, A. M. Hirschl, H. Nemec, K. Schutze, M. Taufer, and H. Wurzer.** 1993. Effect of ranitidine and amoxicillin plus metronidazole on the eradication of *Helicobacter pylori* and the recurrence of duodenal ulcer. *N. Engl. J. Med.* **328:**308–312.

28. **Hirschl, A. M., G. Brandstätter, B. Dragosics, E. Hentschel, M. Kundi, M. L. Rotter, K. Schutze, and M. Taufer.** 1993. Kinetics of specific IgG antibodies for monitoring the effect of anti-*Helicobacter pylori* chemotherapy. *J. Infect. Dis.* **168:**763–766.

29. **Hopkins, R. J., and J. G. Morris, Jr.** 1994. *Helicobacter pylori*: the missing link in perspective. *Am. J. Med.* **97:**265–277.

30. **Josenhans, C., A. Labigne, and S. Suerbaum.** 1995. Comparative ultrastructural and functional studies of *Helicobacter pylori* and *Helicobacter mustelae* flagellin mutants: both flagellin subunits, FlaA and FlaB, are necessary for full motility in *Helicobacter* species. *J. Bacteriol.* **177:**3010–3020.

31. **Klein, P. D., D. Y. Graham, A. R. Opekun, and E. O'Brian-Smith.** 1991. Water source as a risk factor for *Helicobacter pylori* infection in Peruvian children. *Lancet* **337:**1503–1506.

32. **Krajden, S., and P. M. Sherman.** 1990. *Helicobacter* (*Campylobacter*) *pylori* and acid peptic diseases. *Can. J. Gastroenterol.* **4:**237–242.

33. **Kuipers, E. J., A. S. Peña, G. van Camp, A. M. Uyterlinde, G. Pals, N. F. M. Pels, E. Kurz-Pohlmann, and S. G. M. Meuwissen.** 1993. Seroconversion for *Helicobacter pylori*. *Lancet* **342:**328–331.

34. **Kuipers, E. J., J. C. Thijs, and P. M. Festen.** 1995. The prevalence of *Helicobacter pylori* in peptic ulcer disease. *Aliment. Pharmacol. Ther.* **9**(Suppl.):59–69.

35. **Kurata, J. H., and B. M. Haile.** 1984. Epidemiology of peptic ulcer disease. *Clin. Gastroenterol.* **13:**289–307.

36. **Lage, A. P., E. Godfroid, A. Fauconnier, A. Burette, J.-P. Butzler, A. Bollen, and Y. Glupczynski.** 1995. Diagnosis of *Helicobacter pylori* infection by PCR: comparison with other invasive techniques and detection of *cagA* gene in gastric biopsy specimens. *J. Clin. Microbiol.* **33:**2752–2756.

37. **Lanas, A. I., B. Remacha, F. Esteva, and R. Sainz.** 1995. Risk factors associated with refractory peptic ulcers. *Gastroenterology* **109:**1124–1133.

38. **Lee, A.** 1985. Neglected niches: the microbial ecology of the gastrointestinal tract. *Adv. Microb. Ecol.* **8:**115–162.

39. **Lee, A., and M. Chen.** 1994. Successful immunization against gastric infection with *Helicobacter* species: use of a cholera toxin B-subunit–whole-cell vaccine. *Infect. Immun.* **62:**3594–3597.

40. **Lee, A., S. L. Hazell, J. O'Rourke, and S. Kourpach.** 1988. Isolation of a spiral-shaped bacterium from the cat stomach. *Infect. Immun.* **56:**2843–2850.

41. **Levine, M. S., and S. E. Rubesin.** 1995. The *Helicobacter pylori* revolution: radiologic perspective. *Radiology* **195:**593–596.

42. **Leying, H., S. Suerbaum, G. Geis, and R. Haas.** 1992. Cloning and genetic characterization of a *Helicobacter pylori* flagellin gene. *Mol. Microbiol.* **6:**2863–2874.

43. **Loffeld, R. J., I. Willems, J. A. Flendrig, and J. W. Arends.** 1990. *Helicobacter pylori* and gastric carcinoma. *Histopathology* **17:**537–541.

44. **Logan, R. P. H., K. D. Bardham, and L. R. Celestin.** 1995. Eradication of *Helicobacter pylori* and prevention of recurrence of duodenal ulcer: a randomized, double blinded, multi-center trial of omeprazole with or without clarithromycin. *Aliment. Pharmacol. Ther.* **9:**417–424.

45. **Logan, R. P. H., R. J. Polson, J. J. Misiewicz, G. Rao, N. Q. Karim, D. Newell, P. Johnson, J. Wadsworth, M. M. Walker, and J. H. Baron.** 1991. Simplified single sample ^{13}carbon urea breath test for *Helicobacter pylori*: comparison with histology, culture, and ELISA serology. *Gut* **32:**1461–1464.

46. **Luck, J. M., and T. N. Seth.** 1924. Gastric urease. *Biochem. J.* **18:**1227–1231.

47. **Marshall, B. J.** 1983. Unidentified curved bacilli on gastric epithelium in active chronic gastritis. *Lancet* **i:**1273–1275. (Letter.)

48. **Marshall, B. J., J. A. Armstrong, D. B. McGechie, and R. J. Glancy.** 1985. Attempts to fulfill Koch's postulates for pyloric *Campylobacter*. *Med. J. Aust.* **142:**436–439.

49. **Marshall, B. J., and J. R. Warren.** 1984. Unidentified curved bacilli in the stomach of patients with gastritis and peptic ulceration. *Lancet* **i:**1311–1313.

50. **Marshall, B. J., J. R. Warren, E. D. Blincow, M. Phillips, C. S. Goodwin, R. Murray, S. J. Blackbourn, T. E. Waters, and C. R. Sanderson.** 1988. Prospective double-blind trial of duodenal ulcer relapse after eradication of *Campylobacter pylori*. *Lancet* **ii:**1437–1442.

51. **Megraud, F.** 1993. Duodenal ulcer disease: a new infectious disease. *Eur. J. Gastroenterol. Hepatol.* **5:**17–22.

52. **Megraud, F.** 1993. Epidemiology of *Helicobacter pylori* infection. *Gastroenterol. Clin. North Am.* **22:**73–88.

53. **Michetti, P., I. Corthésy-Theulaz, C. Davin, R. Haas, A.-C. Vaney, M. Heitz, J. Bille, J.-P. Kraehenbuhl, E. Saraga, and A. L. Blum.** 1994. Immunization of BALB/c mice against *Helicobacter felis* infection with *H. pylori* urease. *Gastroenterology* **107:**1002–1011.

54. **Neale, K. R., and R. P. H. Logan.** 1995. The epidemiology and transmission of *Helicobacter pylori* infection in children. *Aliment. Pharmacol. Ther.* **9**(Suppl.)**:**77–84.

55. **NIH Consensus Conference.** 1994. *Helicobacter pylori* in peptic ulcer disease. NIH Consensus Development Panel on *Helicobacter pylori* in Peptic Ulcer Disease. *JAMA* **272:**65–69.

56. **Palmer, E. D.** 1940. Investigation of the gastric spirochetes in human gastric mucosa. *Am. J. Dig. Dis.* **7:**443–445.

57. **Parsonnet, J.** 1995. The incidence of *Helicobacter pylori* infection. *Aliment. Pharmacol. Ther.* **9**(Suppl.)**:**45–51.

58. **Parsonnet, J., S. Hansen, L. Rodriguez, A. B. Gelb, R. A. Warnke, E. Jellum, N. Orentreich, J. H. Vogleman, and G. D. Friedman.** 1994. *Helicobacter pylori* infection and gastric lymphoma. *N. Engl. J. Med.* **330:**1267–1271.

59. **Peterson, W. L.** 1991. *Helicobacter pylori* and peptic ulcer disease. *N. Engl. J. Med.* **324:**1043–1048.

60. **Peterson, W. L., C. C. Barnett, D. J. Evans, M. Feldman, T. Carmody, C. Richardson, J. Walsh, and D. Y. Graham.** 1993. Acid secretion and serum gastrin in normal subjects and patients with duodenal ulcer: the role of *Helicobacter pylori. Am. J. Gastroenterol.* **88:**2038–2043.

61. **Rautelin, H., and T. U. Kosunen.** 1991. *Helicobacter pylori* and associated gastroduodenal diseases. *APMIS* **99:**677–695.

62. **Rogge, J. D., D. R. Wagner, R. J. Carrico, E. A. Glowinski, S. J. Mahoney, R. C. Bogulashi, and R. M. Genta.** 1995. Evaluation of a new urease reagent strip for detection of *Helicobacter pylori* in gastric biopsy specimens. *Am. J. Gastroenterol.* **90:**1965–1968.

63. **Salomen, H.** 1986. Ueber das Spirillum des Saugetiermagens und sein Verhalten zu den Belegzellen. *Zentralbl. Bakteriol. Mikrobiol. Hyg.* **19:**433–443.

64. **Schembri, M. A., S. K. Lin, and J. R. Lamber.** 1993. Comparison of diagnostic tests for *Helicobacter pylori* antibodies. *J. Clin. Microbiol.* **31:**2621–2624.

65. **Sherman, P. M.** 1994. Peptic ulcer disease in children. Diagnosis, treatment and implication of *Helicobacter pylori. Gastroenterol. Clin. North Am.* **23:**707–725.

66. **Sherman, P. M., and B. D. Gold.** 1993. Pathogenesis of *Helicobacter pylori* infection. *Can. J. Gastroenterol.* **7:**395–405.

67. **Silverstein, M. D., T. Petterson, and N. J. Talley.** 1996. Initial endoscopy or empirical therapy with or without testing for *Helicobacter pylori* for dyspepsia: a decision analysis. *Gastroenterology* **110:**72–83.

68. **Sipponen, P., K. Seppälä, M. Äärynen, T. Helske, and P. Kettunen.** 1989. Chronic gastritis and gastroduodenal ulcer: a case control study on risk of coexisting duodenal or gastric ulcer in patients with gastritis. *Gut* **30:**922–929.

69. **Staat, M. A., D. Kruszon-Moran, and R. A. Kaslow.** 1994. Analysis of seroprevalence and risk factors for *Helicobacter pylori* (Hp) infection in children and adolescents in the United States. *Am. J. Gastroenterol.* **89:**1396 (A445).

70. **Steer, H. W., and D. G. Colin-Jones.** 1975. Mucosal changes in gastric ulceration and their response to carbenoxolone sodium. *Gut* **16:**590–597.

71. **Strickland, R. G., and J. R. Mackay.** 1973. A reappraisal of the nature and significance of chronic atrophic gastritis. *Am. J. Dig. Dis.* **18:**426–440.

72. **Taylor, D. E., N. Chang, N. S. Taylor, and J. G. Fox.** 1994. Genome conservation in *Helicobacter mustelae* as determined by pulsed-field gel electrophoresis. *FEMS Microbiol. Lett.* **118:**31–36.

73. **Taylor, D. E., M. Eaton, N. Chang, and S. Salama.** 1992. Construction of a *Helicobacter pylori* genome map and demonstration of diversity at the genome level. *J. Bacteriol.* **174:**6800–6806.

74. **Tomkins, L. S., and S. Falkow.** 1995. The new path to preventing ulcers. *Science* **267:**1621–1622.

75. **Tytgat, G. N. J., A. Lee, D. Y. Graham, M. F. Dixon, and T. Rokkas.** 1993. The role of infectious agents in peptic ulcer disease. *Gastroenterol. Int.* **6:**76–89.

76. **Tytgat, N. J., L. Noach, and E. A. J. Rauws.** 1991. *Helicobacter pylori. Scand. J. Gastroenterol.* **26**(Suppl.)**:**1–8.

77. **Vandamme, P., E. Falsen, R. Rossau, B. Hoste, P. Segers, R. Tytgat, and J. De Ley.** 1991. Revision of *Campylobacter, Helicobacter,* and *Wolinella* taxonomy: emendation of generic descriptions and proposal of *Arcobacter* gen. nov. *Int. J. Syst. Bacteriol.* **41:**88–103.

78. **Vandenplas, Y., U. Blecker, T. Devreker, E. Keppens, J. Nijs, S. Cadrane, M. Pipeleers-Marichal, A. Goossens, and S. Lauwers.** 1992. Contribution of the ^{13}C-urea breath test to the detection of *Helicobacter pylori* gastritis in children. *Pediatrics* **90:**608–611.

79. **Van Zanten, S. J. O. V., P. T. Pollak, L. M. Best, G. S. Bezanson, and T. Marrie.** 1994. Increasing prevalence of *Helicobacter pylori* infection with age: continuous risk of infection in adults rather than cohort effect. *J. Infect. Dis.* **169:**434–437.

80. **van Zwet, A. A., J. C. Thijs, A. M. D. Kooistra-Smid, J. Schirm, and J. A. M. Snijder.** 1993. Sensitivity of culture compared with that of polymerase chain reaction for detection of *Helicobacter pylori* from antral biopsy specimens. *J. Clin. Microbiol.* **31:**1918–1920.

81. **Veldhuyzen van Zanter, S. J., and P. M. Sherman.** 1994. *Helicobacter pylori* infection as a cause of gastritis, duodenal ulcer, gastric cancer, and nonulcer dyspepsia: a systematic overview. *Can. Med. Assoc. J.* **150:**177–185.

82. **Walsh, J. H., and W. L. Peterson.** 1995. The treatment of *Helicobacter pylori* infection in the management of peptic ulcer disease. *N. Engl. J. Med.* **333:**984–991.

83. **Webb, P. M., T. Night, S. Greaves, A. Wilson, D. G. Newell, J. Elder, and D. Forman.** 1994. Relation between infection with *Helicobacter pylori* and living-conditions in childhood: evidence for person-to-person transmission in early life. *Br. Med. J.* **308:**750–753.

84. **Xiang, Z., S. M. Censini, P. Bayeli, J. L. Telford, N. Figura, R. Rappuoli, and A. Coracci.** 1995. Analysis of expression of CagA and VacA virulence factors in 43 strains of *Helicobacter pylori* reveals that clinical isolates can be divided into two major types and that CagA is not necessary for expression of the vacuolating cytotoxin. *Infect. Immun.* **63:**94–98.

85. **Yoshida, N., D. N. Granger, D. J. Evans, Jr., D. G. Evans, D. Y. Graham, D. C. Anderson, R. E. Wolf, and P. R. Kvietys.** 1993. Mechanisms involved in *Helicobacter*-induced inflammation. *Gastroenterology* **105:**1431–1440.

chapter 13

Cryptosporidiosis

David G. Addiss, Dennis D. Juranek, and David A. Schwartz

*C*ryptosporidium parvum, a coccidian protozoan, has been recognized as a human pathogen only since 1976. *Cryptosporidium* oocysts measure 4 to 6 μm in diameter and are highly resistant to most commonly used disinfectants, such as chlorine. Symptoms of *Cryptosporidium* infection generally begin within 3 to 12 (median, 5 to 7) days after ingestion of oocysts. In immunocompetent persons, cryptosporidiosis causes an acute, self-limiting diarrheal illness which lasts a median of 5 to 10 days and which is often accompanied by nausea, vomiting, abdominal cramps, and low-grade fever. In patients with AIDS, diarrhea can be prolonged, voluminous, debilitating, and, not infrequently, fatal.

Cryptosporidiosis is caused by the protozoan C. *parvum*, a member of the phylum *Apicomplexa*, suborder *Eimeriorina*. It is widespread in the environment and infects the gastrointestinal tracts of a variety of hosts, including fish, birds, reptiles, and mammals (12). The parasite is phylogenetically related to two other human pathogens, *Isospora belli* and *Toxoplasma gondii*. In-

David G. Addiss and Dennis D. Juranek, Division of Parasitic Diseases, National Center for Infectious Diseases, Centers for Disease Control and Prevention, 4770 Buford Highway, Mailstop F-22, Atlanta, GA 30341. **David A. Schwartz,** Department of Pathology and Division of Infectious Diseases, Emory University School of Medicine, Atlanta, GA 30303, and National Center for Infectious Diseases, Centers for Disease Control and Prevention, Atlanta, GA 30333.

Pathology of Emerging Infections
Edited by C. Robert Horsburgh, Jr., and Ann Marie Nelson
© 1997 American Society for Microbiology, Washington, DC 20005-4171

fection begins when oocysts are ingested and encyst in the small intestine. The four sporozoites which are released from each oocyst initiate the asexual cycle by invading the microvillous border of the enterocytes, where they develop into type 1 and type 2 meronts. Each type 1 meront releases six to eight merozoites, which reinvade the host cells and initiate another cycle of merogony. Type 2 meronts release four merozoites, which initiate the sexual stage of development by developing into microgametocytes and macrogametocytes. Motile, aflagellar microgametes fertilize the macrogametes, which subsequently develop into oocysts and complete the cycle. Both sexual and asexual stages of development can occur in the gastrointestinal tract, and the infectious, fully sporulated oocysts are passed in the feces. Humans may become infected by ingesting oocysts from a variety of environmental sources.

In the past few years, *C. parvum* has emerged as the leading known cause of waterborne disease outbreaks in the United States (6), an important opportunistic infection in persons with AIDS, and a significant cause of outbreaks of diarrhea in child day care centers (11). In March and April 1993, the largest documented waterborne disease outbreak in U.S. history occurred in Milwaukee, Wis. An estimated 403,000 people developed watery diarrhea after drinking municipal water contaminated with *C. parvum* (32). The magnitude of this outbreak and its association with a municipal water plant that was operating within existing state and federal regulatory standards heightened public concern about the quality of drinking water in the United States, highlighted the need for improved surveillance and coordination between public health agencies and water utilities, and revitalized efforts to develop regulatory standards for cryptosporidium in drinking water.

> *In the past few years, C. parvum has emerged as the leading known cause of waterborne disease outbreaks in the United States*

Epidemiology

Waterborne Cryptosporidiosis

Cryptosporidium oocysts are ubiquitous in surface waters such as lakes and rivers, are highly resistant to disinfectants commonly used in municipal water treatment, and are incompletely removed by conventional water treatment that includes filtration. Small numbers of oocysts have been detected in samples of drinking water in 17 to 55% of U.S. cities with surface water supplies (28, 38). The extent to which low levels of oocysts in drinking water cause human infections which are not associated with recognized outbreaks (sporadic infections) is unknown. Further, current laboratory methods to detect oocysts in water are cumbersome, time-consuming, and inefficient, and they do not reliably discriminate between oocysts that are viable or infectious and those that are not. Concern about the possibility of *Cryptosporidium* transmission through drinking water has prompted several recent community-wide "boil water advisories" in cities across the United States.

There have been seven well-documented outbreaks of cryptosporidiosis attributable to drinking water in the United States, including two that have occurred since the large Milwaukee outbreak in 1993. Two common features of the outbreaks involving surface water sources were that water treatment included both chlorination and filtration and that the finished water quality met existing state and federal standards. In terms of its implications for prevention, the most disturbing recent outbreak occurred in Clark County, Nev., in 1994 (18). Seventy-eight laboratory-confirmed cases occurred, mostly in persons with human immunodeficiency virus (HIV) infection, despite pristine source water (Lake Mead), a state-of-the-art water treatment plant, and extremely low turbidity of both the raw and finished water. A case-control study showed that persons who drank unboiled tap water were four times more likely than persons who drank only bottled water to have had cryptosporidiosis. Among persons with CD4 counts of less than 100, persons who drank unboiled tap water were 13 times more likely than persons who drank only bottled water to have had cryptosporidiosis (18).

Household Transmission

Although high levels of secondary household transmission were associated with outbreaks among children attending day care centers (12 to 40%) (11), studies during and after the Milwaukee outbreak documented household attack rates of about 5% when the index case was an adult (32, 35). Thus, risk of household transmission of *Cryptosporidium* infection appears to be inversely related to age, which is most likely a proxy for hygiene. These findings suggest that the risk of person-to-person transmission is low in settings where good hygiene is practiced and exposure to feces is limited.

Infection and Disease in Immunocompromised Persons

Preliminary data from a prospective study of persons with HIV infection in Atlanta, Ga., suggest that 5 to 10% of these persons can be expected to develop *Cryptosporidium* infection annually. Initial detection of oocysts in stool did not always correlate with new onset of diarrhea. Growing experience with *Cryptosporidium* surveillance suggests that for persons with AIDS, it is often not possible to identify or recall a specific date of onset of cryptosporidial diarrhea. These findings suggest that case-control studies to assess risk factors for cryptosporidiosis among persons who are immunosuppressed may be difficult.

5 to 10% of HIV-infected persons can be expected to develop Cryptosporidium infection annually

The issue of whether cryptosporidiosis in persons with AIDS represents new infection or reactivation of previous infection remains unsettled. Individual observations and case reports (23) suggest that reactivation of old infection may occur as the CD4 cell count decreases. This is an issue that needs clarification, as it has important implications for prevention of cryptosporidiosis in persons with AIDS. If reactivation accounts for even a modest proportion of cases in persons with AIDS, prevention of exposure to cryptosporidia after the diagnosis of AIDS has been made will have limited impact on reducing cryptosporidium-related disease in this population.

A survey of HIV-infected persons in Milwaukee after the outbreak revealed that the attack rate among these persons during the outbreak appeared to be no greater than that among the general population, regardless of CD4 count. However, increasing severity of illness was associated with decreasing CD4 counts (16), as had been previously documented (14).

Another study of HIV-infected persons during the Milwaukee outbreak documented the high proportion of patients with biliary tract involvement, particularly among those with low CD4 counts (41). Among those with biliary tract involvement, 1-year mortality was 83%. Extraintestinal cryptosporidiosis has been documented previously in persons with AIDS, with the principal sites being the bile ducts, pancreas, and lung. Other than severity of immunosuppression, risk factors for extraintestinal disease are not well defined.

Recent outbreaks of cryptosporidiosis in the United States have also been associated with swimming pools, lakes, water slides, and recreational water parks (5, 31, 33). In only a few of these instances were fecal accidents actually observed. Because oocysts are highly resistant to disinfection by chlorine and because most recreational water filtration units are not effective in removing oocysts, it is likely that recreational waterborne outbreaks of cryptosporidiosis will continue to occur.

Recent outbreaks of cryptosporidiosis in the United States have also been associated with swimming pools, lakes, water slides, and recreational water parks

Pathology

Developmental stages of cryptosporidia can be identified at all levels of the gastrointestinal tract. Although the jejunum is usually the most heavily infected site, parasites are often found throughout the length of the colon, as well as the duodenum, including the ampulla of Vater, ileum, gall bladder, bile ducts, and pancreatic ducts. In the small intestine and colon, the infection may produce no histologic abnormalities. In some patients, however, cryptosporidial infection may be associated with a histologic acute enteritis or colitis, increased inflammatory cells in the lamina propria, or small intestinal villous blunting.

Cryptosporidial organisms are easily identified by light microscopy in biopsy and autopsy tissue sections stained with hematoxylin and eosin, and special stains are unnecessary for detection of the organisms. The trophozoites and schizonts of cryptosporidia appear as small, 2- to 6-µm-diameter, blue- to pink-staining spherical structures which are most frequently present on the apical border of the epithelial lining cells of the involved organ (Fig. 13.1 and 13.2). Frequently, internal structures can be vaguely seen within the organisms by using high magnification. Because of their small size and indistinct structure by light microscopy, they can be easily confused with cellular debris or mucous drops. Although cryptosporidia appear to be extracellular by projecting into the lumen from the apex of infected cells, electron microscopic examination reveals that, in fact, all developmental stages are intracellular, with the organisms covered by a thin membrane of host cell origin (Fig. 13.3 and 13.4). In some organisms, a membranous zone formed by parallel folds of the cryptosporidial double unit membrane, or pellicle, develops adjacent to the attachment site with the host cell membrane. When there is any doubt as to the diagnosis, antisera are available for use in formalin-fixed and paraffin-embedded tissues (Fig. 13.5). Electron microscopy is useful for the confirmation of cryptosporidial infection in cases in which the organisms cannot be reliably distinguished from fat droplets or other material. Ultrastructural evaluation will demonstrate the various developing stages of cryptosporidia (Fig. 13.3 and 13.4), including macrogametes, microgametes, schizonts, and trophozoites. Electron microscopy can also be useful for identifying the presence of protozoal coinfections, especially those with microsporidia (*Enterocytozoon bieneusi* and *Septata intestinalis*) and *Giardia* spp. (27). The histologic findings for gastric cryptosporidiosis are similar to those seen in the colon. Developing stages of the organism are present on the lining epithelium and may extend into the gastric glands (Fig. 13.6). Infection can be associated with active gastritis and with a lymphoplasmacellular infiltrate in the lamina propria.

Hepatobiliary tract infection is a frequent complication of intestinal cryptosporidiosis. The most severe extraintestinal complications of cryptosporidiosis in patients with AIDS are secondary to infection of the gall bladder, biliary tract, and pancreatic ducts. The organisms are believed to infect these structures following direct extension from the duodenum through the major pancreatic and biliary ducts. It has been estimated that up to 15% of AIDS patients with intestinal cryptosporidiosis have hepatobiliary tract infection (36). Cryptosporidial infection of the gall bladder is often diagnosed following cholecystectomy for acalculous cholecystitis. The organisms are seen lining the gall bladder epithelium and extending into the Rokitansky-Aschoff sinuses associated with chronic cholecystitis. Sclerosing cholangitis can result from cryptosporidial infection of the intra- or extrahepatic bile ducts.

Hepatobiliary tract infection is a frequent complication of intestinal cryptosporidiosis

The spectrum of microscopic features resulting from cryptosporidial infection of the respiratory tract is largely unknown, as only a few case reports have described the pathologic findings from biopsy or autopsy specimens. In one report of a patient with AIDS, transbronchial biopsy revealed cryptosporidia on the luminal surface of bronchial lining epithelial cells; there were metaplastic changes but no inflammatory reaction (15). Following the death of this patient, autopsy examination revealed cryptosporidial infection of the tracheal mucosa as well. There has been one report of cryptosporidial involvement of the tracheal glands and mucosa, which was identified at the time of autopsy of a 12-year-old boy with hypogammaglobulinemia (2). In addition to a report finding cryptosporidia on the surface of the superficial epithelial lining cells of the tracheo-bronchial mucosa, there has been one report of cryptosporidial organisms identified within the alveolar inflammatory exudate in an open lung biopsy from an AIDS patient with interstitial pneumonitis (4). However, microbiological cultures of this specimen were positive for cytomegalovirus and *Mycobacterium avium-Mycobacterium intracellulare*, and a subsequent autopsy revealed cytomegalovirus inclusions in the lung. Thus, the clinical and pathological findings in the lungs of this patient could be explained by viral or mycobacterial infection, and pulmonary disease could not be definitively attributed to *Cryptosporidium* spp. Several additional patients with respiratory tract cryptosporidiosis have been reported (26); however, some were diagnosed using sputum cytology (19, 34), tracheal aspirates (20), or bronchoalveolar lavage (25), and thus the histologic findings and distribution of respiratory infection in these cases remain unknown.

Diagnosis

Intestinal cryptosporidiosis is most commonly detected by finding the characteristic sporulated oocysts (4 to 6 μm in diameter) in stool. Because the organisms are not easily visible when the stool is processed for the routine ovum and parasite exam, special stains must be performed. The most frequently performed staining method for stool specimens is a modification of the acid-fast technique. The oocysts stain pink to bright red and often contain prominent black granules (Fig. 13.7). Although the trichrome stain is not the technique of choice for demonstrating cryptosporidial infection because it does not consistently stain the organisms, occasional well-stained sporocysts containing four sporozoites are sometimes seen (17, 29).

Almost all patients with extraintestinal cryptosporidiosis are initially diagnosed with intestinal infection. Diagnosis of pulmonary infection can been made by using either sputum or transbronchial or bronchoalveolar lavage specimens. Cytologic specimens of sputum and bronchoalveolar lavage fluid should be stained with the modified acid-fast stain (25, 34) for the diagnosis of cryptosporidiosis. As in other pulmonary infections in immunocompromised patients, diagnosis of respiratory tract cryptosporidiosis should first be attempted using sputum cytology, the safest and least invasive method. Open biopsies of organs, including the lung and liver, suspected of being infected should be performed only in cases in which cytologic and endoscopic techniques fail to identify an etiologic process.

Evidence for the low sensitivity of available diagnostic tests for cryptosporidia in stool continues to accumulate. In the Milwaukee outbreak (30), as in earlier waterborne outbreaks (22), cryptosporidia were detected in <40% of stool specimens submitted by persons with watery diarrhea (i.e., clinical cryptosporidiosis). In the volunteer study by Dupont et al., in which samples of every stool specimen were examined in triplicate by using a comparatively sensitive direct immunofluorescence assay, *Cryptosporidium* oocysts were detected in only 62% of stool specimens submitted by infected persons on days when they were known to be shedding oocysts (i.e., at least one of their specimens submitted on the same day was positive for cryptosporidia) (8).

Other studies have shed light on how detection of infection might be improved, given existing laboratory tests. Perhaps most importantly, examination of multiple stool specimens increases sensitivity (10). Among children evaluated at Wisconsin Children's Hospital during the Milwaukee outbreak, those who tested positive for cryptosporidia submitted more stool specimens and submitted them later during the course of their illness (median, 8 days after onset of diarrhea) than did children who tested negative (median, 4 days) (9). Thus, collection of specimens towards the end of the first week of illness may improve detection of the organism.

Two recent studies highlighted the fact that stools submitted for testing for ova and parasites in U.S. diagnostic laboratories are infrequently tested for cryptosporidia. In a national survey, Boyce et al. (3) found that only 5% of laboratories routinely perform tests for this organism. A survey of Connecticut laboratories further suggested that physicians may not be selecting the patients most likely to have *Cryptosporidium* infection; in laboratories that tested for cryptosporidia only on physician request, 2.8% of stool specimens were positive for cryptosporidia, compared with 5.8% for laboratories that also used other testing criteria (37). Development and evaluation of selective screening criteria for this organism are needed.

Cyclospora cayetanensis is a newly described intestinal coccidian parasite of humans. It produces a nonsporulated oocyst which is shed in the feces and which also stains positively in stools when the modified acid-fast method is used. However, these oocysts are larger (10 µm in diameter) than those produced by cryptosporidia (Fig. 13.8). *C. cayetanensis* develops within an intracytoplasmic vacuole at the apical portion of the lining enterocytes, unlike the brush border location where *C. parvum* develops.

Clinical Features

Infectious Dose, Asymptomatic Infections, and Oocyst Shedding

In a remarkable recent study, Dupont and colleagues infected 29 human volunteers with various numbers (30 to 1,000,000) of *Cryptosporidium* oocysts (13). Of these, 18 persons became infected (had oocysts recovered in the stool); only 7 (39%) of these developed gastrointestinal symptoms. One volunteer who received 30 oocysts became infected; the mean infectious dose was estimated to be 132 oocysts. Data from animal studies suggest that as few as 2 to 10 oocysts may be enough to establish infection.

In this same study, patterns of oocyst shedding were associated with the presence of symptoms but not with the number of oocysts ingested (8). Volunteers with diarrheal illness shed numbers of oocysts 50-fold higher than those shed by volunteers who developed other mild symptoms or remained asymptomatic. In addition, persons with diarrhea were more likely to shed oocysts consistently, i.e., on consecutive days. Thus, parasitologic confirmation of *Cryptosporidium* infection may be particularly difficult in persons with mild symptoms.

Before the Milwaukee outbreak, intermittent diarrhea or a "waxing and waning" pattern of cryptosporidiosis had been described, primarily in immunosuppressed patients. However, MacKenzie et al. (32) reported that 39% of immunocompetent persons with laboratory-confirmed cryptosporidiosis experienced a return of watery diarrhea after at least 2 days of normal stools (interval range, 2 to 14 days). Six percent had recurrence after at least 5 days of normal stools. Similar patterns among visitors who were infected in Milwaukee and returned home were observed, so this recurrent pattern could not easily be explained by reinfection. Intermittent cryptosporidial diarrhea has implications for transmission in child day care centers, public swimming pools, and other settings.

Intermittent cryptosporidial diarrhea has implications for transmission in child day care centers, public swimming pools, and other settings

Treatment

Treatment of cryptosporidiosis remains unsatisfactory. Paromomycin appears to be the current drug of choice, and many patients respond with improvement in diarrhea and decreased shedding of organisms (1) but not parasitologic cure. In phase I studies, letrazuril resulted in improvement of diarrhea in 50% of patients (21).

Prevention

Because of the important public health implications of possible transmission of cryptosporidia through drinking water, particularly for immunosuppressed persons, considerable effort has been directed towards defining this risk. Studies to assess this risk are difficult to perform, particularly given the inaccuracies of existing methods for detecting and quantifying cryptosporidia in water. Efforts to develop less labor-intensive and more efficient methods for detecting *Cryptosporidium* oocysts in water and environmental and stool samples are under way. New methods for detecting serum antibody to cryptosporidia are also in progress.

A workshop to assess the public health threat associated with waterborne cryptosporidiosis and to bring all interested parties together was held at the Centers for Disease Control in September 1994. To effectively deal with this emerging disease, it was recognized that communication and advance planning were needed among public health agencies, water utilities, and other groups, such as physicians and representatives of immunosuppressed persons. The report of this workshop provided guidance for immunosuppressed persons and outlined a framework for future research and public health action (7). The workshop also led to the establishment of the Waterborne Cryptosporidiosis Working Group, a national group that meets every 2 weeks by teleconference to discuss emerging issues and to develop information and guidelines regarding cryptosporidia for public health departments, physicians, water utility officials, immunosuppressed persons, and other groups. The Working Group is developing a series of documents that hopefully will be widely distributed during 1997. These efforts are being mirrored at the state and local levels, as public health agencies, water utilities, and other groups begin to come together to develop effective public education messages and guidelines for prevention and early identification of outbreaks of waterborne cryptosporidiosis.

Prevention guidelines for cryptosporidia that are based on existing knowledge have been published (24), and an informational pamphlet on cryptosporidiosis for persons with AIDS has been developed. The Council of State and Territorial Epidemiologists recently established cryptosporidiosis as a nationally notifiable disease; this action will facilitate and stimulate public health surveillance for this condition. Much work remains to be done. Studies to assess the magnitude of risk for *Cryptosporidium* infection associated with drinking municipal water and other exposures are just getting under way. More rapid and sensitive serologic and molecular diagnostic techniques are needed for detection of cryptosporidia in humans and environmental sources. Prevention strategies resulting from current studies will need to be evaluated, and more effective drugs are urgently needed to treat the infection in immunosuppressed persons.

> *To effectively deal with this emerging disease, communication and advance planning are needed among public health agencies, water utilities, and other groups, such as physicians and representatives of immunosuppressed persons*

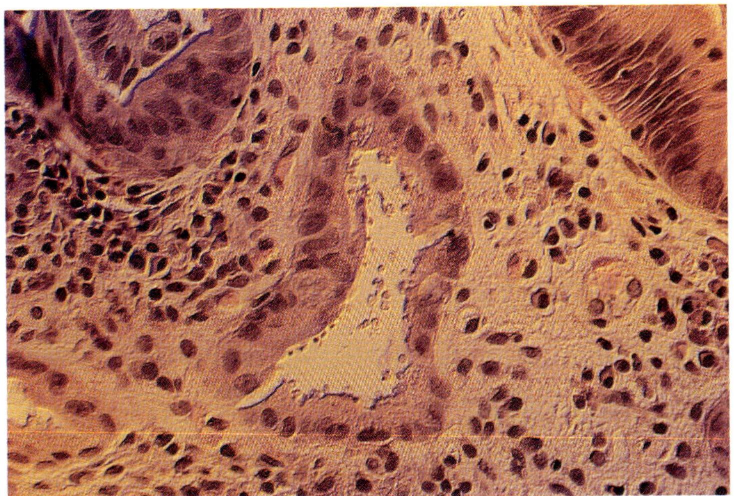

Figure 13.1 Cryptosporidia line the surface of epithelial cells in an intestinal gland (Nomarski interference contrast, hematoxylin and eosin; original magnification, ×400). From reference 39 with permission.

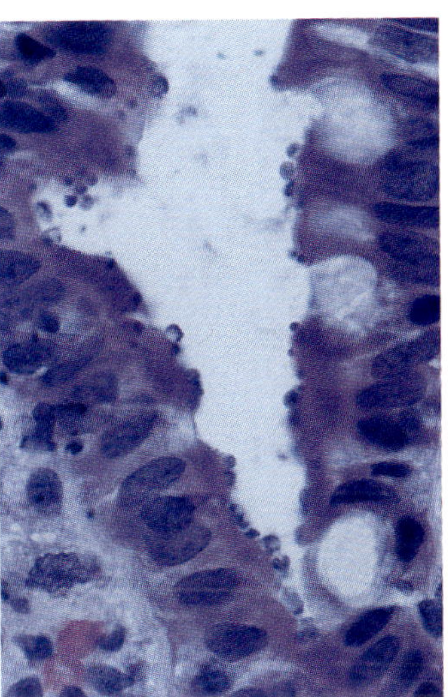

Figure 13.2 Numerous cryptosporidia on the apical surface of intestinal epithelial cells from an AIDS patient with chronic diarrhea. The various stages of cryptosporidial development cannot be distinguished by light microscopy (hematoxylin and eosin; original magnification, ×1,000).

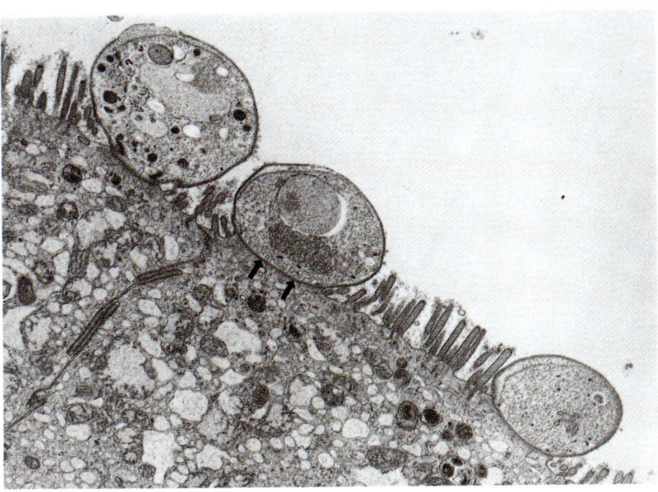

Figure 13.3 Typical ultrastructural appearance of cryptosporidia lining the luminal surface of the intestinal epithelium. The attachment of the organisms by means of a highly folded parasite pellicle is seen (arrows). Original magnification, ×8,000.

Figure 13.4 *Cryptosporidium* schizonts containing merozoites (asterisks) are present in the intestinal lumen. Original magnification, ×10,000.

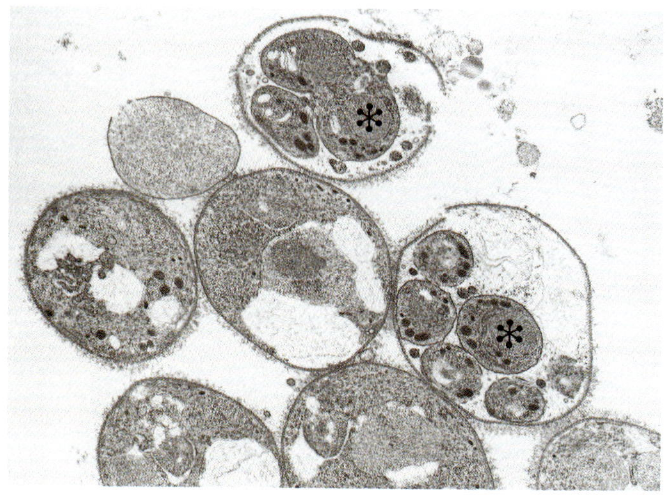

Figure 13.5 Immunofluorescence shows numerous brightly fluorescent cryptosporidia lining the epithelial cell surfaces in a small intestinal biopsy from an AIDS patient with diarrhea (fluorescent antibody to *C. parvum*; original magnification, ×400). From reference 40 with permission. Photograph courtesy of G. S. Visvesvara, Centers for Disease Control and Prevention, Atlanta, Ga.

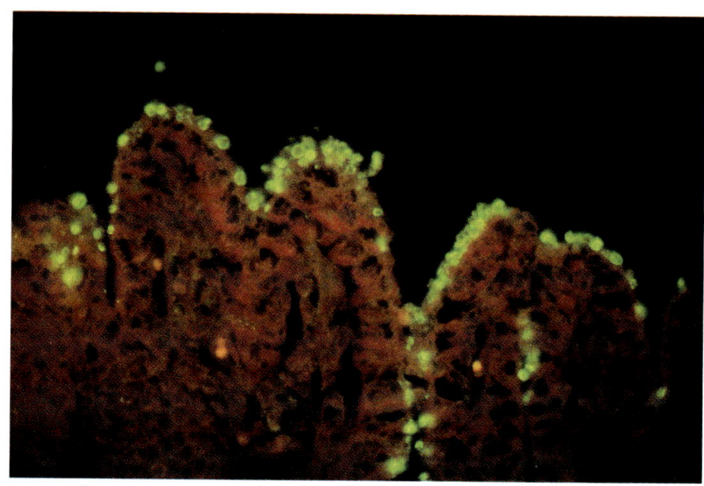

Figure 13.6 Cryptosporidial gastritis. Organisms are extensively parasitizing one gastric gland in this figure (hematoxylin and eosin; original magnification, ×400).

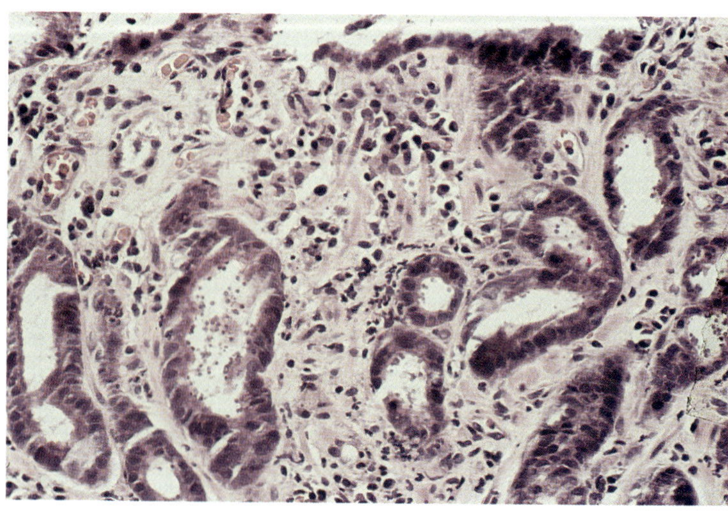

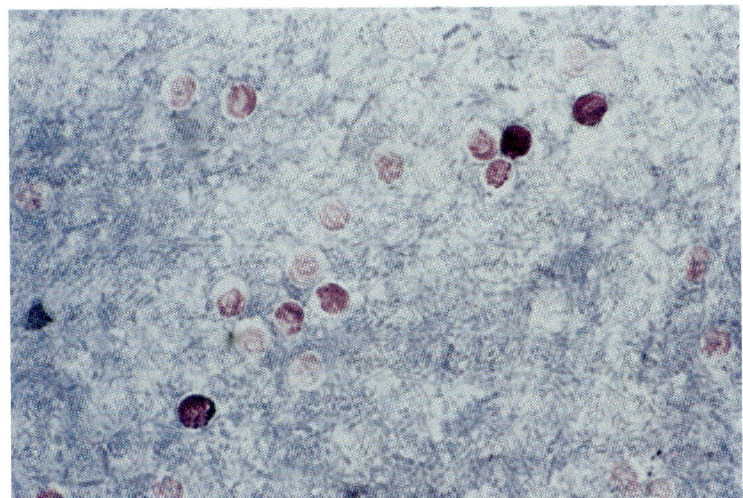

Figure 13.7 Stool smear stained with the modified acid-fast technique. Cryptosporidial oocysts stain pink to bright red (modified acid-fast stain; original magnification, ×1,000).

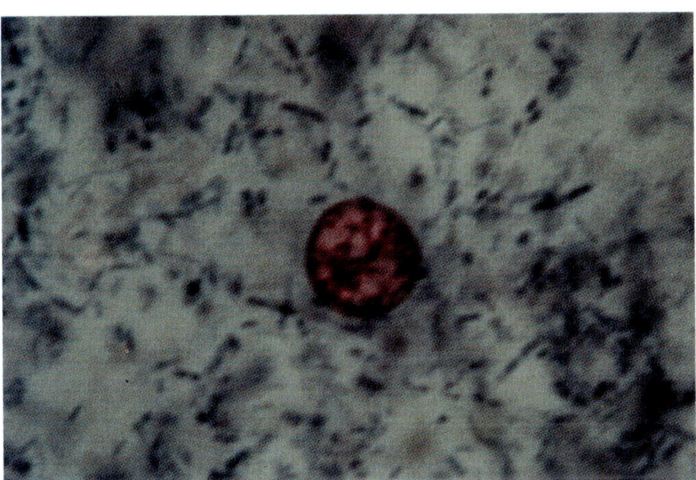

Figure 13.8 Nonsporulated oocyst of *C. cayetanensis* in stool. These oocysts are much larger than those of *C. parvum* (modified acid-fast stain; original magnification, ×1,600). Photograph courtesy of Molly Eaton, Emory University, Atlanta, Ga.

References

1. **Bissuel, F., L. Cotte, M. Rabodonirina, P. Rougier, M. A. Piens, and C. Trepo.** 1994. Paromomycin: an effective treatment for cryptosporidial diarrhea in patients with AIDS. *Clin. Infect. Dis.* **18:**447-449.

2. **Booth, C. C., G. Slavin, and R. R. Dourmashkin.** 1980. Immunodeficiency and cryptosporidiosis. *Br. Med. J.* **281:**1123-1127.

3. **Boyce, T. G., A. G. Pemberton, and D. G. Addiss.** 1996. *Cryptosporidium* testing practices among clinical laboratories in the United States. *Pediatr. Infect. Dis. J.* **15:**87-88.

4. **Brady, E. M., M. L. Margolis, and O. M. Korzeniowski.** 1984. Pulmonary cryptosporidiosis in acquired immune deficiency syndrome. JAMA **252:**89-90.

5. **Centers for Disease Control.** 1993. *Cryptosporidium* infections associated with swimming pools—Dane County, Wisconsin, 1993. *Morbid. Mortal. Weekly Rep.* **43:**561-563.

6. **Centers for Disease Control.** 1993. Surveillance for waterborne disease outbreaks—United States, 1991-1992. *Morbid. Mortal. Weekly Rep.* **42**(SS-5):1-22.

7. **Centers for Disease Control and Prevention.** 1995. Assessing the public health threat associated with waterborne cryptosporidiosis: report of a workshop. *Morbid. Mortal. Weekly Rep.* **44**(RR-6):1-19.

8. **Chappell, C. L., P. C. Okhuysen, C. R. Sterling, and H. L. DuPont.** 1996. *Cryptosporidium parvum*: intensity of infection and oocyst excretion patterns in healthy volunteers. *J. Infect. Dis.* **173:**232-236.

9. **Cicirello, H. G., K. S. Kehl, D. G. Addiss, M. J. Chusid, R. I. Glass, J. P. Davis, and P. L. Havens.** Cryptosporidiosis in children during a massive waterborne outbreak in Milwaukee, Wisconsin: clinical, laboratory, and epidemiologic findings. *Epidemiol. Infect.*, in press.

10. **Clavel, A., A. C. Arnal, and E. C. Sanchez.** 1995. Evaluation of the optimal number of faecal specimens in the diagnosis of cryptosporidiosis in AIDS and immunocompetent patients. *Eur. J. Clin. Microbiol. Infect. Dis.* **14:**46-49.

11. **Cordell, R. L., and D. G. Addiss.** 1994. Cryptosporidiosis in child care settings: a review of the literature and recommendations for prevention and control. *Pediatr. Infect. Dis. J.* **13:**310-317.

12. **Current, W. L., N. C. Reese, J. V. Ernst, W. S. Bailey, M. B. Heyman, and W. M. Weinstein.** 1983. Human cryptosporidiosis in immunocompetent and immunodeficient persons. Studies of an outbreak and experimental transmission. *N. Engl. J. Med.* **308:**1252-1257.

13. **Dupont, H. L., C. L. Chappell, C. R. Sterling, P. C. Okhuysen, J. B. Rose, and W. Jakubowski.** 1995. Infectivity of *Cryptosporidium parvum* for adult humans. *N. Engl. J. Med.* **332:**855-859.

14. **Flanigan, T., C. Whalen, J. Turner, R. Soave, J. Toerner, D. Havlir, and D. Kotler.** 1992. *Cryptosporidium* infection and CD4 counts. *Ann. Intern. Med.* **116:**840-842.

15. **Forgacs, P., A. Tarshis, P. Ma, M. Federman, L. Mele, M. L. Silverman, and J. A. Shea.** 1983. Intestinal and bronchial cryptosporidiosis in an immunodeficient homosexual man. *Ann. Intern. Med.* **99:**793-794.

16. **Frisby, H.** Unpublished data.

17. **Garcia, L. S., D. A. Bruckner, T. C. Brewer, and R. Y. Shimizu.** 1983. Techniques for the recovery and identification of *Cryptosporidium* oocysts from stool specimens. *J. Clin. Microbiol.* **18:**185-190.

18. **Goldstein, S. T., D. D. Juranek, O. Ravenholt, A. W. Hightower, D. G. Martin, J. L. Mesnik, S. D. Griffiths, A. J. Bryant, R. R. Reich, and B. L. Herwaldt.** 1996. Cryptosporidiosis: an outbreak associated with drinking water despite state-of-the-art water treatment. *Ann. Intern. Med.* **124:**459-468.

19. **Gross, T. L., J. Wheat, M. Bartlett, and K. W. O'Connor.** 1986. AIDS and systemic involvement with *Cryptosporidium. Am. J. Gastroenterol.* **81:**456-458.

20. **Harari, M. D., B. West, and B. Dwyer.** 1986. *Cryptosporidium* as a cause of laryngotracheitis in an infant. *Lancet* **ii:**1207.

21. **Harris, M., G. Deutsch, J. D. MacLean, and C. M. Tsoukas.** 1994. A phase I study of letrazuril in AIDS-related cryptosporidiosis. *AIDS* **8:**1109-1113.

22. **Hayes, E. B., T. D. Matte, T. R. O'Brien, T. W. McKinley, G. S. Logsdon, J. B. Rose, B. L. Ungar, D. M. Word, P. F. Pinsky, M. L. Cummings, et al.** 1989. Large community outbreak of cryptosporidiosis due to contamination of a filtered water supply. *N. Engl. J. Med.* **320:**1372-1376.

23. **Holley, H. P., and B. H. Thiers.** 1986. Cryptosporidiosis in a patient receiving immunosuppressive therapy: possible activation of latent infection. *Dig. Dis. Sci.* **31:**1004-1007.

24. **Juranek, D. D.** 1996. Cryptosporidiosis—sources of infection and guidelines for prevention. *Clin. Infect. Dis.* **21**(Suppl.)1:S57-S61.

25. **Kibbler, C. C., A. Smith, S. J. Hamilton-Dutoit, H. Milburn, J. K. Pattinson, and H. G. Prentice.** 1987. Pulmonary cryptosporidiosis occurring in a bone marrow transplant recipient. *Scand. J. Infect. Dis.* **19:**581-584.

26. **Kocoshis, S. A., M. L. Cibull, T. E. Davis, J. T. Hinton, M. Seip, and J. G. Banwell.** 1984. Intestinal and pulmonary cryptosporidiosis in an infant with severe combined immune deficiency. *J. Pediatr. Gastroenterol. Nutr.* **3:**149-157.

27. **Kotler, D. P., and J. M. Orenstein.** 1994. Prevalence of intestinal microsporidiosis in HIV-infected individuals referred for gastroenterological evaluation. *Am. J. Gastroenterol.* **89:**1998-2002.

28. **LeChevallier, M. W., and W. D. Norton.** 1995. Occurrence of *Giardia* and *Cryptosporidium* in raw and finished drinking water. *J. Am. Water Works Assoc.* **87:**54-68.

29. **Ma, P., and R. Soave.** 1983. Three-step stool examination for cryptosporidiosis in 10 homosexual men with protracted watery diarrhea. *J. Infect. Dis.* **147:**824-828.

30. **MacKenzie, W. R., N. J. Hoxie, M. E. Proctor, M. S. Gradus, K. A. Blair, D. E. Peterson, J. J. Kazmierczak, D. G. Addiss, K. R. Fox, J. B. Rose, et al.** 1994. A massive waterborne outbreak of cryptosporidium infection transmitted through the public water supply. *N. Engl. J. Med.* **331:**161-167.

31. **MacKenzie, W. R., J. J. Kazmierczak, and J. P. Davis.** 1995. An outbreak of cryptosporidiosis associated with a resort swimming pool. *Epidemiol. Infect.* **115:**545-553.

32. **MacKenzie, W. R., W. L. Schell, K. A. Blair, D. G. Addiss, D. E. Peterson, N. J. Hoxie, J. J. Kazmierczak, and J. P. Davis.** 1995. Massive waterborne outbreak of cryptosporidiosis, Milwaukee, Wisconsin: recurrence of illness and risk of secondary transmission. *Clin. Infect. Dis.* **21:**57-62.

33. **McAnulty, J. M., D. W. Fleming, and A. H. Gonzalez.** 1994. A community-wide outbreak of cryptosporidiosis associated with swimming at a wave pool. *JAMA* **272:**1597-1600.

34. **Miller, R. A., J. N. Wasserheit, J. Kirihara, and M. B. Coyle.** 1984. Detection of *Cryptosporidium* oocysts in sputum during screening for mycobacteria. *J. Clin. Microbiol.* **20:**1192-1193.

35. **Osewe, P., D. G. Addiss, K. A. Blair, A. Kamb, A. W. Hightower, and J. P. Davis.** 1996. Cryptosporidiosis in Wisconsin: a case-control study of risk factors for post-outbreak transmission. *Epidemiol. Infect.* **117:**297-304.

36. **Peterson, C.** 1994. Cryptosporidiosis, p. 6.18-1-10. *In* P. T. Cohen, M. A. Sande, and P. A. Volberding (ed.), *The AIDS Knowledge Base*, 2nd ed. Little, Brown & Co., Boston.

37. **Roberts, C. L., C. Morin, D. G. Addiss, S. P. Wahlquist, P. A. Mshar, and J. L. Hadler.** 1996. Factors influencing *Cryptosporidium* testing in Connecticut. *Am. J. Clin. Microbiol.* **34:**2292-2293.

38. **Rose, J. B., C. P. Gerba, and W. Jakubowski.** 1991. Survey of potable water supplies for *Cryptosporidium* and *Giardia*. *Environ. Sci. Technol.* **25:**1393-1399.

39. **Schwartz, D. A., R. T. Bryan, and J. M. Hughes.** 1995. Pathology and emerging infections: quo vadimus? *Am. J. Pathol.* **147:**1525–1533.

40. **Schwartz, D. A., and R. T. Bryan.** 1996. Infectious disease pathology and emerging infections: are we prepared? *Arch. Pathol. Lab. Med.* **120:**117–124.

41. **Vakil, N. B., S. M. Schwartz, B. P. Buggy, C. F. Brummitt, M. Kherellah, D. M. Letzer, I. H. Gilson, and P. G. Jones.** 1996. Biliary cryptosporidiosis in HIV-infected people after the waterborne outbreak of cryptosporidiosis in Milwaukee. *N. Engl. J. Med.* **334:**19–23.

chapter 14

Pathogenic and Opportunistic Free-Living Amebae

Govinda S. Visvesvara, Ronald C. Neafie, and A. Julio Martinez

Small free-living amebae belonging to the genera *Naegleria* and *Acanthamoeba* and the recently discovered genus *Balamuthia* (previously identified as leptomyxid amebae) have been known to cause a fatal disease of the central nervous system (CNS) in humans. Among the several species of *Naegleria*, only one species, *Naegleria fowleri*, causes an acute and a rapidly fatal (within 10 days) primary amebic meningoencephalitis (PAM). Several species of *Acanthamoeba* (*A. castellanii*, *A. culbertsoni*, *A. rhysodes*, *A. polyphaga*, *A. divionensis*, and *A. healyi*) and *Balamuthia mandrillaris* cause a chronic and usually fatal granulomatous amebic encephalitis (GAE) that may last for several weeks or even months (1, 4, 7, 17, 18).

In 1958, Culbertson and colleagues isolated *Acanthamoeba* sp. strain A-1 (now designated *A. culbertsoni*) from tissue culture medium thought to contain an unknown simian virus (2). They also demonstrated that these ame-

Govinda S. Visvesvara, Host/Parasite Biology Section, Biology and Diagnostics Branch, Division of Parasitic Diseases, National Center for Infectious Diseases, Centers for Disease Control and Prevention, 4770 Buford Highway, Mailstop F-13, Atlanta, GA 30341-3724. **Ronald C. Neafie,** Parasitic Disease Pathology Branch, Geographic Pathology Division, Department of Infectious and Parasitic Disease Pathology, Armed Forces Institute of Pathology, Washington, DC 20306-6000. **A. Julio Martinez,** Neuropathology Section, Room 586, Presbyterian University Hospital and University of Pittsburgh, Pittsburgh, PA 15213.

Pathology of Emerging Infections
Edited by C. Robert Horsburgh, Jr., and Ann Marie Nelson
© 1997 American Society for Microbiology, Washington, DC 20005-4171

bae, on intracerebral inoculation in immunosuppressed monkeys and mice, caused death of these animals, and they hypothesized that similar strains might exist in nature and may infect humans. Fowler and Carter (3a) described the first fatal CNS infection caused by a free-living ameba in an Australian boy. Butt (1a) described the first case of *N. fowleri* infection in the United States and coined the term "primary amebic meningoencephalitis" (7, 9, 18).

Epidemiology and Ecology

Both Naegleria and Acanthamoeba spp. occur worldwide and are commonly found in soil, freshwater, sewage and sludge

Both *Naegleria* and *Acanthamoeba* spp. occur worldwide and are commonly found in soil, freshwater (including tap water), sewage and sludge, dust in the air, thermal effluents of power plants, swimming pools, and hot springs. Additionally, *Acanthamoeba* spp. have also been isolated from brackish water and seawater; ocean sediments; frozen water; bottled water; heating, ventilating, and air conditioning units; bacterial, mycotic, and mammalian cell cultures; vegetables and mushrooms; the human nose and throat; dental units; catheters; contact lens paraphernalia, corneal smears, and corneal biopsy material; human skin ulcers; and the CNS. *B. mandrillaris*, however, has not been isolated from nature to date (7, 9, 17, 18).

Isolation and Culture

To isolate the etiologic agents, cerebrospinal fluid (CSF) or small pieces of brain, lungs, skin, or corneal biopsy or autopsy material must be obtained aseptically. The specimens may be kept at 4°C for short periods of time but should never be frozen. The CSF should be centrifuged at 250 × g for about 10 min, the supernatant should be aspirated, and the sediment should be inoculated onto the center of a nonnutrient agar plate that has been coated with bacteria (e.g., *Escherichia coli*) and incubated at 37°C. Small pieces of tissue (brain or lung biopsy or autopsy material) should be triturated in a small amount (0.5 ml) of ameba saline, placed in the center of the agar plate, and incubated as described above (7, 9).

Both *Naegleria* and *Acanthamoeba* spp. can be easily cultivated in this way and, with periodic transfers, maintained indefinitely. After 2 to 3 days of incubation, amebae will begin to encyst. If a plate is examined after 4 to 5 days of incubation, trophozoites as well as cysts will be seen. *B. mandrillaris* cannot be cultured on agar plates. It can, however, be cultivated on mammalian cell cultures and the recently developed complex chemical medium (11).

Identification of the amebae to the genus level is based on characteristic patterns of locomotion, morphologic features of the trophic and cyst forms, and enflagellation experiments. In the enflagellation experiment, amebae growing on agar are scraped from the agar and inoculated into a sterile tube containing sterile distilled water. If *Naegleria* spp. are present, biflagellated organisms will be seen within 10 min to 1 h. Flagellated stages are not present in *Acanthamoeba* and *B. mandrillaris* (7, 9, 17).

Morphology and Life Cycle

N. *fowleri* has three stages in its life cycle: trophozoite, cyst, and flagellate. The trophozoite is limax-like and measures 9 to 14 µm. It is uninucleate, and the nucleus has a large, centrally located, densely staining nucleolus. A contractile vacuole is often seen. Under certain conditions, such as a change in the ionic concentration in the environment, the trophozoite transforms into a pear-shaped biflagellated stage which usually reverts back to the trophic stage. The trophozoite also differentiates into smooth-walled spherical cysts measuring 7 to 15 µm (7, 10, 12).

Acanthamoeba trophozoites measure 15 to 45 µm and produce fine, tapering, spinelike projections (acanthopodia) from the surface of the body. Periodically, a contractile vacuole may also be seen rupturing at the surface of the body. The trophozoites are usually uninucleate, and the nucleus has a large, dense nucleolus. *Acanthamoeba* spp. do not have a flagellate stage; rather, they differentiate into cysts during adverse conditions. The cysts are uninucleate, with an outer wrinkled ectocyst and an inner oval, stellate, or polygonal endocyst. Pores or ostioles are present at the point of contact between the ecto- and endocyst and are usually covered by an operculum. On the basis of the size and morphology of the cysts, *Acanthamoeba* spp. can be divided into three groups, each group with many species (10).

Primary Amebic Meningoencephalitis (PAM)

Clinical Syndrome

PAM is an acute fulminating infection with an abrupt onset and is characterized by severe headache, fever, nausea, vomiting, stiff neck, positive Kernig's and Brudzinski's signs, photophobia, confusion, delirium, seizures, coma, and death. PAM usually occurs in previously healthy children and young adults with a history of recent contact with freshwater. The portal of entry is the nasal passages, and the incubation period is usually between 3 and 8 days. PAM may resemble acute bacterial leptomeningitis in the early stages.

*P*AM *is an acute fulminating infection with an abrupt onset*

Pathophysiology

The salient feature of PAM is an acute hemorrhagic necrosis of the olfactory bulbs associated with inflammatory infiltrate consisting of polymorphonuclear leukocytes, eosinophils, macrophages, and occasional lymphocytes. The cerebral cortex is also affected, with pockets of amebic trophozoites within edematous and hemorrhagic CNS tissue (Fig. 14.1). Large numbers of amebic trophozoites may also be seen deep in the Virchow-Robin spaces and around blood vessels but with minimal or no inflammatory response. *N. fowleri* is not generally known to produce cysts in CNS tissue. As of December 1996, more than 175 cases (81 in the United States) of PAM have been reported worldwide and only a few patients have survived this disease (7, 9).

Laboratory Diagnosis

PAM resembles acute pyogenic or bacterial meningoencephalitis, having an elevated peripheral leukocyte count and a predominance of polymorphonuclear leukocytes, an elevated CSF pressure, low CSF glucose, and high protein. CSF pleocytosis is seen and may be mistaken for bacterial infection (7, 9). It is therefore recommended that a history of freshwater contact within the past 2 weeks is ascertained and that a wet mount of a CSF preparation is examined under the microscope for the presence of amebae. *N. fowleri* trophozoites, measuring 9 to 14 μm with active directional movement, may easily be distinguished from the host cells in the wet mount. CSF smears should also be stained, preferably with trichrome stain, for the presence of trophozoites with the characteristic nuclear morphology (Fig. 14.2).

Treatment

Only a few patients have survived PAM to date. One of the U.S. patients who survived this disease was treated with intravenous and intrathecal amphotericin B and miconozole and oral rifampin (12).

Granulomatous Amebic Encephalitis (GAE)

Clinical Syndrome

GAE due to *Acanthamoeba* spp. is a chronic illness with an insidious onset that occurs primarily in immunosuppressed, chronically ill, or otherwise debilitated persons with no history of exposure to freshwater. GAE is a slowly progressive CNS disease with no clear-cut incubation period and may last from a few days to several weeks or months. It usually manifests with focal neurologic deficits, signs of increased intracranial pressure, and neuro- and radiographic features suggestive of an expanding space-occupying mass. Therefore, in the differential diagnosis, a brain tumor, abscess, or intracerebral hematoma should be considered (4, 8, 9). Common clinical symptoms are headache, irritability, confusion, seizures, dizziness, drowsiness, and behavioral changes. Less common symptoms include diplopia, aphasia, ataxia, altered mental status, lethargy, and hemiparesis (8). In GAE there is moderate edema and hemorrhagic softening of some areas in the cerebral cortex (Fig. 14.3). Modest purulent exudate may be detected in the affected areas (4, 7, 9).

Pathophysiology

The CNS lesions consist of hemorrhagic necrosis of the CNS parenchyma, with variable amounts of subacute and chronic inflammatory reaction and with amebic trophozoites and cysts around and within blood vessel walls (Fig. 14.4). Multinucleated giant cells may be present (4, 7, 9). Some patients, especially those with human immunodeficiency virus and/or AIDS, develop abscesses, erythematous nodules, or skin lesions containing trophozoites and cysts of amebae (4, 7, 13, 18; Fig. 14.5 and 14.6). The portal of entry is probably through the lower respiratory tract, ulceration of the skin or mucosa, or open wounds. CNS disease is a secondary feature and is probably due to hematogenous spread from a primary site (9). Amebae may also be found in the liver, lungs, kidneys, prostate, lymph nodes, skin, and other organs, suggesting probable premortem hematogenous dissemination. As of December 1996, more than 100 cases of GAE due to *Acanthamoeba* spp. have been recorded worldwide; 73 of these cases have occurred in the United States (more than 50 in patients with AIDS).

Diagnosis

Unlike *N. fowleri*, *Acanthamoeba* spp. have only rarely been isolated from the CSF. However, *Acanthamoeba* spp. have been isolated quite readily from skin abscesses as well as from brain biopsies. Amebae and cysts can be identified by their characteristic morphology.

Acanthamoeba spp. have been isolated from skin abscesses as well as from brain biopsies

Treatment

GAE usually results in death, as there is no good treatment for this disease (4, 7-9). However, patients with amebic skin abscesses may not develop CNS disease if they are diagnosed early and treated with a combination of topical chlorhexidine gluconate and intravenous pentamidine (13).

Acanthamoeba Keratitis

Clinical Syndrome

Acanthamoeba keratitis is a painful, vision-threatening disease of the cornea which may lead to a chronic ulceration of the cornea, loss of visual acuity, and eventually blindness and enucleation (7, 14, 15). More than 700 cases of *Acanthamoeba* keratitis have been reported worldwide. It is believed that as of 1 December 1996, more than 500 cases of *Acanthamoeba* keratitis have occurred in the United States. The first case was reported in 1973 in a south Texas rancher with a history of trauma to his right eye. *A. polyphaga* was repeatedly cultured from the corneal scrapings and biopsy specimens (6). Although the number of *Acanthamoeba* keratitis cases increased gradually to 31 between 1973 and 1984, a dramatic increase in the number of cases occurred from August 1984 to June 1985, and by July 1988, 208 cases had been diagnosed. On the basis of an in-depth epidemiologic and case-control study, the use of soft contact lenses along with the use of homemade saline was determined to be the principal risk factor associated with *Acanthamoeba* keratitis (14, 15).

Laboratory Diagnosis

Corneal scrapings smeared on microscope slides may be fixed with methanol and stained with Hemacolor stain or trichrome stain (7).

Treatment

Acanthamoeba spp., especially in the cyst stage, are resistant to commonly used chemotherapeutic agents, even at very high concentrations. However, some patients with *Acanthamoeba* keratitis have been treated successfully with topical applications of a variety of drugs, including propamidine isethionate (Brolene), neosporin suspensions, clotrimazole, and, more recently, polyhexamethylene biguanide (3, 5, 7, 19).

GAE Due to *Balamuthia* (Leptomyxid) Ameba

Clinical Syndrome

Until recently, it was believed that all cases of GAE were caused by *Acanthamoeba* spp. However, in 1986, *B. mandrillaris* was isolated into culture and definitively identified as another agent that causes GAE (16, 17). As of 1 December 1996, more than 60 cases (30 in the United States) of *B. mandrillaris* GAE have occurred worldwide.

Pathophysiology

The pathology and pathogenesis of *Balamuthia* GAE are similar to those of *Acanthamoeba* GAE. Both trophozoites and cysts are found in the CNS tissue, and their sizes overlap with those of *Acanthamoeba* spp. (Fig. 14.7).

Laboratory Diagnosis

It is difficult to differentiate *Balamuthia* from *Acanthamoeba* spp. in tissue sections on the basis of light microscopic morphology. However, *Balamuthia* trophozoites may have more than one nucleolus in the nucleus (Fig. 14.8). In such cases, it may be possible to distinguish *Balamuthia* from *Acanthamoeba* amebae on the basis of the nuclear morphology, since *Acanthamoeba* trophozoites have only one nucleolus. Cysts of *Balamuthia* spp. are also seen in tissue sections, but it is difficult to distinguish these cysts from those of *Acanthamoeba* spp. at the light microscope level (Fig. 14.7). Ultrastructurally, however, the cysts of *Balamuthia* spp. are characterized by three layers in the cyst wall: an outer wrinkled ectocyst, a middle structureless mesocyst, and an inner thin endocyst (Fig. 14.9). *Balamuthia* amebae are antigenically distinct from those of *Acanthamoeba* spp.; they can be easily distinguished by immunofluorescence assay. Therefore, electron microscopy, immunohistochemical technique, or both are necessary to identify *Balamuthia* organisms in tissue sections (1, 4, 16–18).

Treatment

There is no known treatment for GAE due to *Balamuthia* spp.

It is difficult to differentiate Balamuthia from Acanthamoeba spp. in tissue sections on the basis of light microscopic morphology

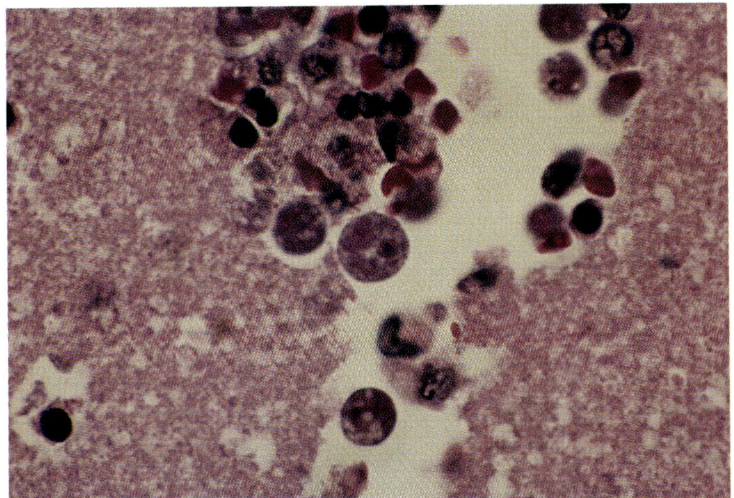

Figure 14.1   Brain section of a 4-year-old boy from North Carolina who died of PAM 7 days after swimming in a freshwater lake. Many rounded *N. fowleri* trophozoites measuring 8 to 11 µm were seen in the brain section (hematoxylin and eosin stain; original magnification, ×330).

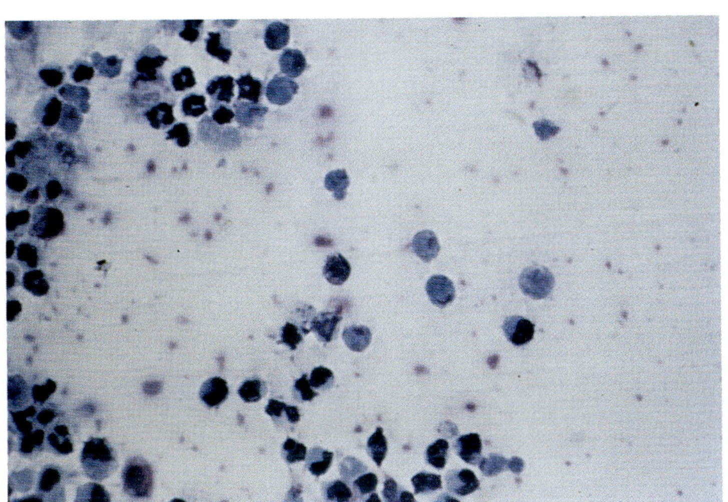

Figure 14.2   CSF smear of a PAM patient. Note rounded *N. fowleri* trophozoites in the midst of polymorphonuclear leukocytes (Giemsa stain; original magnification, ×160).

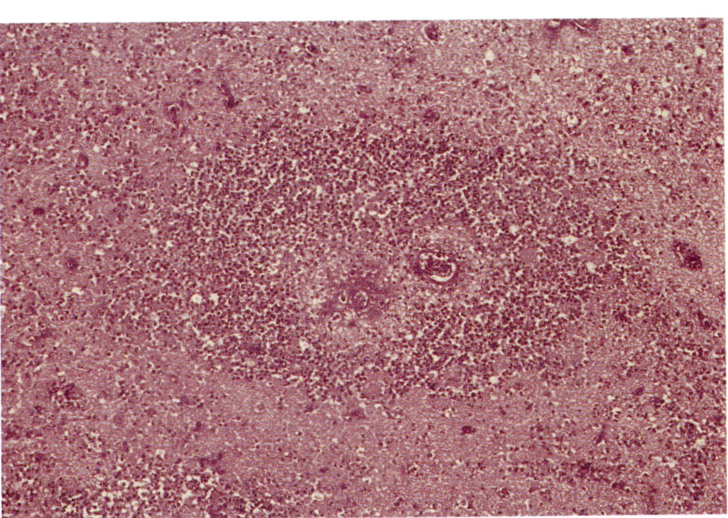

Figure 14.3   Brain section of a 27-year-old woman with GAE due to *A. culbertsoni.* Low-power view of a section with multiple areas of necrosis containing histiocytes, neutrophils, and numerous amebae (hematoxylin and eosin stain; original magnification, ×33).

Figure 14.4 Higher magnification (×330) of the same section shown in Fig. 14.3, showing rounded amebae 7 to 12 μm in diameter with foamy cytoplasm.

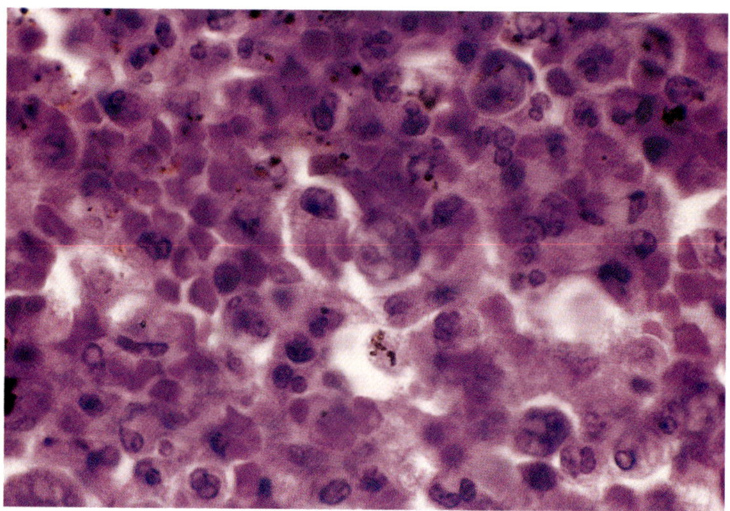

Figure 14.5 Section of the skin on the upper arm of an AIDS patient who had multiple nodular masses on his arms and legs. Note many cysts of *Acanthamoeba* spp. in the necrotic panniculus. The cysts measure 12 to 18 μm and possess an outer wrinkled ectocyst and an inner polygonal endocyst. Original magnification, ×250.

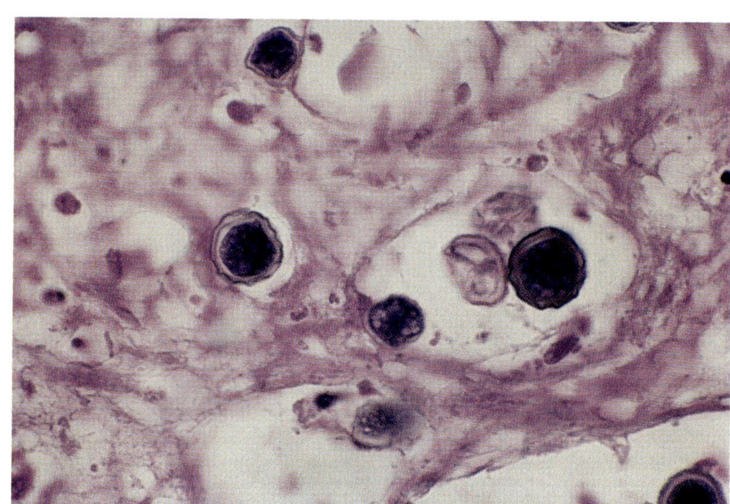

Figure 14.6 Immunofluorescence patterns of *Acanthamoeba* spp. in a skin biopsy of an AIDS patient with disseminated infection. Note large numbers of amebae showing apple-green fluorescence. Original magnification, ×40.

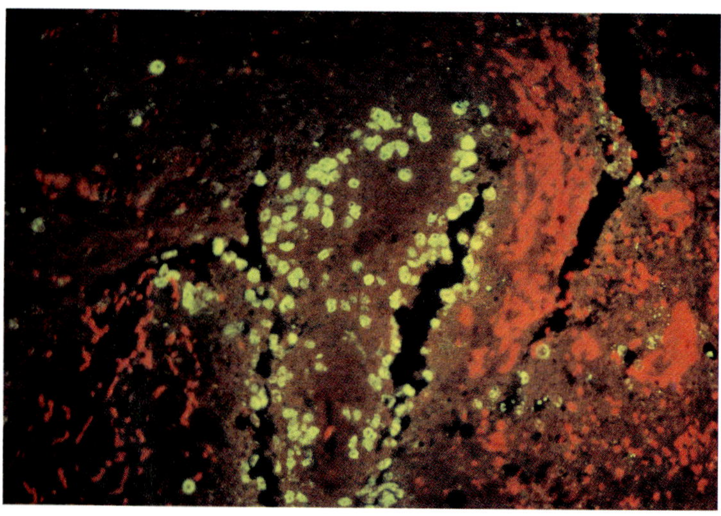

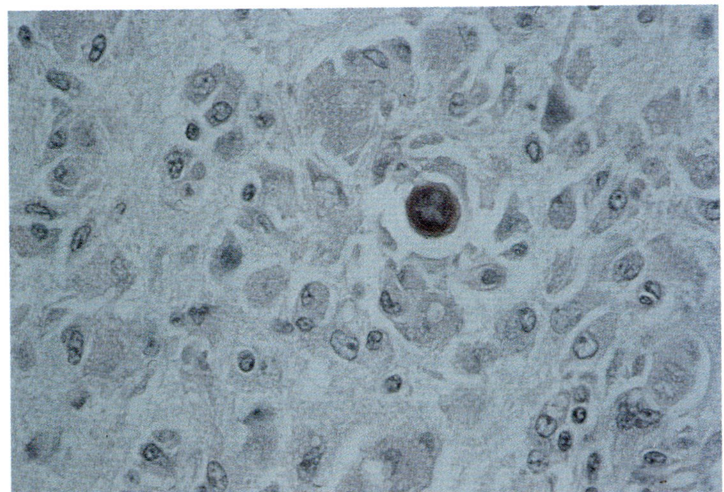

Figure 14.7 CNS section of an AIDS patient with *B. mandrillaris*. Note many trophozoites and a cyst interspersed within the brain tissue (periodic acid-Schiff stain; original magnification, ×240).

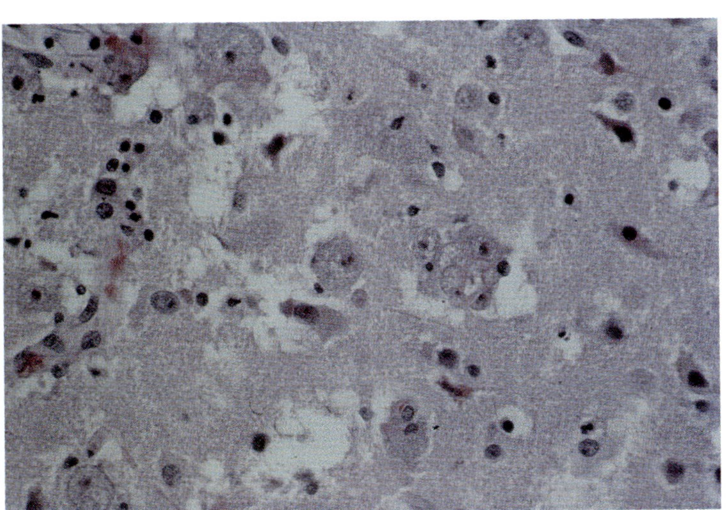

Figure 14.8 *B. mandrillaris* trophozoites in a CNS section of a patient with GAE. Note the presence of multiple nucleolar elements within the nucleus (hematoxylin and eosin stain; original magnification, ×400).

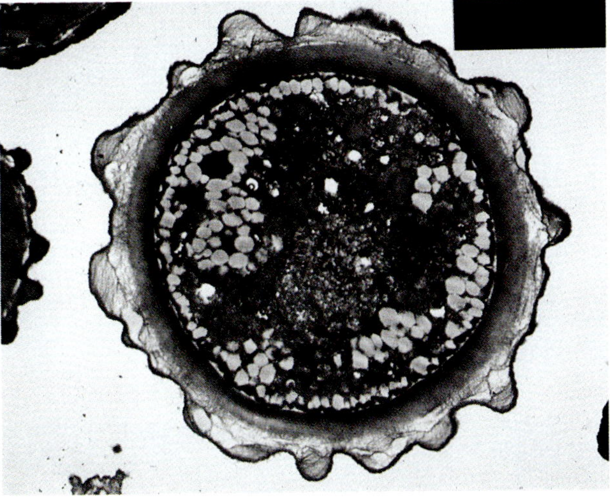

Figure 14.9 Electron micrograph of a cyst of *B. mandrillaris*. Note the tripartite cyst wall. Original magnification, ×7,500.

References

1. **Anzil, A. P., C. Rao, M. A. Wrozlek, G. S. Visvesvara, J. H. Sher, and P. B. Kozlowski.** 1991. Amebic meningoencephalitis in a patient with AIDS caused by a newly recognized opportunistic pathogen: leptomyxid ameba. *Arch. Pathol. Lab. Med.* **115**:21–25.

1a. **Butt, C. G.** 1966. Primary amebic meningoencephalitis. *N. Engl. J. Med.* **274**:1473–1476.

2. **Culbertson, C. G., J. W. Smith, and J. R. Minner.** 1958. *Acanthamoeba*: observations on animal pathogenicity. *Science* **127**:1506.

3. **Driebe, W. T. , G. A. Stern, R. J. Epstein, G. S. Visvesvara, M. Adi, and T. Komadina.** 1991. Potential role for topical clotrimazole in combination chemotherapy. *Arch. Ophthalmol.* **106**:1196–1201.

3a. **Fowler, M., and R. F. Carter.** 1965. Acute pyrogenic meningitis probably due to *Acanthamoeba* sp.: a preliminary report. *Br. Med. J.* **ii**:740–742.

4. **Gordon, S. M., J. P. Steinberg, M. DuPuis, P. Kozarsky, J. F. Nickerson, and G. S. Visvesvara.** 1992. Culture isolation of *Acanthamoeba* species and leptomyxid amebas from patients with amebic meningoencephalitis, including two patients with AIDS. *Clin. Infect. Dis.* **15**:1024–1030.

5. **Hay, J., C. M. Kirkness, D. V. Seal, and P. Wright.** 1994. Drug resistance and *Acanthamoeba* keratitis: the quest for alternative antiprotozoal chemotherapy. *Eye* **8**:555–563.

6. **Jones, D. B., G. S. Visvesvara, and N. M. Robinson.** 1975. *Acanthamoeba polyphaga* keratitis and *Acanthamoeba uveitis* associated with fatal meningoencephalitis. *Trans. Ophthalmol. Soc. UK* **95**:221–232.

7. **Ma, P., G. S. Visvesvara, A. J. Martinez, F. H. Theodore, P.-M. Daggett, and T. K. Sawyer.** 1990. Naegleria and Acanthamoeba infections: review. *Rev. Infect. Dis.* **12**: 490–513.

8. **Martinez, A. J.** 1980. Is *Acanthamoeba* encephalitis an opportunistic infection? *Neurology* **30**:567–574.

9. **Martinez, A. J.** 1985. *Free-Living Amebas: Natural History, Prevention, Diagnosis, Pathology, and Treatment of the Disease.* CRC Press, Inc., Boca Raton, Fla.

10. **Page, F. C.** 1985. *A New Key To Fresh Water and Soil Gymnamoebae.* Fresh Water Biological Association, Cumbria, England.

11. **Schuster, F. L., and G. S. Visvesvara.** 1996. Axenic growth and drug sensitivity studies of *Balamuthia mandrillaris*, an agent of amebic meningoencephalitis in humans and other animals. *J. Clin. Microbiol.* **34**:385–388.

12. **Seidel, J. S., P. Harmatz, G. S. Visvesvara, A. Cohen, J. Edwards, and J. Turner.** 1982. Successful treatment of primary amebic meningo-encephalitis. *N. Engl. J. Med.* **306**:346–348.

13. **Slater, C. A., J. Z. Sickel, G. S. Visvesvara, R. C. Pabico, and A. A. Gaspari.** 1994. Successful treatment of disseminated Acanthamoeba infection in an immunocompromised patient. *N. Engl. J. Med.* **331**:85–87.

14. **Stehr-Green, J. K., T. M. Bailey, F. H. Brandt, J. H. Carr, W. W. Bond, and G. S. Visvesvara.** 1987. *Acanthamoeba* keratitis in soft contact lens wearers. A case-control study. *JAMA* **258**:57–60.

15. **Stehr-Green, J. K., T. M. Bailey, and G. S. Visvesvara.** 1990. The epidemiology of *Acanthamoeba* keratitis in the United States. *Am. J. Ophthalmol.* **107:**331–336.

16. **Visvesvara, G. S., A. J. Martinez, F. L. Schuster, G. J. Leitch, S. V. Wallace, T. K. Sawyer, and M. Anderson.** 1990. Leptomyxid ameba, a new agent of amebic meningoencephalitis in humans and animals. *J. Clin. Microbiol.* **28:**2750–2756.

17. **Visvesvara, G. S., F. L. Schuster, and A. J. Martinez.** 1993. *Balamuthia mandrillaris*, new genus, new species, agent of amebic meningo-encephalitis in humans and animals. *J. Eukaryot. Microbiol.* **40:**504–514.

18. **Visvesvara, G. S., and J. K. Stehr-Green.** 1990. Epidemiology of free-living ameba infections. *J. Protozool.* **37:**25S–33S.

19. **Wright, P., D. Warhurst, and B. R. Jones.** 1985. *Acanthamoeba* keratitis successfully treated medically. *Br. J. Ophthalmol.* **69:**778–782.

Lyme Borreliosis

Carlos del Rio, Scott R. Granter, and Paul H. Duray

Lyme disease was first described in 1977 after a clustering of what appeared to be cases of juvenile rheumatoid arthritis occurred among children in the town of Old Lyme, Conn. (63). Lyme disease is now recognized as a multistage, systemic illness caused by a tick-transmitted spirochete, *Borrelia burgdorferi* (61). The disease had been previously recognized in Europe and given different names, including Bannwarth syndrome, acrodermatitis chronica atrophicans, and erythema chronicum migrans (43).

Three genera of spirochetes cause the major human spirochetal infections: *Treponema*, *Leptospira*, and *Borrelia*. Unlike the other two groups, borreliae are transmitted primarily by ticks, both hard and soft bodied. Borrelia infections are epizoonoses, in that reservoir animal hosts maintain the spirochete between tick stages. The spirochetes heavily colonize the tick vectors and are maintained in low numbers in the mammalian hosts.

Carlos del Rio, Department of Medicine, Division of Infectious Diseases, Emory University School of Medicine, 69 Butler Street, S.E., Atlanta, GA 30303. **Scott R. Granter,** Brigham and Women's Hospital, Harvard Medical School, Boston, MA 02115. **Paul H. Duray,** Department of Pathology, National Cancer Institute, National Institutes of Health, 9000 Rockville Pike, Bethesda, MD 20201.

Pathology of Emerging Infections
Edited by C. Robert Horsburgh, Jr., and Ann Marie Nelson
© 1997 American Society for Microbiology, Washington, DC 20005-4171

Etiologic Agent

The genus *Borrelia* belongs to the family *Treponemataceae*, which includes all spirochetal pathogens (the genera *Treponema* and *Leptospira* are also in this family). The causative agent of Lyme disease is *B. burgdorferi*, first identified in 1982 when Burgdorfer identified spirochetes in the midgut of the adult deer tick (8). Subsequently, spirochetes were cultured from blood and skin lesions of patients with erythema migrans (13, 14). In 1984, this new spirochete was named *B. burgdorferi*. *Borrelia* spp. are longer and more loosely coiled than other spirochetes, and their outer membrane is unique in that the genes encoding it are located in linear plasmids, which may enable *Borrelia* spp. to express protective antigenic variation. *B. burgdorferi* is the longest and narrowest of all *Borrelia* spp., with 7 to 11 flagella and over 30 different immunogenic proteins. *B. burgdorferi* grows best at 33°C in Barbour-Stoenner-Kelly (BSK) medium, but it can also grow on a variety of solid media.

B. burgdorferi sensu lato is now classified phylogenetically into three major genospecies on the basis of nucleotide analysis of 16S rRNA sequences (36). B31 is the prototypic reference strain from Shelter Island, N.Y. Some sensu lato isolates in Europe are now called *Borrelia garinii*, sp. nov., and *Borrelia afzelii* (36). These nucleotide 16S rRNA genospecies correlate with different epitopes on the OspA proteins that are all recognized by a panel of monoclonal antibodies, thus permitting an OspA serotype classification.

The relapsing fever borrelia (*Borrelia hermsii*) and *B. burgdorferi* have roughly 70% DNA homology. Both have an extrachromosomal large plasmid that harbors the genes coding for the bulk of the surface membrane proteins. Both genes are co-located within a 1-kb segment and act at the molecular level as a single operon (29). This permits rapid gene activations, temporary rearrangements, and single-base changes that lead to minor but significant changes in the translated protein in the outer membrane (9).

The single borrelia chromosome is about 1 Mb, with molecular size variation occurring among the diverse strains in different geographic regions. The chromosome is linear with covalently closed ends; the genomic DNA is surrounded by multiple plasmid DNA particles which for the most part are coiled. The genes that code for the cell wall and surface proteins are found on these plasmids outside the chromosome. In the Lyme spirochete, the OspA and OspB genes are co-located on a large hairpin-shaped, open-looped 49-kb plasmid. This is unusual for bacterial DNA construction and is more likely to be found in viruses. In the case of the relapsing fever spirochete, *B. hermsii*, the variation in surface protein antigenic epitopes is linked to the transposition of genes to an expression sequence.

The surface proteins in all strains are OspA (31 to 32 kDa), OspB (34 kDa), and OspC (17 kDa). OspC, found in some American isolates but predominantly found in European strains, was recently mapped to a 26-kb circular plasmid; it is the first gene to be mapped to one of the multiple coiled plasmids found exterior to the single 1-Mb chromosome (37). The operon of OspA and OspB is found on a single, 49-kb, open-ended linear plasmid.

> *B. burgdorferi sensu lato is now classified phylogenetically into three major genospecies on the basis of nucleotide analysis of 16S rRNA sequences*

Epidemiology and Ecology

Lyme disease occurs throughout the temperate northern hemisphere and is now the most common vector-borne infectious disease reported in the United States, with approximately 10,000 cases reported to the Centers for Disease Control and Prevention each year (19). Areas of endemicity include North America, the British Isles, parts of the Russian Federation (from the Baltic States to the far east), western and central Europe, Scandinavia, and northeastern China. In the United States, Lyme disease occurs in three principal foci: the Northeast, the upper Midwest, and the Pacific Coast. The emergence of areas of high endemicity, particularly in the northeastern United States, makes Lyme disease a serious health concern in those areas (18). Also of concern have been the rapid extension of the disease in some regions and the identification of *B. burgdorferi* in ticks and small mammals in regions where human cases of Lyme disease are thought not to occur from indigenous exposures (16, 67, 69).

The incidence of Lyme disease in the United States was 4.4 cases per 100,000 population in 1995 (19), but the highest density of cases comes from the three regions of endemicity previously mentioned: the northeastern states (New York, New Jersey, Connecticut, Maryland, Massachusetts, Rhode Island, and Pennsylvania), the upper Midwest (Wisconsin and Minnesota), and northern California. Incidence is correlated with the density of *Ixodes* ticks in the environment and can be as high as 450 cases per 100,000 (19). There is only a rough correlation between incidence in a given region and the infection rate of *Ixodes* ticks by *B. burgdorferi* (31). Rates of infection of vector ticks range from as high as 50% in areas of high endemicity to 0% in regions of the southern United States (10). Workers who spend substantial amounts of time outdoors appear to be at increased risk (16, 57). The ticks that transmit *B. burgdorferi* can also transmit *Ehrlichia* spp., *Babesia microti*, rickettsiae, viruses, and perhaps other microorganisms. Concurrent infection with *B. microti* leading to a fatal outcome has been described (38).

The range of *B. burgdorferi* in the United States extends from the northeastern states to as far south as Georgia and Florida (45) and as far west as northern California (17). It is unclear whether *B. burgdorferi* has spread from the northeastern states to other regions or whether it has been present in the southern and western states for many years, as has been recently suggested (44–46). Lower rates of infection in some parts of the United States may be attributed to the preference of *Ixodes pacificus* for feeding on lizards, which are not susceptible to infection and thus do not serve as reservoirs of *B. burgdorferi* (30). It has been suggested that the emergence and spread of Lyme disease may be related to reforestation of land and the resultant reintroduction and population increase in deer, mice, and parasite populations (11). Another factor in the increasing incidence of Lyme disease in humans may be the increasing participation in outdoor activities or in occupations that are carried out mostly outdoors (57).

The vectors of Lyme borreliosis are several closely related hard ticks that are part of the *Ixodes ricinus* complex. In the United States, *B. burgdorferi* is transmitted to humans by *Ixodes scapularis* (also called *I. dammini*) in the

Lyme disease occurs throughout the temperate northern hemisphere and is now the most common vector-borne infectious disease reported in the United States

Northeast and Midwest and *I. pacificus* in northern California. While *I. scapularis* may be recovered from many species of birds and mammals (6), the usual mammalian reservoirs for larval and nymphal ixodid ticks are small mammals, especially the white-footed mouse (*Peromyscus leucopus*) in the eastern United States. In the western United States, the dusky footed wood rat (*Neotoma fuscipes*) and California kangaroo rat (*Dipodomys californicus*) are usual hosts. It has been proposed that migrating birds play a role in the establishment of new enzootic foci (5) and in the rapid spread of the infection. The white-tailed deer (*Odocoileus virginianus*) is the usual maintenance host for the adult ticks (70). Deer do not serve as reservoir hosts, but they are critical for the survival of the ticks (27). Humans are incidental hosts of *B. burgdorferi*, and dogs are a potential reservoir (40). In the Pacific Coast focus, *Ixodes noetomae* transmits *B. burgdorferi* between rodents but does not feed on humans (17). Recently, an enzoonotic cycle involving *B. burgdorferi*, the Mexican wood rat (*Neotoma mexicana*), and the *Ixodes spinipalpis* tick has been described in northern Colorado, an area where Lyme disease is not endemic (41). Transovarial passage of *B. burgdorferi* occurs at an insignificant rate, and essentially all ticks become infected after feeding on spirochetemic animals, typically a small mammal, during the larval and nymphal stages. Humans are usually infected following a nymphal stage tick bite in the spring or summer. Rarely, adult ticks feeding in the fall and winter transmit the disease. Animal models have demonstrated that transmission is unlikely to occur before a minimum of 36 h of tick attachment and feeding.

Pathogenesis

The location of the surface-membrane-protein-encoding genes on plasmids and not within the genomic DNA may confer an advantage for *B. burgdorferi* by allowing easier conditional gene transposition from silent to expression sites. In this way, borreliae may have a mechanism to change protein epitopes on short notice, which could confuse or mask an immunologic response (9).

Both humoral and cell-mediated immunity occur in Lyme borreliosis, although the responses vary greatly from patient to patient. The inflammatory deposits, when present, consist of B and T lymphocytes (CD3 and -4 in the skin), mononuclear phagocytes, and, in some lesions, many mast cells (26). B lymphoblasts are increased in response to OspA, but greater responses occur with blastogenic doses of spirochete membrane fragments containing DNA (blebs) than with full-length OspA proteins. Elevations in serum immunoglobulin M (IgM) peak within 30 days, and this peak is followed by the appearance of IgG antibodies to many of the *B. burgdorferi* proteins over a period of weeks to months; these may persist for several years.

Evidence that molecular mimicry and immunologic cross-reactivity (autoreactivity) occur in the tissues of Lyme disease patients is increasing (1, 51, 55, 54). Patient serum can cross-react with the peripheral nerve, synovium, and myocardium (1). Major histocompatibility complex class II-restricted autoreactive interleukin-2-responsive T cells occur in greater frequency in blood and synovial fluid from patients with arthritis (patients with rheumatoid and Lyme disease) than in blood and synovial fluid from controls (52). Immune sera from patients with neurologic Lyme disease will cross-react with heterologous nerve axons and will also bind to *B. burgdorferi* (55). Cells secreting IgG to myelin basic protein have been isolated from cerebrospinal fluid of patients with neuroborreliosis in Sweden and have correlated with severity of disease.

Histopathology

The inflammatory infiltrate in most lesions consists of mixed T and B cells, mast cells, and macrophages (22). The infiltrate is largely perivascular. Plasma cells are plentiful in tissues, with the exception of the central nervous system, where microglial cells are more abundant. In chronic infections and in long-standing lesions, the vascular lumens are obliterated in the skin, soft tissues, and joint synovia. However, there is no evidence of active vasculitis, proteinaceous (fibrinoid) deposits, nuclear debris, or necrosis, as seen in polyarteritis nodosa and Wegener's granulomatosis. Plasma cell vasculitis and granulomatous inflammation of the type seen in syphilis patients have also not been encountered in Lyme disease infection. Dermal eosinophils can occur at the site of tick attachment but are not noticeable in other sites. T cells of the skin and synovia are CD3+, CD4+, and CD8– and are accompanied by an approximately equal number of B cells and plasma cells, especially in the synovia (52). Large and sometimes atypical-appearing B lymphoblastoid cells are seen in high numbers in the lymph nodes and soft tissues and the spleen. These are similar in appearance to neoplastic lymphoid cells in the cerebrospinal fluid. The currently recognized pathologic lesions associated with Lyme disease are summarized in Table 15.1.

B. burgdorferi is found only in very small numbers if the patient is immunologically intact. In the presence of immunodeficiency, spirochetes may present in greater numbers, but data are lacking. The organisms, when present, can be visualized best with a modified Dieterle stain (21, 24); they have long and short forms, some with curved or tapered ends (2). Prolonged search for these forms may be required and is beyond the scope of routine pathology practice. If clinically indicated, routine histopathology revealing the characteristic, but nonspecific, infiltrates, along with a positive DNA amplification by polymerase chain reaction (PCR), would be supportive evidence of Lyme disease (25, 68).

B. burgdorferi organisms, when present, can be visualized best with a modified Dieterle stain

Clinical Manifestations

Lyme disease is a multisystem infectious disease with protean clinical manifestations that may closely mimic other systemic diseases, making clinical diagnosis extremely difficult in some cases (58). Several analogies between the clinical aspects of Lyme disease and syphilis have been made: both diseases have distinct clinical stages and both are characterized by early dermatological manifestations that are followed by multisystem involvement. Erythema migrans is the hallmark of Lyme disease. This characteristic skin

Table 15.1 Summary of pathologic lesions in Lyme disease

A. Cutaneous
    1. Acute
        a. Erythema migrans
        b. Disseminated erythema migrans
    2. Intermediate
        a. Lymphocytoma cutis
        b. Morpheaform
    3. Chronic
        a. Acrodermatitis chronica atrophicans
B. Soft tissue
    1. Diffuse fasciitis with or without peripheral eosinophilia
    2. Nodular and septal panniculitis
    3. Forearm subcutaneous fibrous nodules
    4. Tenosynovitis and carpal tunnel syndrome lesions
    5. Ligamentous inflammation and sclerosis
    6. Nodular myositis
C. Lymphoreticular
    1. Regional lymphadenopathy
    2. Follicular hyperplasia, histiocytic hyperplasia with plasma cells
    3. Mild splenomegaly with B lymphoblasts
    4. Marrow lymphoblasts
D. Cardiovascular
    1. Endocarditis, transmural interstitial myocarditis of lymph nodes and plasma cells
    2. Rarely, fibrinous pericarditis
    3. Occlusive microvasculopathy: synovia, acrodermatitis chronica atrophicans
E. Central nervous system/peripheral nervous system
    1. Meningoencephalitis
    2. Mild gliosis, spongiosis
    3. Ganglionitis
    4. Axonal degeneration: perivascular infiltrates in peripheral nerves
F. Placental
    1. Chronic villitis

lesion begins at the site of a tick bite after 3 to 32 days and occurs in 60 to 80% of patients. The lesion is a centrifugally expanding erythematous macule or papule, often with central clearing. The lesion is often asymptomatic and may be missed (7).

Early in the course of infection, the spirochete may disseminate, causing myriad clinical symptoms; however, many patients will have no symptoms following the early localized rash. Some patients experience general malaise, fatigue, fever, headache, arthralgias, and myalgias; this constellation of findings is often attributed to a flu-like illness by patient or physician. Some of these symptoms, particularly the arthritis, myalgias, and headache, are characteristically intermittent, lasting from hours to days. The arthritis is typically migratory (59). Acute, nondisseminated infection due to B. *burgdorferi* consists of the rash, with or without fatigue and headache. For reasons that are unclear, many patients control the infection with no further apparent sequelae. However, there may be an intervening period of apparent return to the usual state of health which is followed months to years later by musculoskeletal and/or peripheral or central nervous system involvement (4). Acute disseminated disease is defined as disease in visceral or secondary cutaneous sites occurring less than 6 weeks after acquisition. Examples are lymphadenopathy, cranial neuritis, aseptic meningitis and meningoencephalopathy, nodular myositis (50), and cardiac junctional conduction disturbances (66). The same lesions can occur in an intermediate stage over months and then abruptly end with or without treatment. Chronic dissemination refers to initial infection that has progressed longer than a year and is usually manifested as intermittent oligoarthritis, encephalopathic syndromes (47), and a variety of skin and soft tissue lesions (23).

Dermatologic Manifestations

Because skin involvement is usually the earliest clinical manifestation of Lyme disease, recognition of cutaneous involvement is critical to making an early diagnosis and allowing prompt therapy. More than two-thirds of patients develop erythema migrans, the characteristic erythematous rash seen in early stages of infection (12). The rash usually occurs a few days to a few weeks after a tick bite. The initial rash occurs at the site of the bite as a solitary expanding annular lesion with an erythematous outer border and central clearing. Occasionally, concentric rings of alternating erythema and clearing create a target-like appearance. The lesions vary from only a few to over 50 cm in diameter. Some patients develop secondary lesions that tend to resemble erythema migrans but that may be smaller and may have less central pallor. Several to dozens of secondary lesions may develop. Secondary lesions may occur at nearly any site but tend to spare acral regions.

Because skin involvement is usually the earliest clinical manifestation of Lyme disease, recognition of cutaneous involvement is critical to making an early diagnosis

Neurologic Manifestations

Approximately 15 to 20% of untreated patients develop neurologic symptoms, most commonly meningitis, cranial neuritis (commonly seventh-nerve palsy), and radiculoneuritis (48, 49). Unusual neurologic manifestations in early infection include mononeuritis multiplex, chorea, cerebellar ataxia, atypical Guillain-Barré syndrome, Brown-Sequard syndrome, optic neuritis, and myelitis (3, 28, 32, 33). Estimates of central nervous system involvement by spirochetes determined by using clinical criteria are low compared with those determined by identification of *B. burgdorferi* DNA by PCR. In a small study, two-thirds of patients with acute disseminated infection had *B. burgdorferi* DNA detected in their spinal fluid by PCR (33). Neurologic manifestations are often associated with pleocytosis of the cerebrospinal fluid (3).

Cardiac Manifestations

Cardiac manifestations are uncommon early in disease, but they do occur in 4 to 8% of untreated patients (60). The abnormalities include heart block and myocarditis (56). A case of fatal pancarditis in a patient who had concomitant babesiosis has been reported (38).

Musculoskeletal Manifestations

Musculoskeletal involvement, particularly arthritis, is a common clinical characteristic of Lyme disease (59). The clinical picture is that of intermittent attacks of oligoarticular arthritis, which primarily involves large joints

(64). The knee is the joint most commonly affected and is often associated with significant effusion. The diagnosis is usually based on the clinical picture, history of exposure in an area of endemicity, and an elevated IgG antibody response to *B. burgdorferi*. Recently, *B. burgdorferi* DNA has been detected in joint fluid of patients with Lyme arthritis by PCR (42).

Diagnosis

A complicating factor in the diagnosis of Lyme disease is the limited accuracy of currently available serologic tests, resulting in both over- and underdiagnosis (67). Extreme caution must be used in the interpretation of these tests, as patients in early stages of disease may be nonreactive by the enzyme-linked immunosorbent assay (ELISA) (15).

Diagnosis is not difficult in patients who are living in or visiting areas of endemicity and who develop the classic erythema migrans rash following a tick bite. However, in patients with vague symptoms and absence of the characteristic rash, confirmation of the diagnosis is difficult, and clinical and laboratory data must be carefully evaluated before rendering a definitive diagnosis. Both overdiagnosis and underdiagnosis of Lyme disease are serious concerns. While it is difficult to estimate the frequency of underdiagnosis, overdiagnosis seems to be common. In one study, of 788 patients referred to a Lyme disease clinic over a 4.5-year period, 452 (57%) were believed to have been misdiagnosed (65). Many of these patients were referred for lack of improvement with antibiotic therapy. Because this study was performed at a referral clinic, the percentage of complicated and atypical cases was probably high. Nevertheless, overdiagnosis seems to be a serious problem. Definitive diagnosis in such cases relies on demonstration of organisms in tissue biopsies by light microscopic, immunohistochemical, or biochemical methods. ELISA followed by Western blot is the recommended procedure for serological evaluation of borderline and positive reactions (19). Because of the possibility of false-positive results with the ELISA, it is extremely important to perform a confirmatory Western blot. False-positive ELISA results have been associated with connective tissue disease, viral illnesses, Rocky Mountain spotted fever, and infections with spirochetes other than *B. burgdorferi* (35). In addition, a positive ELISA result in patients without clinical evidence of disease may occur. Because of the possibility of both false-positive and false-negative results, serologic evidence of infection can be supportive but must be carefully evaluated within the clinical context (e.g., positive serologic studies may indicate inactive past infection).

Treatment

Treatment for Lyme disease depends on the stage of disease and the clinical manifestations; however, the efficacy of treatment of late disease and of patients with a complicated clinical course is controversial. When patients are diagnosed early in the course of disease, oral antibiotics are effective treatment (39). In patients who are diagnosed later in the course of infection, longer courses of oral antibiotics and/or intravenous antibiotics are often

> *A complicating factor in the diagnosis of Lyme disease is the limited accuracy of currently available serologic tests, resulting in both over- and underdiagnosis*

used; however, the most effective treatment protocol in such situations has not been established (62). In patients who do not respond to antibiotic therapy, other etiologies for the patient's symptoms should be carefully considered.

Acute Lyme disease without dissemination responds to treatment with doxycycline (100 mg orally twice a day) or amoxicillin (500 mg orally three times a day) for 3 to 4 weeks. Erythromycin, cephalosporins, and newer macrolides are also effective. Treatment regimens for disseminated disease have been less well studied. Acute Lyme arthritis also responds to the oral regimens noted above, but central nervous system disease or carditis is usually treated with courses of intravenous antibiotics, such as ceftriaxone or high-dose penicillin G (20).

Prevention

In areas of endemicity, personal protective measures, such as avoiding tick-infested areas, wearing light-colored clothing and long pants tucked into socks or rubber boots, and inspecting for ticks following outdoor activity and promptly removing any ticks found, are useful. Repellents containing DEET (*N,N*-diethyl-*m*-toluamide) applied to the skin and clothing or clothing impregnated with acaricides and repellents may also afford some protection.

The use of antimicrobial prophylaxis following tick bites has been studied (34, 53). One study has suggested that even in many areas of endemicity, the risk of infection following a tick bite is so low that prophylactic antibiotics are not indicated unless the probability of *B. burgdorferi* infection after a bite is 3.6% or higher (34). Factors such as duration of tick attachment, presence of tick engorgement, and stage of tick development may be important. However, such factors are often difficult to ascertain, and this method of protection has limited utility.

Recombinant OspA vaccines that are safe and immunogenic have been developed (71). These vaccines act principally by producing antibodies that kill *B. burgdorferi* within the midgut of feeding ticks. Phase III field trials of these vaccines have been conducted with over 20,000 participants, and results are anticipated by late 1997.

> *In areas of endemicity, personal protective measures, such as avoiding tick-infested areas and wearing light-colored clothing and long pants tucked into socks or rubber boots, are useful*

Figure 15.1   Classic erythema migrans lesion in a patient with Lyme disease.

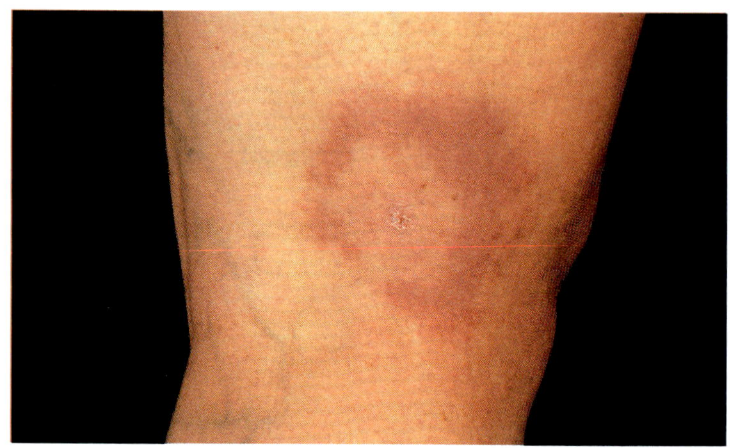

Figure 15.2   *B. burgdorferi* spirochete dividing into two daughter cells in mouse tissue (modified Steiner stain; original magnification, ×1,000).

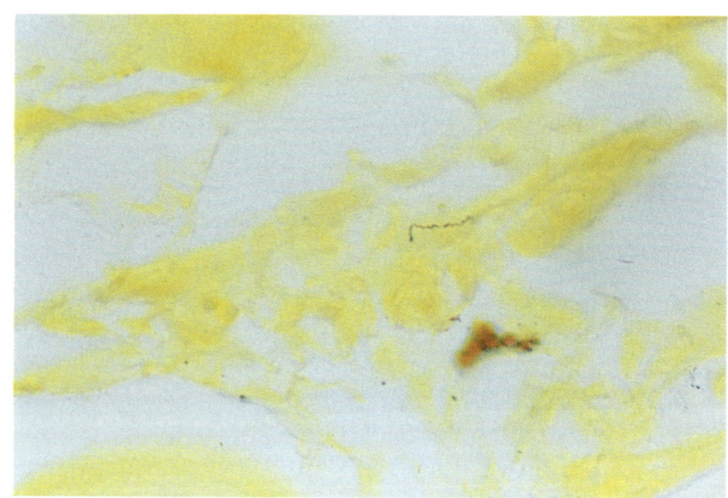

Figure 15.3   Cerebrospinal fluid from a patient with Lyme disease and meningoencephalitis. The pleocytosis in Lyme disease can be confused with a lymphoproliferative disorder.

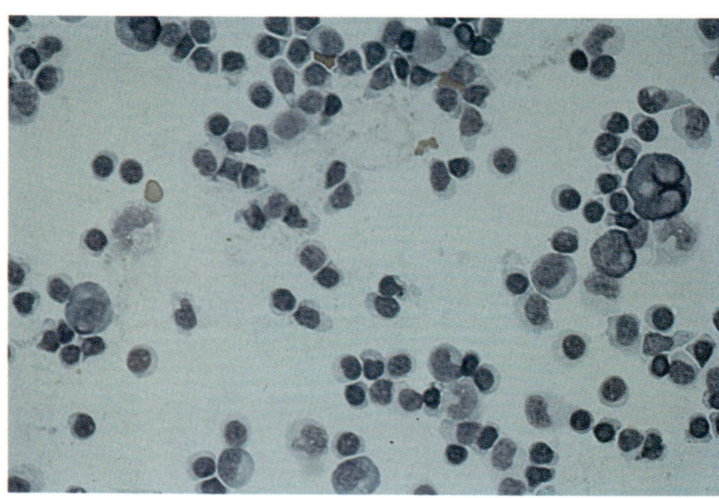

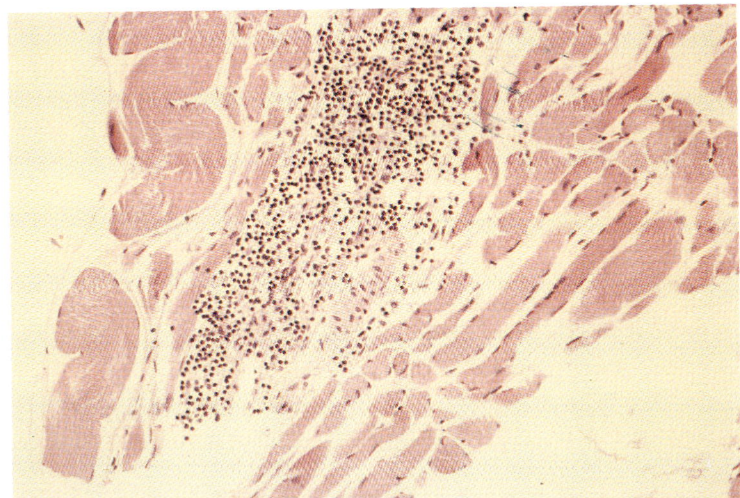

Figure 15.4 Deep thigh muscle biopsy showing nodular myositis, which can accompany Lyme arthritis.

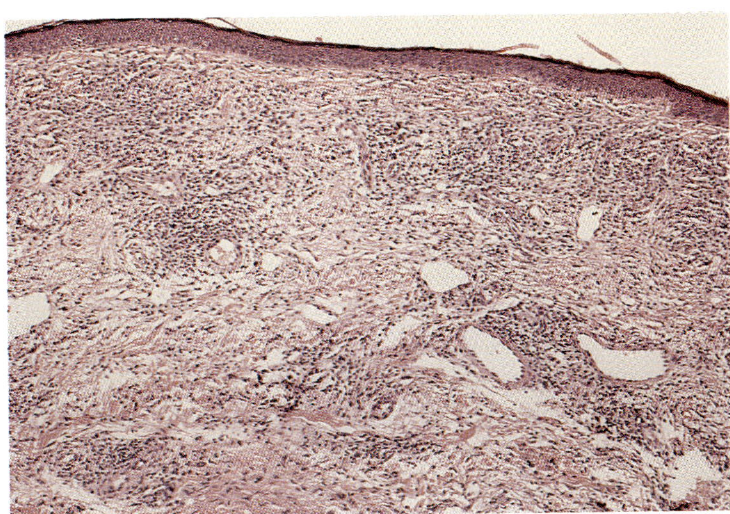

Figure 15.5 Classic histology of acrodermatitis chronica atrophicans.

References

1. **Aberer, E., C. Brunner, G. Suchanek, H. Klade, A. Barbour, G. Stanek, and H. Lassmann.** 1989. Molecular mimicry and Lyme borreliosis: a shared antigenic determinant between B. burgdorferi and human tissue. *Ann. Neurol.* **26:**732–737.

2. **Aberer, E., and P. H. Duray.** 1991. Morphology of *Borrelia burgdorferi*: structural patterns of cultured borreliae in relation to staining methods. *J. Clin. Microbiol.* **29:**764–772.

3. **Ackermann, R., P. Horstrup, and R. Schmidt.** 1984. Tick-borne meningopolyneuritis (Garin-Bujadoux, Bannwarth). *Yale J. Biol. Med.* **57:**485–490.

4. **Ackermann, R., B. Rehse-Kupper, E. Gollmer, and R. Schmidt.** 1988. Chronic neurologic manifestations of erythema migrans borreliosis. *Ann. N.Y. Acad. Sci.* **539:**16–23.

5. **Anderson, J. F.** 1985. Mammalian and avian reservoirs for *Borrelia burgdorferi*. *Ann. N.Y. Acad. Sci.* **539:**180–191.

6. **Anderson, J. F.** 1989. Epizootiology of *Borrelia* in tick vectors and reservoir hosts. *Rev. Infect. Dis.* **11:**S1451–S1458.

7. **Åsbrink, E., and A. Hovmark.** 1990. Lyme borreliosis: aspects of tick-borne *Borrelia burgdorferi* infection from a dermatologic viewpoint. *Semin. Dermatol.* **9:**277–291.

8. **Barbour, A. G.** 1984. Isolation and cultivation of Lyme disease spirochetes. *Yale J. Biol. Med.* **57:**521–525.

9. **Barbour, A. G.** 1988. Antigenic variation of surface proteins of Borrelia species. *Rev. Infect. Dis.* **10**(Suppl.)**:**S399–S402.

10. **Barbour, A. G.** 1996. Does Lyme disease occur in the south? A survey of emerging tick-borne infections in the region. *Am. J. Med. Sci.* **311:**34–40.

11. **Barbour, A. G., and D. Fish.** 1993. The biological and social phenomenon of Lyme disease. *Science* **260:**1610–1616.

12. **Berger, B. W.** 1984. Erythema chronicum migrans of Lyme disease. *Arch. Dermatol.* **120:**1017–1021.

13. **Berger, B. W., O. J. Clemmensen, and G. J. Gottlieb.** 1982. Spirochetes in lesions of erythema chronicum migrans. *Am. J. Dermatopathol.* **4:**455–456.

14. **Berger, B. W., M. H. Kaplan, I. R. Rothenberg, and A. G. Barbour.** 1985. Isolation and characterization of the Lyme disease spirochete from the skin of patients with erythema chronicum migrans. *J. Am. Acad. Dermatol.* **13:**444–449.

15. **Berger, B. W., A. B. MacDonald, and J. L. Benach.** 1988. Use of an autologous antigen in the serologic testing of patients with erythema migrans of Lyme disease. *J. Am. Acad. Dermatol.* **18:**1243–1246.

16. **Bowen, S. G., T. L. Schultze, C. Hayne, and W. E. Parkin.** 1984. A focus of Lyme disease in Monmouth County, New Jersey. *Am. J. Epidemiol.* **120:**387–394.

17. **Brown, R. N., and R. S. Lane.** 1992. Lyme disease in California: a novel enzootic transmission cycle of *Borrelia burgdorferi*. *Science* **256:**1439–1442.

18. **Carter, M. L., P. Mshar, and J. L. Hadler.** 1989. The epidemiology of Lyme disease in Connecticut. *Conn. Med.* **53:**320–323.

19. **Centers for Disease Control and Prevention.** 1996. Lyme disease—United States, 1995. *Morbid. Mortal. Weekly Rep.* **45:**481–484.

20. **Dattwyler, R. J., J. J. Halperin, D. Volkman, and B. J. Luft.** 1988. Treatment of late Lyme borreliosis—randomized comparison of ceftriaxone and penicillin. *Lancet* **i:**1191–1194.

21. **de Koning, J., R. B. Bosma, and J. A. Hoogkamp-Korstanje.** 1987. Demonstration of spirochaetes in patients with Lyme disease with a modified silver stain. *J. Med. Microbiol.* **23:**261–267.

22. **Duray, P. H.** 1987. The surgical pathology of human Lyme disease: an enlarging picture. *Am. J. Surg. Pathol.* **11**(Suppl.):47–60.

23. **Duray, P. H., E. Åsbrink, and K. Weber.** 1989. The cutaneous manifestations of human Lyme disease: a widening spectrum. *Adv. Dermatopathol.* **4:**255–276.

24. **Duray, P. H., A. Kusnitz, and J. Ryan.** 1985. Demonstration of the Lyme spirochete by a modification of the Dieterle stain. *Lab. Med.* **16:**685–687.

25. **Duray, P. H., and A. C. Steere.** 1986. The spectrum of organ and systems pathology in human Lyme disease. *Zentralbl. Bakteriol. Mikrobiol. Hyg. Ser. A* **263:**169–178.

26. **Duray, P. H., and A. C. Steere.** 1988. Clinical pathologic correlations of Lyme disease by stage. *Ann. N.Y. Acad. Sci.* **539:**65–79.

27. **Evans, J.** 1995. Lyme disease. *Curr. Opin. Rheumatol.* **7:**322–328.

28. **Halperin, J. J.** 1995. Neuroborreliosis. *Am. J. Med.* **98**(Suppl. 4A):52S–56S.

29. **Howe, T. R., F. W. LaQuier, and A. G. Barbour.** 1986. Organization of genes encoding two outer membrane proteins of the Lyme disease agent *Borrelia burgdorferi* within a single transcriptional unit. *Infect. Immun.* **54:**207–212.

30. **Lane, R. S., and P. E. Lavoire.** 1988. Lyme borreliosis in California: acarological, clinical and epidemiological studies. *Ann. N.Y. Acad. Sci.* **539:**192–203.

31. **Lane, R. S., J. Pierman, and W. Burgdorfer.** 1991. Lyme borreliosis: relation of its causative agent to its vectors and hosts in North America and Europe. *Annu. Rev. Entomol.* **36:**587–609.

32. **Logigian, E. L., R. F. Kaplan, and A. C. Steere.** 1990. Chronic neurologic manifestations of Lyme disease. *N. Engl. J. Med.* **323:**1438–1444.

33. **Luft, B. J., C. R. Steinman, H. C. Neimark, B. Muralidhar, T. Rush, M. F. Finkel, M. Kunkel, and R. J. Dattwyler.** 1992. Invasion of the central nervous system by *Borrelia burgdorferi* in acute disseminated infection. *JAMA* **267:**1364–1367.

34. **Magid, D., B. Schwartz, J. Craft, and J. S. Schwartz.** 1992. Prevention of Lyme disease after tick bites: a cost-effectiveness analysis. *N. Engl. J. Med.* **327:**534–541.

35. **Magnarelli, L. A.** 1995. Current status of laboratory diagnosis for Lyme disease. *Am. J. Med.* **98:**10S–14S.

36. **Marconi, R. T., and C. F. Garon.** 1992. Identification of a third genomic group of *Borrelia burgdorferi* through signature nucleotide analysis and 16S rRNA sequence determination. *J. Gen. Microbiol.* **138:**533–536.

37. **Marconi, R.T., D. S. Samuels, and C. F. Garon.** 1993. Transcriptional analyses and mapping of the *ospC* gene in Lyme disease spirochetes. *J. Bacteriol.* **175:**926–932.

38. **Marcus, L. C., A. C. Steere, P. H. Duray, A. E. Anderson, and E. B. Mahoney.** 1985. Fatal pancarditis in a patient with co-existent Lyme disease and babesiosis. Demonstration of spirochetes in the myocardium. *Ann. Intern. Med.* **103:**374–376.

39. **Massarotti, E. M., S. W. Luger, D. W. Rahn, R. P. Messner, J. B. Wong, R. C. Johnson, and A. C. Steere.** 1992. Treatment of early Lyme disease. *Am. J. Med.* **92:**369–403.

40. **Mather, T. N., D. Fish, and R. T. Coughlin.** 1994. Competence of dogs as reservoirs for Lyme disease spirochetes (*Borrelia burgdorferi*). *JAMA* **205:**186–188.

41. **Maupin, G. O., K. L. Gage, J. Piesman, J. Montenieri, S. L. Sviat, L. VanderZanden, C. M. Happ, M. Dolan, and B. J. Johnson.** 1994. Discovery of an enzootic cycle of *Borrelia burgdorferi* in *Neotoma mexicana* and *Ixodes spinipalpis* from northern Colorado, an area where Lyme disease is nonendemic. *J. Infect. Dis.* **170:**636–643.

42. **Nocton, J. J., F. Dressler, B. Rutledge, P. Rys, D. Persing, and A. Steere.** 1994. Detection of *Borrelia burgdorferi* DNA by polymerase chain reaction in synovial fluid from patients with Lyme arthritis. *N. Engl. J. Med.* **330:**229–234.

43. **Nocton, J. J., and A. C. Steere.** 1995. Lyme disease. *Adv. Intern. Med.* **40:**69–115.

44. **Oliver, J. H.** 1995. Arthropod research in the southeastern US. *J. Agromed.* **2:**79–84.

45. **Oliver, J. H., F. W. Chandler, A. M. James, F. H. Sanders, Jr., H. J. Hutcheson, L. O. Huey, B. S. McGuire, and R. S. Lane.** 1995. Natural occurrence and characterization of the Lyme disease spirochete, *Borrelia burgdorferi*, in cotton rats (*Sigmodon hispidus*) from Georgia and Florida. *J. Parasitol.* **81:**30–36.

46. **Oliver, J. H., F. W. Chandler, M. P. Luttrell, A. M. James, D. E. Stallknecht, B. S. McGuire, H. S. Hutcheson, G. A. Cummins, and R. S. Lane.** 1993. Isolation and transmission of the Lyme disease spirochetes from southeastern United States. *Proc. Natl. Acad. Sci. USA* **90:**7371–7375.

47. **Pachner, A. R., P. H. Duray, and A. C. Steere.** 1989. Central nervous system manifestations of Lyme disease. *Arch. Neurol.* **46:**790–795.

48. **Pachner, A. R., and A. C. Steere.** 1985. The triad of neurologic manifestations of Lyme disease: meningitis, cranial neuritis, and radiculoneuritis. *Neurology* **35:**47–53.

49. **Reik, L., A. C. Steere, N. H. Bartenhagen, R. E. Shope, and S. E. Malawista.** 1979. Neurologic abnormalities of Lyme disease. *Medicine* (Baltimore) **58:**281–294.

50. **Reimers, C. D., D. E. Pongratz, U. Neubert, A. Pilz, G. Hubner, M. Naegele, B. Wilske, P. H. Duray, and J. de Koning.** 1989. Myositis caused by *B. burgdorferi*: report of four cases. *J. Neurol. Sci.* **91:**215–226.

51. **Schlesier, M., G. Haas, G. Wolff-Vorbeck, I. Melchers, and H. H. Peter.** 1989. Autoreactive T cells in rheumatic disease. *J. Autoimmun.* **2:**31–49.

52. **Shanafelt, M. C., H. Yssel, R. Lahesmaa, C. Soderberg, J. Anzola, A. Allsup, C. Turck, P. Hindersson, and G. Peltz.** 1992. T cells in the pathogenesis of Lyme arthritis, p. 189–206. *In* S. E. Schuzter (ed.), *Lyme Disease: Molecular and Immunologic Approaches.* Cold Spring Harbor Laboratory Press, Cold Spring Harbor, New York.

53. **Shapiro, E. D., M. A. Gerber, N. B. Holabird, A. T. Berg, H. M. Feder, Jr., G. L. Bell, P. N. Rys, and D. H. Persing.** 1992. A controlled trial of antimicrobial prophylaxis for Lyme disease after deer-tick bites. *N. Engl. J. Med.* **327:**1769–1773.

54. **Sigal, L., and A. H. Tatum.** 1988. Molecular mimicry in Lyme neurologic disease: cross reactivity between B. burgdorferi and neuronal antigens. *Neurology* **38:**1439.

55. **Sigal, L. H.** 1993. Cross-reactivity between *B. burgdorferi* flagellin and a human axonal 64,000 molecular weight protein. *J. Infect. Dis.* **167:**1372–1378.

56. **Sigal, L. H.** 1995. Early disseminated Lyme disease: cardiac manifestations. *Am. J. Med.* **98**(Suppl. 4A):25S–28S.

57. **Smith, P. F., J. L. Benach, D. J. White, D. F. Stroup, and D. L. Morse.** 1988. Occupational risk of Lyme disease in endemic areas of New York State. *Ann. N.Y. Acad. Sci.* **539:**286–301.

58. **Steere, A. C.** 1989. Lyme disease. *N. Engl. J. Med.* **321:**586–596.

59. **Steere, A. C.** 1995. Musculoskeletal manifestations of Lyme disease. *Am. J. Med.* **98**(Suppl. 4A):44S–48S.

60. **Steere, A. C., W. P. Batsford, M. Weinberg, J. Alexander, H. S. Berger, S. Wolfson, and S. E. Malawista.** 1980. Lyme carditis: cardiac abnormalities of Lyme disease. *Ann. Intern. Med.* **93:**8–16.

61. **Steere, A. C., R. L. Grodzicki, A. N. Kornblatt, J. E. Craft, A. G. Barbour, W. Burgdorfer, G. P. Schmid, E. Johnson, and S. E. Malawista.** 1983. The spirochetal etiology of Lyme disease. *N. Engl. J. Med.* **308:**733–740.

62. **Steere, A. C., R. Levin, P. Molloy, R. A. Kalish, J. H. Abraham, N. U. Liu, and C. H. Schmid.** 1994. Treatment of Lyme arthritis. *Arthritis Rheum.* **37:**878–888.

63. **Steere, A. C., S. E. Malawista, D. R. Snydman, R. E. Shope, W. A. Andiman, M. R. Ross, and F. M. Steele.** 1977. Lyme arthritis: an epidemic of oligoarticular arthritis in children and adults in three Connecticut communities. *Arthritis Rheum.* **20:**7–17.

64. **Steere, A. C., R. T. Schoen, and E. Taylor.** 1987. The clinical evolution of Lyme arthritis. *Ann. Intern. Med.* **107:**725–731.

65. **Steere, A. C., E. Taylor, G. L. McHugh, and E. L. Logigian.** 1993. The overdiagnosis of Lyme disease. *JAMA* **269:**1812–1816.

66. **van der Linde, M. R., H. J. Crijns, J. de Koning, J. A. Hoogkamp-Korstanje, J. J. de Graaf, D. A. Piers, A. van der Galien, and K. I. Lie.** 1990. Range of atrioventricular conducting disturbances in Lyme borreliosis: a report of four cases and review of other published reports. *Br. Heart J.* **63:**162–168.

67. **Walker, D. H., A. G. Barbour, J. H. Oliver, R. S. Lane, S. Dumler, D. T. Dennis, D. H. Persing, A. F. Azad, and E. McSweegan.** 1996. Emerging bacterial zoonotic and vector-borne diseases. *JAMA* **275:**463–469.

68. **Weinecke, R., U. Neubert, and M. Volkenandt.** 1994. Molecular detection of *Borrelia burgdorferi* in formalin fixed, paraffin embedded lesions of lyme disease. *J. Cutaneous Pathol.* **20:**385–388.

69. **White, D. J., H.-G. Chang, J. L. Benach, E. M. Bosler, S. C. Meldrum, R. G. Means, J. G. Debbie, G. S. Birkhead, and D. L. Morse.** 1991. The geographic spread and temporal increase of the Lyme disease epidemic. *JAMA* **266:**1230–1236.

70. **Wilson, M. L., G. H. Adler, and A. Spielman.** 1986. Correlation between abundance of deer and that of the deer tick, Ixodes dammini (acari: Ixodidae). *Ann. Entomol. Soc. Am.* **78:**172–176.

71. **Wormser, G. P.** 1995. Prospects for a vaccine to prevent Lyme disease in humans. *Clin. Infect. Dis.* **21:**1267–1274.

chapter 16

Ebola Virus Infection in Nonhuman Primate Models

Nancy K. Jaax

The recent epidemic of Ebola-Zaire virus in Africa after a nearly 2-decade hiatus has again highlighted the paucity of information available regarding the natural ecology of Ebola virus. Ebola virus has been responsible for acute, explosive, and lethal outbreaks of hemorrhagic fever in both humans and nonhuman primates. There have been over a dozen separate, virus-isolation-confirmed filovirus outbreaks to date, yet nothing about how and where these viruses are maintained in nature has been learned (1, 5, 9, 11, 12, 16, 22, 25, 26, 29, 32, 33, 35–37). This is largely attributable to the typical pattern of disease outbreaks, which are sporadic and, as a rule, widely separated temporally. While the devastating secondary outbreaks of infections with Ebola-Zaire and Ebola-Sudan viruses have been traced to a single source (a health care worker), that individual can be positively identified only as the index case for the secondary outbreak. Unfortunately, the primary human infection frequently either is unidentified or has died before initial diagnosis of the disease (25). This has made determination of complete and accurate exposure history virtually impossible and has severely hampered ensuing epidemiological studies aimed at elucidating the viral reservoir.

Nancy K. Jaax, Pathology Division, U.S. Army Medical Research Institute of Infectious Diseases, 1425 Porter Street, Fort Detrick, MD 21702-5011.

Pathology of Emerging Infections
Edited by C. Robert Horsburgh, Jr., and Ann Marie Nelson
© 1997 American Society for Microbiology, Washington, DC 20005-4171

In contrast to Ebola-Zaire and Ebola-Sudan viruses, Ebola-Reston virus appears to be a lethal pathogen only for non-human primates

For a variety of reasons, availability of human tissues for complete histologic examination has been limited. However, human isolates of Ebola-Zaire and Ebola-Sudan viruses are highly lethal for nonhuman primates, and as a result, much of what is known about the behavior of the virus and the characteristic lesion patterns has been determined from experimental primate model studies (2–4, 10, 14, 17, 18, 20, 31).

In contrast to Ebola-Zaire and Ebola-Sudan viruses, Ebola-Reston virus appears to be a lethal pathogen only for nonhuman primates (19). Although Ebola-Reston virus infects humans, it does not produce clinical disease (6–8). The most recently characterized Ebola virus isolate, the Ivory Coast strain, was obtained from a human infected while performing a necropsy on a chimpanzee (*Pan troglodytes*) that died from hemorrhagic fever (23). The Ivory Coast isolate is clearly pathogenic for humans, although a lethal human infection has not been reported to date. A new outbreak of Ebola virus infection has also occurred in Gabon; recent information regarding the sequence of this isolate indicates that the Gabon isolate is a variant of the Ebola-Zaire strain.

Microbiology

Ebola virus belongs to a unique family, the *Filoviridae*, order *Mononegavirales*. The only two members of this family, Ebola virus and Marburg virus, are both lethal pathogens. Marburg and Ebola viruses are classified as biosafety level 4 pathogens and require maximum containment facilities for laboratory work. Ebola virus has four subtypes, Zaire, Sudan, Reston, and Ivory Coast. There is no antigenic cross-reactivity between Marburg and Ebola viruses, but the Ebola virus subtypes have both common and unique epitopes.

In most cell culture preparations as well as in tissues examined by electron microscopy, both Marburg and Ebola virions appear as filamentous, pleomorphic forms with a uniform diameter of 80 nm and variations in length (up to 14,000 nm; average, 790 nm), depending on the preparation and stage of infection. Virions have a helical nucleocapsid (50 nm in diameter), an envelope, and a surface projection layer composed of 10-nm-long peplomers (14). Both Marburg and Ebola virions contain one molecule of negative-sense single-stranded RNA. Morphologic differences between Marburg and Ebola viral inclusion bodies and virions are visible by electron microscopy and can be recognized by an experienced microscopist (13, 14); however, confirmation by immunological techniques is recommended (15). Strains of Ebola virus cross-react and require viral sequencing for specific identification.

Both Marburg and Ebola viruses are stable at room temperature. Infectivity is destroyed by UV light, gamma irradiation, lipid solvents, commercial bleach preparations, and phenolic disinfectants, but specific attention must be paid to contact time and required concentration of the disinfecting agent. The mode of entry of Ebola and Marburg viruses into cells is unknown at this time. Once infection occurs, virion assembly involves the budding of preformed nucleocapsids from plasma membranes. Massive amounts of viral nucleocapsid material occur in large, irregularly shaped intracytoplasmic inclusion bodies (14).

In monkeys, onset of viremia occurs between days 2 and 5 postexposure (p.e.) and peak viremia usually occurs on day 7 p.e. (1, 17, 20). Peak viremias are high and range from 7.4 $\log_{10}$ to 7.9 $\log_{10}$. The highest titers are present, in order of prevalence, in the spleen, mandibular lymph nodes, liver, adrenal gland, mesenteric lymph nodes, and femoral bone marrow. In one reported study, titers in the organs of the intramuscularly infected control ranged from 3.9 $\log_{10}$ (in the eyelid) to 7.3 $\log_{10}$ (in the kidney) and were, as a rule, lower than titers in the organs of the conjunctivally or orally infected monkeys (17).

Clinical Illness in Nonhuman Primates

The clinical course of Ebola (Zaire) fever is relatively consistent in all nonhuman primate studies to date, which include rhesus, cynomolgus, and African green monkeys. Clinical signs include anorexia, fever, and lethargy and are consistently present by day 4 postinfection (p.i.), although anorexia and fever are occasionally manifested as early as day 2 p.i. By day 5 p.i., monkeys become moderately to severely depressed. They become passive and relatively nonresponsive to external stimuli (17). They sit in a hunched-over position, with their heads down and with either their arms wrapped around their bodies or their hands holding the back of their necks. As the disease progresses, they become recumbent, fail to respond even if touched, and have shallow, rapid respiration. Vomiting and diarrhea can occur but are relatively infrequent.

A facial and bilaterally symmetrical rash (absent in African green monkeys) in the axillary and inguinal areas usually appears by day 5 and is fully developed by day 7 p.e. (17). There is prolonged bleeding from venipuncture sites and subcutaneous bruising. Epistaxis, frank hemorrhage from body orifices, recurrent vomiting or diarrhea, respiratory distress, and nasal exudate are not consistent clinical features of Ebola-Zaire in nonhuman primates, although they do occur; pulmonary signs appear to be more pronounced in Ebola-Reston (20). Time to death is a relatively constant feature, occurring between days 7 and 9 p.i. in nearly all cases of experimental primate Ebola-Zaire infection (1, 4, 17, 21); time to death with Ebola-Reston virus is somewhat longer (20).

In general, monkeys have moderate leukocytosis with relative lymphopenia; absolute lymphopenia may also be present early in the course of the disease. Leukocytosis is due to a mature neutrophilia, and the hematology may resemble that seen in acute bacterial infections. Platelet counts decrease over time, a finding consistent with disseminated intravascular coagulation (DIC). Clinical chemistry values up to day 5 p.e. are generally not elevated above those seen on day 0 p.e. The 2- to 10-fold elevations in terminal kidney and liver enzyme profiles that occur in infected monkeys are consistent with renal and hepatic failure. Fibrin degradation products (FDPs) are generally elevated by day 5 p.e. and increase dramatically by day 7 p.e. Endotoxin detectable in serum and/or plasma of monkeys prior to day 5 p.e. has

Clinical signs of Ebola (Zaire) fever include anorexia, fever, and lethargy and are consistently present by day 4 postinfection

not been reported. Elevated endotoxin levels have been detected in the terminal serum of infected monkeys, suggesting that levels rise dramatically between days 5 and 7 p.e.; it is likely that endotoxin plays a role in the pathophysiology of the disease (17, 24, 27, 30, 34).

Pathology

Necropsy findings present in Ebola-Zaire-virus-infected monkeys include a cutaneous rash (absent in African green monkeys) involving the axilla, thorax, abdomen, groin, proximal limbs, and face, particularly in the periorbital area; enlarged (1.5 to 3 times the normal size) and reddened mesenteric, mandibular, mediastinal, axillary, and inguinal lymph nodes; periorbital edema; an enlarged, swollen liver with rounded, friable capsular borders and a prominent reticulated pattern; segmental vascular congestion and edema in the ileum; and subcutaneous hemorrhage evident at venipuncture sites and pressure points (17). Other findings may include pharyngitis, conjunctivitis, hemothorax, hemoperitoneum, icterus, pulmonary hemorrhage, a sharply demarcated zone of congestion and/or hemorrhage at the junction of the pylorus and the duodenum, gastrointestinal hemorrhage, and adrenal, ovarian, or urinary bladder hemorrhage. There is no apparent relationship between the exposure method and occurrence or distribution of gross necropsy lesions, with the possible exception of conjunctivitis. A higher incidence of conjunctivitis in monkeys exposed to the virus by conjunctival exposure compared with oral exposure has been reported (17).

Hematopoietic System

The most consistently and strongly immunoreactive cells in experimentally infected monkeys are those of the mononuclear phagocyte system. Virtually all circulating monocytes have an abundant, heavily immunopositive cytoplasm. Aggregates of immunopositive monocytes enmeshed in an antigen-positive network of fibrin often adhere to vascular walls of the circulatory system in all organs; the vascular endothelium adjacent to these aggregates is also immunopositive (17).

Immunocytochemistry findings are confirmed by ultrastructural examination, which shows large amounts of free virus, virus enmeshed in fibrin in blood vessels, and heavily infected monocytes. Large numbers of macrophages in the bone marrow, alveolar macrophages, and macrophages (histiocytes) in the skin, lymph nodes, liver (Kupffer cells), spleen, and other tissues are consistently heavily immunopositive; ultrastructure examination has confirmed the presence of Ebola virus in all immunopositive locations. Lymphocytes and neutrophils in the circulation or in lymph nodes are frequently enmeshed in immunoreactive thrombi, but there is no evidence of intracellular antigen in lymphocytes or neutrophils and viral infections of these cell types have not been verified by ultrastructure, although neutrophils may contain phagocytized portions of virions.

Examination of bone marrow reveals diffuse, mild necrosis. Normal maturational sequences of erythrocytic and granulocytic cells are present. Immunocytochemistry demonstrates abundant free antigen and large numbers

The most consistently and strongly immunoreactive cells in experimentally infected monkeys are those of the mononuclear phagocyte system

of immunoreactive macrophages. Ultrastructural examination confirms immunoreactivity findings in these tissues. Viral replication, demonstrated by intracytoplasmic Ebola virus inclusion material and budding virions, is most prominent in macrophages of the bone marrow, lymph nodes, spleen, and liver (Kupffer cells), but it is also seen in macrophages of all tissues examined. Free virions in demarcation channels of megakaryocytes are occasionally observed, but there are no typical Ebola virus inclusions and they have not been identified in granulocytic or erythrocytic precursors.

Lymph Nodes and Spleen

On hematoxylin and eosin examination, there is depletion and necrosis of all lymphoid germinal centers in the spleen, tonsils, and all peripheral, mediastinal, and mesenteric lymph nodes examined, as well as in the bronchial and gut-associated lymphoid tissue present in sections of the lung and gastrointestinal tract (17, 18, 20).

In the spleen, germinal centers are surrounded by a characteristic mantle zone of hemorrhage and congestion. There is copious deposition of fibrin throughout the red pulp, as well as abundant karyorrhectic cellular debris. Large numbers of macrophages and lesser numbers of neutrophils are also present. Immunoreactive fibrin throughout the red pulp and heavy immunopositive staining within macrophages are seen by immunohistochemistry. No immunoreactivity is associated with the depleted germinal centers, but immunoreactivity is present in macrophages and antigen-presenting cells in the mantle zone.

In the spleen, germinal centers are surrounded by a characteristic mantle zone of hemorrhage and congestion

In the lymph nodes, hemorrhage, diffuse necrosis, and sinus histiocytosis are consistent features, particularly in the tonsils and submandibular and mesenteric lymph nodes. Macrophages and necrotic cellular debris are present in the subcapsular and medullary sinuses of virtually all lymph nodes. The lymph nodes and tonsils have abundant free and macrophage-associated immunoreactivity, with the largest amount occurring in the subcapsular and medullary sinuses. Ultrastructural examination substantiates light microscopy findings.

Circulatory System

Histological evidence of DIC occurs routinely in Ebola-Zaire- and Ebola-Reston-virus-infected primates. Fibrin and fibrinocellular thrombi can be identified in small venules of numerous tissues but are particularly prevalent in the submucosa of the gastrointestinal tract, the renal glomeruli, the renal medulla, and, to a lesser extent, lung (17, 18, 20, 21). Both fibrin thrombi and fibrinocellular thrombi are strongly immunoreactive. The endothelium in muscular arteries and large veins is always immunopositive if it is in contact with an antigen-positive thrombus, but foci of immunoreactivity also occur where no thrombus is present. In these foci, ultrastructural examination reveals typical Ebola virus inclusions within the cytoplasm of some endothelial cells. Endothelial immunoreactivity in capillaries and venules is also present multifocally in the vessels of the brain, heart, and renal medulla. Immunoreactivity of the endothelia of small venules and capillaries in other tissues is difficult to critically evaluate, as extracellular antigen in vessels is abundant and immunopositive thrombi are a consistent feature, particularly in the gastrointestinal tract and kidneys.

Respiratory System

Histologically, monkeys have minimal to mild, multifocal, subacute inflammation in the nares, larynx, and trachea. Regardless of the method of exposure, blood vessels in the nares, larynx, trachea, and bronchial tree are frequently dilated and expanded by immunoreactive aggregates of fibrin and macrophages. Immunoreactivity occurs multifocally in a linear pattern at the junction of the mucosa and submucosa, immediately subjacent to the basement membrane. Multifocal immunoreactivity in mucosal epithelial cells of the nares, larynx, and trachea also occurs.

In the lungs, moderate to severe pulmonary hemorrhage may occur, making other histologic changes difficult to evaluate; the absence of a cellular response in these cases suggests that pulmonary hemorrhage is a terminal event. Pulmonary lesions are generally characterized by a spectrum of mild diffuse interstitial leukocytosis, thrombi, and edema. Alveoli may contain proteinaceous fluid, polymerized fibrin, and large numbers of alveolar macrophages if high levels of circulating endotoxins are present; septal necrosis with associated polymorphonuclear neutrophil accumulation is also present (17).

Digestive System

Histologically, the most severe lesions in the digestive system are present in the liver and small intestine. Sinusoids are dilated and contain fibrin, large numbers of monocytes, and abundant necrotic cellular debris; disseminated foci of hepatocellular necrosis also occur, and the inflammatory response is primarily neutrophilic. Kupffer cells, monocytes, and hepatocytes contain characteristic large (5 to 25 µm), pleomorphic, acidophilic intracytoplasmic inclusions. By immunocytochemistry, copious free and cell-associated immunoreactive material can be seen in the sinusoids; foci of hepatocellular necrosis are also antigen positive. Moderate to severe diffuse vacuolar change may also occur in hepatocytes. Electron microscopy of the liver reveals free virions in sinusoids, the space of Disse, and bile canaliculi. Ebola virus inclusions are seen in Kupffer cells, circulating macrophages, and, less frequently, hepatocytes. Sinusoids contain fibrin, virus particles, and necrotic cellular debris.

The most severe histological lesions in the intestines occur at the gastroduodenal junction, in the proximal duodenum, and in the ileum near the ileocecocolic junction. Erosive lesions in the jejunum and cecum also occur, but the colon is generally spared. Multifocally, in the small intestine, there is moderate to severe hemorrhage in the submucosa and lamina propria, with mucosal necrosis and/or erosion. Fibrin and fibrinocellular thrombi are present throughout the submucosa and lamina propria, suggesting that the necrosis and erosion of the mucosa are secondary to microthrombosis. Abundant immunoreactivity in macrophages in the submucosa and the lamina propria throughout the small and large intestines, with occasional immunoreactivity in enterocytes, can be seen by immunohistochemistry.

> *In the lungs, moderate to severe pulmonary hemorrhage may occur, making other histologic changes difficult to evaluate*

Ultrastructurally, virus-infected macrophages and occasional fibroblasts are observed in the lamina propria and submucosa but not in enterocytes. Minimal to mild glossitis, pharyngitis, esophagitis, sialoadenitis, and/or gastritis (consisting of multifocal accumulations of neutrophils, lymphocytes, and few macrophages in the submucosa) are also consistent findings.

Urinary System

Infected monkeys have histological lesions compatible with DIC. Fibrin thrombi are seen in the glomeruli and/or venules and intertubular capillaries of the kidney. Tubules usually contain proteinaceous and cellular casts, and tubular epithelial cells are frequently degenerated, a finding consistent with nephrosis; renal cortical necrosis secondary to thrombosis also occurs. Free Ebola virions are frequently interspersed among aggregates of fibrin, and virus replication occurs in interstitial macrophages and fibroblasts (17).

Reproductive System

Immunohistochemistry of ovarian sections reveals strong, diffuse immunoreactivity in the follicular cells and multifocal positivity in the stromal cells of all animals. Immunohistochemistry of uterine sections of female primates shows moderate to heavy immunoreactivity in the stromal cells and strong multifocal immunoreactivity of the oviduct epithelium. Electron microscopy of the ovary confirms immunohistochemistry findings, demonstrating Ebola virus inclusions in the stromal macrophages, fibroblasts, and follicular cells (17).

Skin and Adnexa

Sections of skin from the mucocutaneous junction of the nose, lip, eyelids, and haired skin from the chest have been examined. Blood vessels are dilated and contain fibrinocellular thrombi. Immunoreactivity is present in the fibrinocellular thrombi of dermal blood vessels and macrophages in the dermis, particularly at the dermal/epidermal junction and in the connective tissue adjacent to hair follicles, sebaceous glands, and apocrine glands. The acinar and ductular epithelium of apocrine glands, the bulbs of hair follicles, the nasal and oral epithelia, and the epidermis are also occasionally multifocally immunopositive (17).

Endocrine Gland, Central Nervous System, and Eye

The adrenal glands have moderate disseminated multifocal necrosis, primarily limited to the zona fasiculata. Characteristic intracytoplasmic inclusion bodies are also present in adrenal cells. By immunocytochemistry, copious free antigen throughout the adrenal gland can be seen. Immunoreactivity is also present in macrophages and cortical cells and is associated with foci of adrenal cell necrosis. The thyroid and parathyroid glands are histologically normal; however, there is multifocal immunoreactivity in thyroid interstitial cells and there are minimal numbers of immunopositive thyroid follicular epithelial cells. In the parathyroid glands, chief cells are also occasionally immunopositive. Hematoxylin and eosin-stained central nervous system tissues are frequently normal, with the exception of dilation

The adrenal glands have moderate disseminated multifocal necrosis, primarily limited to the zona fasiculata

of perivascular spaces, which is suggestive of edema. Malacic change has been reported, as have focal meningitis and multifocal acute ependymitis. Immunocytochemistry reveals that immunoreactivity is limited to circulating monocytes, multifocal endothelial cells, and multifocal ependymal cells of the choroid plexus. Antigen-positive macrophages are also present in the ciliary body of the eye; immunoreactivity has not been reported in other cell types (17).

Conclusion

Ultrastructural examination has failed to detect any viral replication in any hematopoietic cells other than monocytes

Several points regarding the pathology of Ebola virus in nonhuman primates are of interest. Although extracellular virus is in intimate and sustained contact with all leukocyte types as well as the vascular endothelium, ultrastructural examination has failed to detect any viral replication in any hematopoietic cells other than monocytes. Examination of bone marrow has failed to show replicating virus in megakaryocytes or granulocytic or erythrocytic precursors. Virus present in bone marrow is either free or associated with macrophages. While infection of the endothelium does occur, it is multifocal and is most commonly associated with macrophage adhesion to the endothelial surface.

As indicated by histological lesions and clinical chemistry results, hepato-renal failure is a late event, and renal lesions are consistent with sequelae to DIC. Although replicating virus is present in hepatocytes and adrenal cortical cells, particularly in foci of necrosis, these cells do not appear to be the primary target of the virus. Much higher numbers of Kupffer cells, monocytes, and interstitial macrophages are infected (17).

Although viral titers in the lungs are high and viral antigen is found to be abundant by immunocytochemistry, immunoreactivity in the lungs usually occurs primarily within vascular structures. These findings have been confirmed by ultrastructural examination. However, in monkeys with high levels of endotoxin, severe pulmonary edema is present; alveoli are filled with proteinaceous fluid, fibrin, and large numbers of immunopositive macrophages (17). Immunopositive exudate is also present in bronchioles. On the basis of these findings, such monkeys would be a more likely source of infectious aerosol or droplets than others. This suggests that there may be a percentage of clinical cases that have infectious viral particles in the upper airway, making them a potential aerosol or droplet hazard. This finding has been documented in the primate epizootics of Ebola-Reston in 1989 and 1990.

The relationship between endotoxemia and pulmonary damage in humans and a variety of animal species is well established. Elevated endotoxin levels result in damage to the epithelial mucosa of the gut and loss of mononuclear phagocyte system cell function in the liver and spleen. Breakdown of both the intestinal mucosal barrier and the mononuclear phagocyte system capacity can result in systemic endotoxemia (28, 30). Elevated endotoxin levels in Ebola-infected primates may contribute to the development of pulmonary lesions and presence of intra-alveolar virus.

Endotoxemia is closely associated with the development of adult respiratory distress syndrome and multiple-system organ failure. In the complex series of events leading to acute lung injury in gram-negative sepsis, endotoxin is the proximal mediator. Although endotoxin may be capable of causing direct injury to the pulmonary endothelium, its primary role is in activating inflammatory mediators, neutrophils, and platelets and inducing the production of cytokines and arachidonic acid metabolites. The gastrointestinal tract is thought to be the source of endotoxemia and the first step of a gut-liver-lung axis (28). Translocated bacteria and endotoxins activate Kupffer cells and then secrete proinflammatory and hypotensive mediators. In the lung, these mediators cause polymorphonuclear neutrophils to bind to pulmonary endothelial cells and degranulate. These mediators also activate the coagulation cascade and ultimately cause many of the morphological changes observed in early sepsis-induced adult respiratory distress syndrome, which include interstitial and intra-alveolar edema, vascular thrombosis and hemorrhage, and pulmonary leukoaggregation (28, 30).

The final observation is cautionary and relates to the interpretation of necropsy lesions in nonhuman primates. The finding of a sharply demarcated focus of hemorrhage at the gastroduodenal junction has long been considered virtually pathognomonic for simian hemorrhagic fever, caused by a serious primate pathogen that causes no disease in humans, yet this lesion has been observed in numerous monkeys infected with both Ebola and Marburg viruses. In reality, this lesion, as well as others presented in this paper, is likely a sequela to vascular disturbances that occur in hemorrhagic fevers as a group, rather than a specific effect of a particular virus.

Figure 16.1 Typical appearance of the spleen in Ebola-Zaire-virus-infected monkeys, showing depleted and necrotic germinal centers that are surrounded by a characteristic zone of hemorrhage and congestion (hematoxylin and eosin; original magnification, ×20).

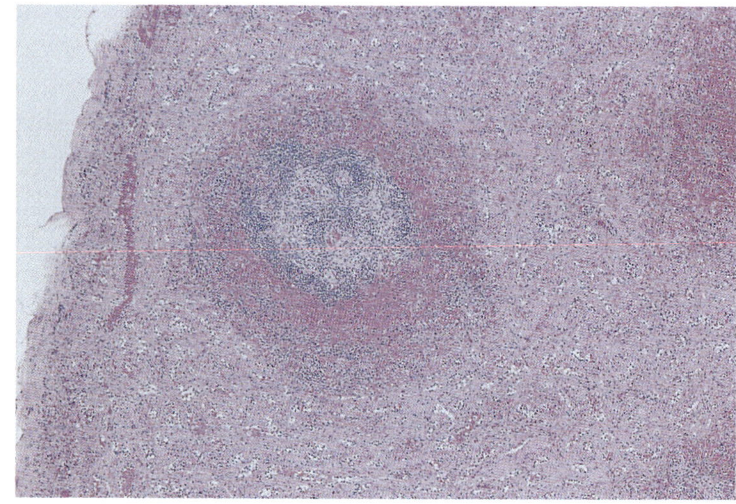

Figure 16.2 Typical appearance of a liver lesion in Ebola-Zaire-virus-infected monkeys, characterized by sinusoidal congestion, multifocal hepatocyte necrosis, and the occurrence of intracytoplasmic inclusion bodies that vary in size and morphology (hematoxylin and eosin; original magnification, ×20).

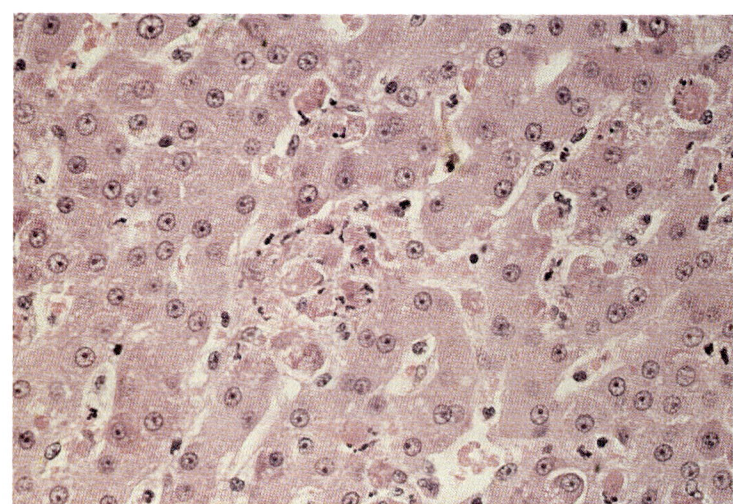

Figure 16.3 Immunocytochemical stain of liver tissue of a monkey infected orally with Ebola-Mayinga virus. The chromogen stains virus-positive cells red. Most immunoreactivity occurs in the sinusoids and Kupffer cells. Multifocally, hepatocytes are also immunopositive, but to a lesser extent. Original magnification, ×40.

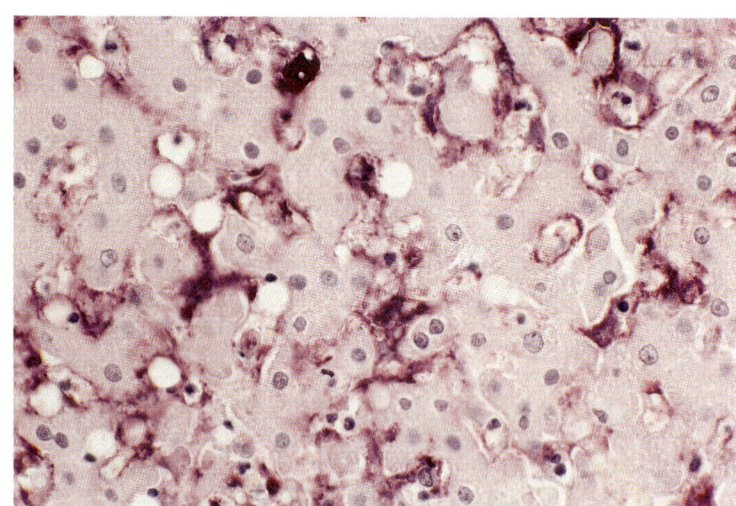

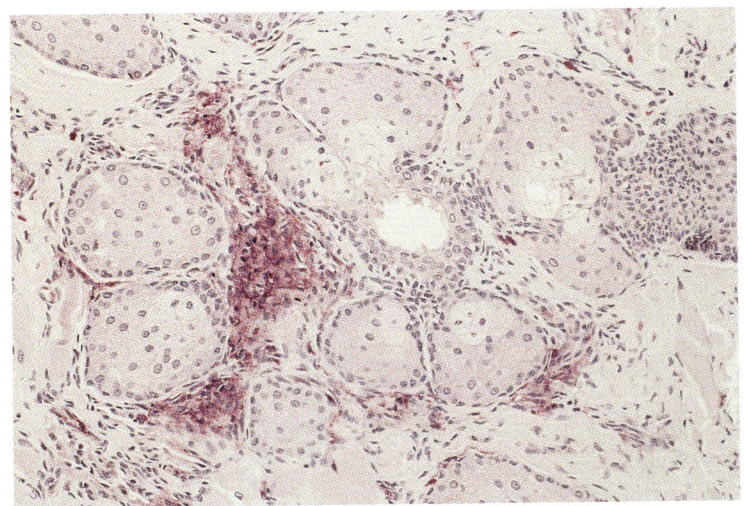

Figure 16.4 Immunocytochemical stain of adnexa from same monkey described in Fig. 16.3. The chromogen stains virus-positive cells red. This section was taken from the axillary skin. There is multifocal immunoreactivity in the interstitial area, which occurs primarily in small capillaries and the interstitial connective tissue. Epithelial cells are infrequently immunopositive. Original magnification, ×50.

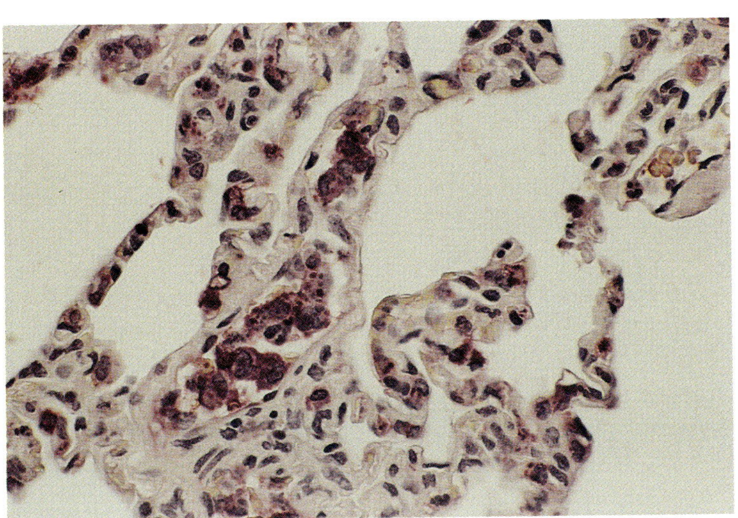

Figure 16.5 Immunocytochemical stain of lung from same monkey described in Fig. 16.3. The chromogen stains virus-positive cells red. Monocytes in pulmonary blood vessels are seen. Note abundant positive staining in the cytoplasm of all monocytes visible in the section. Original magnification, ×50.

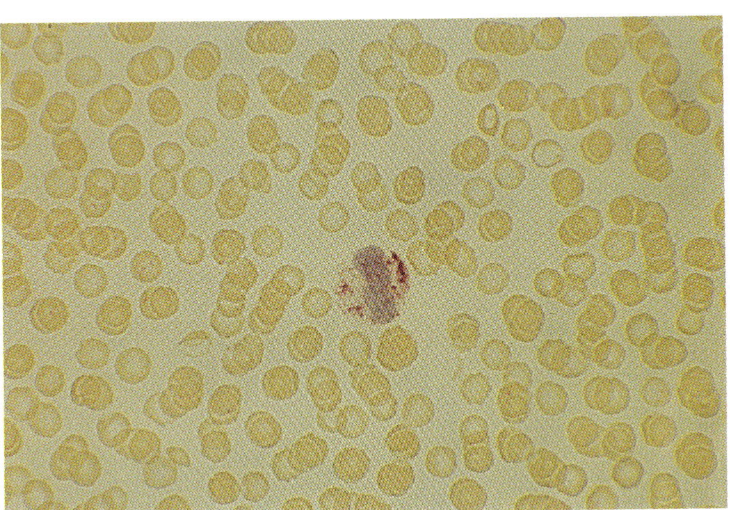

Figure 16.6 Peripheral blood smear from same monkey described in Fig. 16.3. The chromogen stains virus-positive cells red. Positive antigen staining is evident in monocytes. This slide was taken on day 7 p.i. Original magnification, ×250.

References

1. **Baskerville, A., E. T. W. Bowen, G. S. Platt, L. B. McArdell, and D. I. H. Simpson.** 1978. The pathology of experimental Ebola virus infection in monkeys. *J. Pathol.* **125**:131–138.

2. **Baskerville, A., S. P. Fisher-Hoch, G. H. Neild, and A. B. Dowsett.** 1985. Ultrastructural pathology of experimental Ebola haemorrhagic fever virus infection. *J. Pathol.* **147**:199–209.

3. **Bowen, E., G. Platt, G. Lloyd, R. Raymond, and D. Simpson.** 1980. A comparative study of strains of Ebola virus isolated from southern Sudan and northern Zaire in 1976. *J. Med. Virol.* **6**:129–138.

4. **Bowen, E. T. W., G. S. Platt, D. I. H. Simpson, and L. B. McArdell.** 1978. Ebola hemorrhagic fever: experimental infection of monkeys. *Trans. R. Soc. Trop. Med. Hyg.* **72**:188–191.

5. **Bres, P.** 1978. The epidemic of Ebola haemorrhagic fever in Sudan and Zaire, 1976: an introductory note. *Bull. W. H. O.* **56**:245–270.

6. **Centers for Disease Control.** 1990. Update: filovirus infections among persons with occupational exposure to nonhuman primates. *Morbid. Mortal. Weekly Rep.* **39**:266–267.

7. **Centers for Disease Control.** 1990. Update: filovirus infection associated with contact with nonhuman primates or their tissues. *Morbid. Mortal. Weekly Rep.* **39**:404–405.

8. **Centers for Disease Control.** 1990. Update: filovirus infection in animal handlers. *Morbid. Mortal. Weekly Rep.* **39**:221.

9. **Dalgard, D. W., R. J. Hardy, S. L. Pearson, G. J. Pucak, R. V. Quander, P. M. Zack, C. J. Peters, and P. B. Jahrling.** 1992. Combined simian hemorrhagic fever and Ebola virus infection in cynomolgus monkeys. *Lab. Anim. Sci.* **42**:152–157.

10. **Fisher-Hoch, S. P., T. L. Brammer, S. G. Trappier, L. C. Hutwagner, B. B. Farrar, S. L. Ruo, B. G. Brown, L. M. Hermann, G. I. Perez-Oronoz, C. S. Goldsmith, M. A. Hanes, and J. B. McCormick.** 1992. Pathogenic potential of filoviruses: role of geographic origin of primate host and virus strain. *J. Infect. Dis.* **166**:753–763.

11. **Francis, D. P., D. H. Smith, R. B. Highton, D. I. H. Simpson, P. Lolik, I. M. Deng, A. L. Gillo, A. A. Idris, and B. E. Tahir.** 1978. Ebola fever in the Sudan 1976: epidemiological aspects of the disease, p. 129–136. *In* S. R. Pattyn (ed.), *Ebola Virus Hemorrhagic Fever.* Elsevier/North-Holland Biomedical Press, New York.

12. **Gear, J. S. S., G. A. Cassel, A. J. Gear, B. Trappler, L. Clausen, A. M. Meyers, M. C. Kew, T. H. Bothwell, R. Sher, G. B. Miller, J. Schneider, H. J. Koornhof, E. D. Gomperts, M. Isaacson, and J. H. Gear.** 1975. Outbreak of Marburg virus disease in Johannesburg. *Br. Med. J.* **4**:489–493.

13. **Geisbert, T. W.** 1992. Association of Ebola-related Reston virus particles and antigen with tissue lesions of monkeys imported to the United States. *J. Comp. Pathol.* **106**:137–152.

14. **Geisbert, T. W., and P. Jahrling.** 1995. Differentiation of filoviruses by electron microscopy. *Virus Res.* **39**:129–150.

15. **Geisbert, T. W., and P. B. Jahrling.** 1990. Use of immunoelectron microscopy to show Ebola virus during the 1989 United States epizootic. *J. Clin. Pathol.* **43**:813–816.

16. **Heyman, D., P. Weisfeld, P. Webb, K. Johnson, T. Cairns, and H. Berquist.** 1980. Ebola hemorrhagic fever: Tandala, Zaire, 1977–78. *J. Infect. Dis.* **142:**372–376.

17. **Jaax, N., K. Davis, and T. Geisbert.** 1996. Lethal experimental infection of rhesus monkeys with Ebola-Zaire (Mayinga) virus by the oral and conjunctival route of exposure. *Arch. Pathol. Lab. Med.* **120:**140–155.

18. **Jaax, N., P. Jahrling, T. Geisbert, J. Geisbert, K. Steele, K. McKee, D. Nagley, E. Johnson, G. Jaax, and C. Peters.** 1995. Preliminary report: natural transmission of Ebola virus (Zaire strain) to monkeys in a biocontainment laboratory. *Lancet* **346:**1669–1670.

19. **Jahrling, P. B., T. W. Geisbert, D. W. Dalgard, E. D. Johnson, T. G. Ksiazek, W. C. Hall, and C. J. Peters.** 1990. Preliminary report: isolation of Ebola virus from monkeys imported to USA. *Lancet* **335:**502–505.

20. **Jahrling, P. B., T. Geisbert, N. Jaax, M. Hanes, T. Ksiazek, and C. Peters.** 1996. Experimental infection of cynomolgus macaques with Ebola-Reston filovirus from the 1989–90 epizootic. *Arch. Virol.* **11(Suppl.):**115–134.

21. **Johnson, E., N. Jaax, J. White, and P. Jahrling.** 1995. Lethal experimental infections of rhesus monkeys by aerosolized Ebola virus. *Int. J. Exp. Pathol.* **76:**227–236.

22. **Johnson, K. M., C. L. Scribner, and J. B. McCormick.** 1981. Ecology of Ebola virus: a first clue? *J. Infect. Dis.* **143:**749–751.

23. **LeGuenno, B., P. Formentry, M. Wyers, P. Gounon, F. Walker, and C. Boesch.** 1995. Isolation and partial characterization of a new strain of Ebola virus. *Lancet* **345:**1271–1274.

24. **Martin, M. A., and H. J. Silverman.** 1992. Gram-negative sepsis and the adult respiratory distress syndrome. *Clin. Infect. Dis.* **14:**1213–1228.

25. **Martini, G. A.** 1971. *Marburg Virus Disease: Clinical Syndrome*, p. 1–9. Springer Verlag, New York.

26. **Martini, G. A., H. G. Knouff, H. A. Schmidt, G. Mayer, and G. Baltzer.** 1968. A hitherto unknown infectious disease contracted from monkeys. *Germ. Med. Monthly* **13:**457–470.

27. **Nakao, A., S. Taki, M. Yasui, Y. Kimura, T. Nonami, A. Harada, and H. Takagi.** 1994. The fate of intravenously injected endotoxin in normal rats and in rats with liver failure. *Hepatology* **19:**1251–1256.

28. **Pugin, J., and J. C. Chevrolet.** 1991. The intestine-liver-lung axis in septic syndrome. *Schweiz. Med. Wochenschr.* **121:**1538–1544.

29. **Sanchez, A., T. Ksiazek, P. Rollin, D. I. H. Simpson, P. Lolik, I. M. Derg, A. L. Gillo, A. Idris, and B. El Tahir.** 1995. Reemergence of Ebola virus in Africa. *Emerg. Infect. Dis.* **1:**129–136.

30. **Simons, R., R. Maier, and C. Ey.** 1991. Pulmonary effects of continuous endotoxin infusion in the rat. *Circ. Shock.* **33:**233–243.

31. **Simpson, D., E. Bowen, and W. Bright.** 1968. Vervet monkey disease: experimental infection of monkeys with the causative agent and antibody studies in wild caught monkeys. *Lab. Anim.* **75.**

32. **Smith, D. H., D. Francis, D. I. H. Simpson, and R. B. Highton.** 1978. The Nzara outbreak of viral hemorrhagic fever, p. 137–141. *In* S. P. Pattyn (ed.), *Ebola Virus Hemorrhagic Fever.* Elsevier/North Holland Biomedical Press, New York.

33. **Smith, D. H., B. K. Johnson, M. Isaacson, R. Swanapoel, K. M. Johnson, M. Killey, A. Bagshawe, T. Siongok, and W. K. Keruga.** 1982. Marburg virus disease in Kenya. *Lancet* **i:**816–820.

34. **Van Leeuwen, P. A., M. A. Boermeester, A. P. Houdijk, C. C. Ferwerda, M. A. Cuesta, S. Meyer, and R. I. Wesdorp.** 1994. Clinical significance of translocation. *Gut* **35:**S28–S34.

35. **World Health Organization.** 1978. Ebola haemorrhagic fever in Sudan. *Bull. W. H. O.* **56:**247–270.

36. **World Health Organization.** 1978. Ebola haemorrhagic fever in Zaire, 1976. *Bull. W. H. O.* **56:**271–293.

37. **World Health Organization.** 1979. Ebola hemorrhagic fever—Southern Sudan. *Morbid. Mortal. Weekly Rep.* **28:**557–559.

chapter 17

Ebola Virus Hemorrhagic Fever

Sherif R. Zaki and Peter H. Kilmarx

Ebola virus causes an illness classified as a hemorrhagic fever. The term hemorrhagic fever refers to conditions characterized, as the name suggests, by fever and hemorrhage. Hemorrhagic fever of infectious origin may be caused by diverse pathogens, such as viruses, rickettsia, bacteria, and protozoa (49). However, the term "hemorrhagic fever viruses" is reserved for a special group of viruses transmitted to humans by arthropods and rodents (Table 17.1).

Ebola hemorrhagic fever was first recognized in concurrent outbreaks in Zaire and Sudan in 1976 (38, 39). There were a few outbreaks identified following that, including two sporadic cases and a smaller outbreak (2, 19); in the mid-1990s, there have been several outbreaks, including a large outbreak in Zaire in 1995 which captured the attention of the popular press (7). The causative agent, Ebola virus, is named after a small river near the site of the 1976 epidemic in Zaire.

Sherif R. Zaki, Infectious Disease Pathology Activity, Division of Viral and Rickettsial Diseases, National Center for Infectious Diseases, Centers for Disease Control and Prevention, 1600 Clifton Road, N.E., Mailstop G-32, Atlanta, GA 30333. **Peter H. Kilmarx,** Epidemic Intelligence Service, Epidemiology Program Office, and Epidemiology and Surveillance Branch, Division of STD Prevention, National Center for HIV, STD, and TB Prevention, Centers for Disease Control and Prevention, Atlanta, GA 30333, and The HIV/AIDS Collaboration, P.O. Box 8 Lanna Station, Chiang Rai 57001, Thailand.

Pathology of Emerging Infections
Edited by C. Robert Horsburgh, Jr., and Ann Marie Nelson
© 1997 American Society for Microbiology, Washington, DC 20005-4171

Table 17.1 Hemorrhagic fever viruses

Virus	Disease name[a]	Case-fatality rate (%)	Vertebrate host	Arthropod vector
Arenaviruses				
Junin	Argentine HF	15–30	Rodents (*Calomys musculinus*)	None
Machupo	Bolivian HF	15–30	Rodents (*Calomys callosus*)	
Guanarito	Venezuelan HF	15–30	Rodents (*Zygodontomys brevicauda*)	None
Sabia	Brazilian HF	15–30	Presumably an unidentified rodent	None
Lassa	Lassa fever	~15	Rodents (*Mastomys* spp.)	None
Bunyaviridae				
Rift Valley fever	Rift Valley fever	~50	Vertebrates (sheep, cattle)	Mosquito, *Aedes* spp., and others
Crimean Congo HF	Crimean Congo HF	15–30	Vertebrates (birds, hares, large ungulates)	Ticks, especially *Hyalomma* spp.
Hantaan, Seoul, Puumala, and others	HF with renal syndrome	1–15	Rodents	None
Sin Nombre, Black Creek Canal, and others	Hantavirus pulmonary syndrome	50	Rodents	None
Filoviridae				
Marburg	Marburg HF	25	Unknown	Unknown
Ebola	Ebola HF	50–90	Unknown	Unknown
Flaviviridae				
Yellow fever	Yellow fever	20	Primates	Mosquito, especially *Aedes* spp.
Dengue	Dengue HF, dengue shock syndrome	<1	Primates	Mosquito, especially *Aedes aegypti*
Kyasanur Forest disease	KFD	0.5–9	Rodents	Ticks
Omsk HF	OHF	0.5–9	Rodents	Ticks

[a] HF, hemorrhagic fever; KFD, Kyasanur Forest disease; OHF, Omsk hemorrhagic fever.

Virology

Ebola and Marburg viruses are members of a unique RNA virus family, the *Filoviridae* (33). Filoviruses constitute the third family of negative-strand RNA viruses, along with the *Paramyxoviridae* and *Rhabdoviridae*, within the order *Mononegavirales* (27). Ebola virus has five known subtypes (Zaire, Sudan, Côte-d'Ivoire, Gabon, and Reston); there are no known subtypes of Marburg virus. Marburg virus and Ebola virus subtypes Zaire, Sudan, Côte-d'Ivoire, and Gabon are highly pathogenic for humans, causing a hemorrhagic fever with high mortality rates. Reston virus does not appear to cause disease in humans, although it is highly pathogenic in nonhuman primates (32). The subtypes of Ebola virus have common as well as unique epitopes, while Ebola and Marburg viruses show no antigenic cross-reactivity. Because of the extreme pathogenicity of certain strains and the lack of a protective vaccine or effective antiviral drug, filoviruses are classified as biosafety level 4 agents.

Because of the extreme pathogenicity of certain strains and the lack of a protective vaccine or effective antiviral drug, filoviruses are classified as biosafety level 4 agents

Morphology

Ebola and Marburg virions are composed of a helical nucleocapsid containing a negative-sense, single-stranded RNA genome surrounded by a lipid envelope. The virions are pleomorphic, sometimes appearing as short U-shaped or circular forms or, more commonly, as long filamentous particles up to 14,000 nm in length with diameters of about 80 nm (Fig. 17.1A and 17.1B). Characteristic viral inclusions are a feature of many infected cells, as seen by thin-section electron microscopy (Fig. 17.1C) (30).

Epidemiology

Ecology

Despite extensive ecologic investigations, the natural reservoir of Ebola virus (where it is propagated between human outbreaks) remains unknown. In both outbreaks in Sudan, the first patients were employed at a textile factory that was colonized by bats (2, 38). No evidence of infection in captured bats was found in subsequent ecologic studies at that site (1); however, bats were recently shown to support replication and circulation of high titers of virus in the laboratory, whereas other animals did not (37). The Reston strain of Ebola virus, which is not associated with human disease, has been isolated from cynomolgus monkeys (*Macaca fascicularis*) imported to the United States (6, 9) and Italy (40) from the Philippines. Contact with dead chimpanzees (*Pan troglodytes*) has been implicated in cases in Côte-d'Ivoire (24) and Gabon (44). In some outbreaks, the putative first case had expired by the time epidemiologic investigations started, making it difficult to assess ecologic exposures. Ecologic investigation underway in the Taï Forest in Côte-d'Ivoire, where chimpanzee troops have been decimated by possible hemorrhagic fever, may yield additional information (24).

Despite extensive ecologic investigations, the natural reservoir of Ebola virus remains unknown

Outbreaks

Three outbreaks of Ebola virus infections were identified in the 1970s, which were followed by a hiatus until 1994, when a Swiss researcher was infected after performing an autopsy on a chimpanzee (Table 17.2) (24). An outbreak in Gabon in 1994 was initially thought to be yellow fever but was retrospectively identified as Ebola infection (17). The more frequent recognition of outbreaks in the 1990s may be due to a true change in the epidemiology, heightened awareness among health care providers and public health authorities, or improvements in communication and diagnostic techniques (41, 42, 44, 45). In 1996, an infected physician flew from Gabon to South Africa, where a nurse who provided care for him became fatally infected (43), highlighting the real potential for international transmission of such pathogens. In the 1995 Zaire outbreak, 80 of the patients were health care workers, which heightens the public health impact of disease in areas which are already medically underserved (22).

Table 17.2 Reported human Ebola hemorrhagic fever outbreaks

Subtype	Year	Location	Cases	Mortality (%)
Zaire	1976	Zaire	318	88
Sudan	1976	Sudan	284	53
Sudan	1976	England	1	0
Zaire	1977	Zaire	1	100
Sudan	1979	Sudan	34	65
Côte-d'Ivoire	1994	Côte-d'Ivoire	1	0
Gabon	1994	Gabon	49	65
Zaire	1995	Zaire	316	79
Côte-d'Ivoire (?)[a]	1995	Liberia	1	0
Gabon	1996	Gabon	37	57
Gabon	1996–7	Gabon	60	75
Gabon	1996	South Africa	1	100

[a] No virologic data, based on serology.

Transmission

Person-to-person transmission occurs with direct contact, which usually occurs while nursing ill, infected persons or preparing cadavers for burial or by reuse of unsterilized needles and syringes. As a result, health care facilities have frequently been the focus of transmission. In the 1976 Zaire epidemic, infection was acquired by receiving an injection at the implicated hospital or by contact with another patient (39). In the 1979 Sudan outbreak, transmission occurred by direct contact in chains of transmission in the family of the first patient and in four other families, each with contact with the local hospital (2). In the 1995 Zaire epidemic, a study of household transmission indicated that Ebola virus is principally transmitted by direct contact with ill persons or their body fluids during the late stages of illness or by preparing the body for burial. Of 78 household members of Ebola patients who did not have direct contact with the patient, none became ill, suggesting that aerosol transmission was not an important mode of transmission (11). Transmission is most likely due to contact with blood or body fluids, mucous membranes, or skin. Ebola virus has been isolated from the semen of convalescent patients, so sexual transmission is also a concern. Transmission to a laboratory worker from an accidental needle stick occurred in England in 1977 (13).

Pathology

Filovirus infections in humans have several pathological features in common with other severe viral hemorrhagic fevers (VHFs), such as Lassa fever, Argentine hemorrhagic fever, and yellow fever (49). However, among the VHFs, the filoviruses cause the most widespread destructive tissue lesions. Gross pathologic findings at autopsy include widespread petechial hemorrhages and ecchymoses involving skin, mucous membranes, and internal organs. The histopathologic changes are similar in Marburg virus (23, 28, 29,

34) and Ebola virus (3, 4, 10, 12, 14, 15, 20, 21, 26, 31, 35, 46, 48) infections, although the latter tends to be more severe. Necrosis is seen in many organs and is maximal in the liver, spleen, kidney, and gonads. The necrosis is both ischemic in nature and related to cytopathic effect of the virus. Characteristic histolopathologic features in the liver are seen, with widespread hepatocellular necrosis, Councilman bodies, microvesicular fatty change, and Kupffer cell hyperplasia. Ebola virus inclusions within the cytoplasm of hepatocytes are seen (Fig. 17.2A). They are usually numerous, eosinophilic, and oval or filamentous and ultrastructurally are seen to be composed of aggregates of viral nucleocapsids (Fig. 17.2B) (18, 21, 46–48). The spleen and lymph nodes show extensive follicular necrosis and necrotic debris. The lungs are usually hemorrhagic and show features of diffuse alveolar damage. Myocardial edema is seen but is not associated with any appreciable inflammatory infiltrates. Electron microscopic studies reveal that viral particles and inclusions are widely distributed in various tissues examined. These are seen primarily within endothelial cells and macrophages and are free within the interstitium. Immunohistochemistry and in situ hybridization studies reveal that the distribution of viral antigens and nucleic acids correlates with ultrastructural localization of virus (Fig. 17.3 and 17.4). Significant injury to the microvasculature and increased endothelial permeability appear to be central to the pathogenesis of the shock syndrome seen in Ebola virus infections. Pharmacological mediators of inflammation, such as tumor necrosis factor, also appear to be responsible for the increased vascular permeability and shock.

Clinical Features

The incubation period ranges from 2 to 21 days, but typically it is between 5 and 10 days. Early symptoms include fever, headache, and weakness and are followed by nausea, vomiting, and diarrhea (Table 17.3) (5, 22, 39). Some patients develop respiratory symptoms, sore throat, dysphagia, or hiccups. Conjunctival injection is occasionally seen, as is gingival hemorrhage. Some, but by no means all, patients develop frank hemorrhage with petechia, gastrointestinal bleeding, or hematoma or bleeding at sites of needle punctures. A morbilliform skin rash has been described, but this may not be evident in dark-skinned individuals. Delirium and depressed consciousness are common and may indicate central nervous system involvement. Laboratory data are limited. Abnormalities identified include proteinuria, thrombocytopenia, and elevation of transaminases. Pregnant women frequently abort, and mortality is high among infants born to mothers who died of hemorrhagic fever (5, 39).

Mortality has ranged from 53 to 88% in large outbreaks, and death usually comes 7 to 10 days after the onset of illness. Multi-organ system failure is evident in terminal patients with coma and oliguria. Convalescent patients regain strength over a period of weeks. Late complications include arthralgia, especially of the large joints; orchitis; parotitis; keratoconjunctivitis with corneal perforation; and hearing loss.

Early symptoms include fever, headache, and weakness and are followed by nausea, vomiting, and diarrhea

Table 17.3 Clinical features of Ebola hemorrhagic fever

Symptom or sign	Percent of cases
Fever	90–100
Headache	40–90
Myalgia/arthralgia	40–80
Weakness	75–95
Sore throat/dysphagia	40–80
Nausea/vomiting	65–75
Abdominal pain	60–80
Diarrhea	75–85
Cough or dyspnea	20–40
Hiccups	5–25
Conjunctival injection	20–50
Gingival bleeding	10–25
Rash	5–20
Petechiae	5–20
Hematemesis	10–40
Lower gastrointestinal bleeding	15–50
Any bleeding	40–70

Diagnosis

Ebola virus infection should be considered as a possible diagnosis in patients who have traveled in the specific local area where an Ebola infection has recently occurred, have had direct contact with body fluids of a person or animal with Ebola infection, or have worked in a laboratory or animal facility that handles Ebola virus. Otherwise, Ebola virus infection is very unlikely, and evaluation for and treatment of other, more likely serious diseases such as malaria or typhoid must not be delayed.

The diagnosis of Ebola virus infection by history and clinical manifestations can also be supported histopathologically. The main pathological differential diagnosis should include viral hepatitis, leptospirosis, malaria, and rickettsial diseases. However, because of the similar pathologic features in VHF and a variety of other viral, rickettsial, and bacterial infections, unequivocal diagnosis can be made only by laboratory tests. Currently, virus-specific laboratory diagnosis and confirmation can be accomplished by the detection of filovirus antigens and antibodies by enzyme-linked immunosorbent assay or immunofluorescence procedures. Diagnosis can also be accomplished by detection of viral RNA by reverse transcriptase-polymerase chain reaction or by isolation of the virus from body fluids (33). Viral particles may be identified by electron and immunoelectron microscopic examination of human tissues. Ebola virus antigens can be detected by immunohistochemical examination of formalin-fixed tissues by using specific polyclonal and monoclonal antibodies. During the recent epidemic in Kikwit, Zaire, a novel immunohistochemical test was developed at the Centers for Disease Control and Prevention by using skin biopsy specimens for the diagnosis of Ebola VHF (16, 25). Formalin-fixed biopsy specimens are not infectious and

Ebola virus antigens can be detected by immunohistochemical examination of formalin-fixed tissues by using specific polyclonal and monoclonal antibodies

may be sent without special precautions or refrigeration and may be taken in the most basic field conditions. This approach therefore has an advantage over viral cultures and fluorescent-antibody tests, which are commonly used for surveillance purposes and require special handling and transport of infectious material and a cold chain. This new diagnostic modality and immunohistochemical findings open the way to a more practical surveillance mechanism and provide new insights into a possible epidemiologic role for contact transmission.

Treatment

Treatment of Ebola hemorrhagic fever is supportive; no specific antiviral drug or vaccine is currently available. In the 1995 Zaire epidemic, patients treated with transfusions from convalescent patients had a high survival rate. However, this may be accounted for by their other favorable prognostic factors, such as infection later in the epidemic, when the mortality rate was lower (36). Most outbreaks have occurred in resource-poor settings, and a higher survival rate may be expected in settings where more intensive care can be provided.

Treatment of Ebola hemorrhagic fever is supportive; no specific antiviral drug or vaccine is currently available

Prevention

Since the natural reservoir of Ebola virus is not known, specific vector control or primary prevention is not feasible. In the United States, imported nonhuman primates are kept under quarantine to prevent spread of Ebola virus (9), and avoidance of direct contact with nonhuman primates in sub-Saharan Africa that may be ill with or deceased from hemorrhagic fever also seems prudent.

Barrier nursing and sterilization of medical instruments are the keys to prevention of secondary human cases and should be practiced routinely to prevent infection with other agents, such as hepatitis B and human immunodeficiency viruses. Once an outbreak is identified, surveillance of infected and exposed individuals should be instituted to prevent additional cases. Ill persons should be cared for in health care settings, where barrier nursing techniques can be ensured (8). The patient should be placed in a private room if available, and a negative-pressure room should be considered, even in early stages, to avoid the need for later transport. Nonessential staff and visitors should not enter the room, and barrier precautions—gloves and gowns—should be worn by those who do enter. Face shields or surgical masks and eyewear should be used for patient contact (coming less than 3 feet from the patient). Patients with prominent cough, vomiting, diarrhea, or hemorrhage should be placed in a negative-pressure room, and personal protective respirators should be worn. Some of these resources, such as negative-pressure rooms or high-efficiency personal respirators, may not be available in outbreak situations in developing countries. Other barriers may be needed, such as leg and shoe coverings if, for example, the patient is vomiting. Barriers should be removed, and soiled shoes should be cleaned and disinfected before entering the hallway. An anteroom is useful for this purpose. Cadavers should be wrapped in sealed leakproof material and cremated or buried promptly.

Education of health care providers and of the general public is essential and should include information about disease recognition, reporting procedures, and barrier precautions. As long as there continue to be insufficient resources for sterilization of medical equipment and for proper nursing barrier practices in sub-Saharan Africa, outbreaks of Ebola hemorrhagic fever are also likely to occur.

> *Education of health care providers and of the general public is essential and should include information about disease recognition, reporting procedures, and barrier precautions*

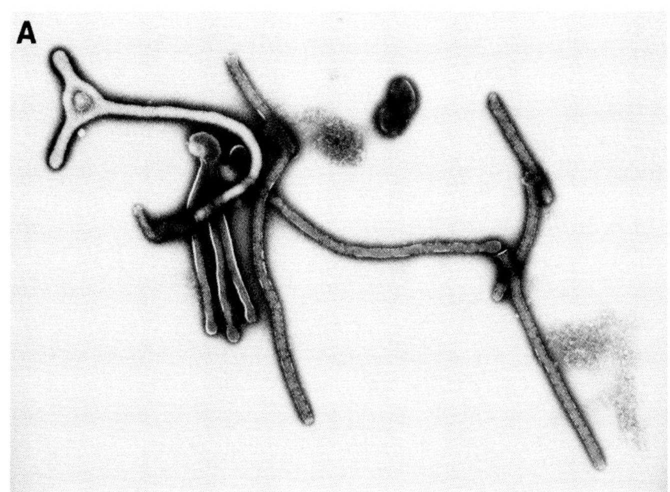

Figure 17.1 Electron micrographs of an Ebola virus isolate. (A) Negative stain of whole virus showing filamentous and irregularly shaped particles; (B) thin section of Ebola virus-infected Vero E6 cells showing virions in longitudinal and cross sections (arrowhead); (C) low-power electron micrograph of Ebola virus-infected Vero E6 cells showing inclusions, which are aggregates of viral nucleocapsids (arrow). (Scale bars: B, 100 nm; C, 1 μm.) Courtesy of Charles Humphrey and Cynthia Goldsmith, Infectious Disease Pathology Activity, Centers for Disease Control and Prevention.

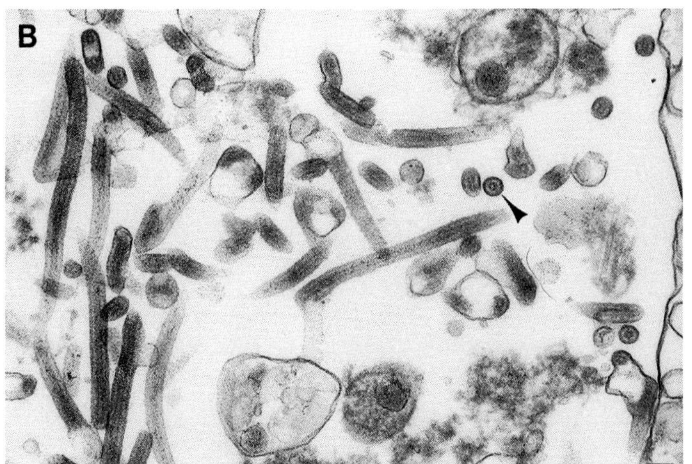

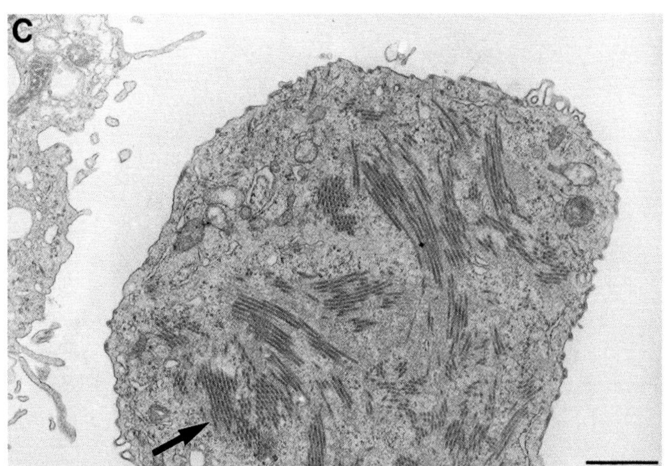

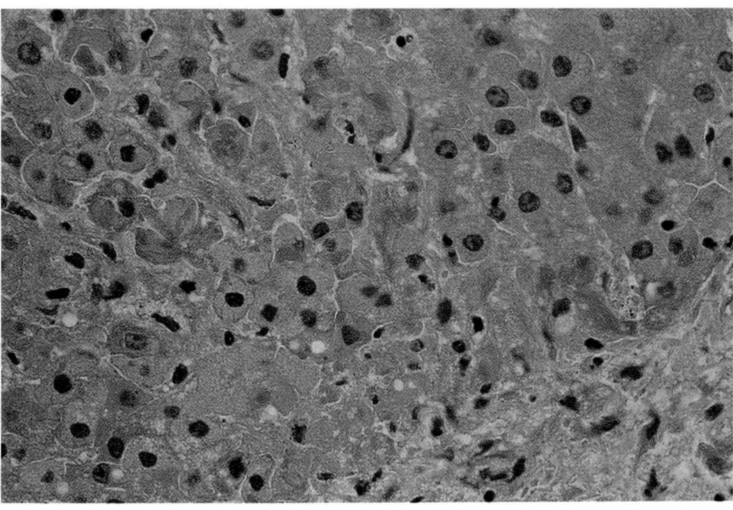

Figure 17.2A Ebola virus hemorrhagic fever. Photomicrograph of liver showing hepatocellular necrosis and numerous Ebola viral inclusions (hematoxylin and eosin; original magnification, ×158).

Figure 17.2B Ebola virus hemorrhagic fever. A large Ebola virus inclusion (arrow) is seen in a thin-section electron micrograph of the liver. Abundant viral particles are also seen within hepatic sinusoids (arrowhead). Scale bar, 1 μm.

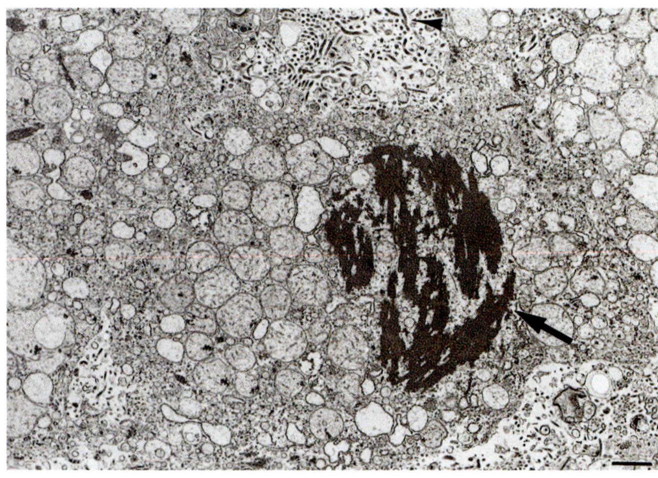

Figure 17.3A Ebola virus hemorrhagic fever. Immunostaining of viral antigens in the liver, as determined by immunohistochemistry. Photomicrograph shows extensive immunostaining of viral antigens; antigens are seen within sinusoidal lining cells and hepatocytes. (Naphthol fast red substrate with light hematoxylin counterstain; original magnification, ×158.)

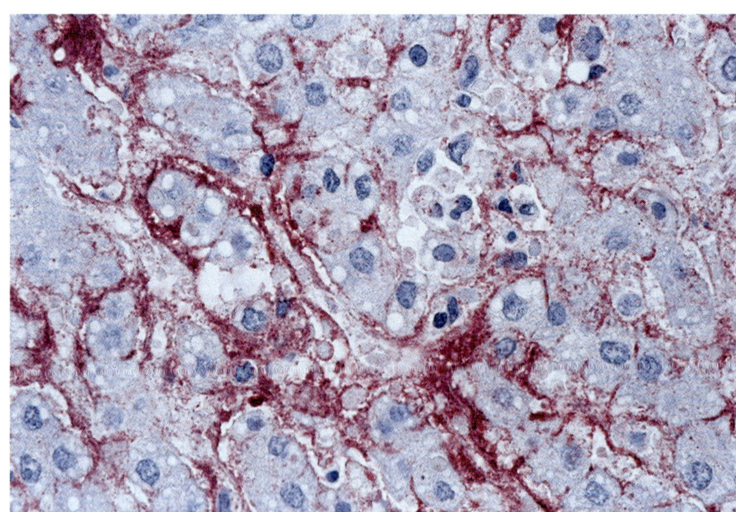

Figure 17.3B Ebola virus hemorrhagic fever. Immunostaining of viral antigens in endothelial cells of skeletal muscle, as determined by immunohistochemistry (naphthol fast red substrate with light hematoxylin counterstain; original magnification, ×158).

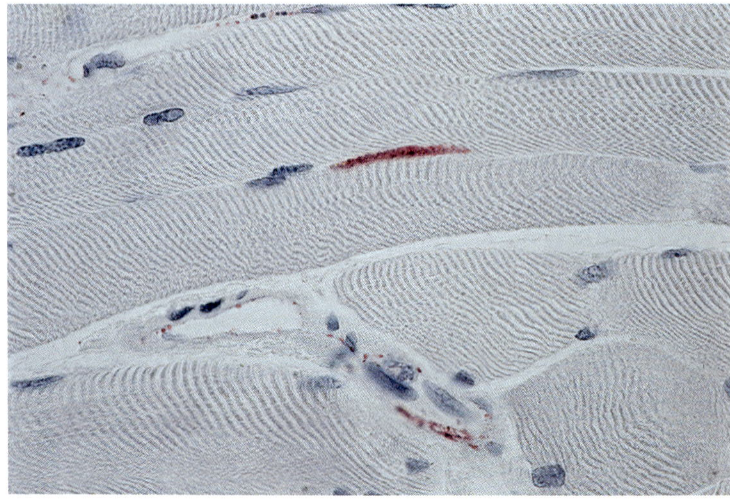

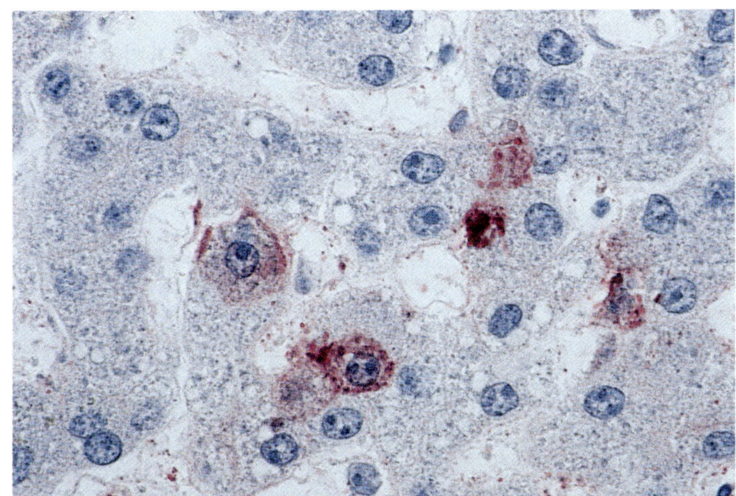

Figure 17.4 Ebola virus hemorrhagic fever. Ebola virus-infected hepatocytes as seen by colorimetric in situ hybridization using digoxigenin-labeled probes (naphthol fast red substrate with light hematoxylin counterstain; original magnification, ×250).

References

1. **Arata, A. A., and B. Johnson.** 1978. Approaches towards studies on potential reservoirs of viral hemorrhagic fever in southern Sudan, p. 191–200. *In* S. R. Pattyn (ed.), *Ebola Virus Haemorrhagic Fever.* Elsevier/North-Holland Biomedical Press, Amsterdam.

2. **Baron, R. C., J. B. McCormick, and O. A. Zubeir.** 1983. Ebola virus disease in southern Sudan: hospital dissemination and intrafamilial spread. *Bull. W. H. O.* **61:**997–1003.

3. **Baskerville, A., E. T. W. Bowen, G. S. Platt, L. B. McArdell, and D. I. H. Simpson.** 1978. The pathology of experimental Ebola virus infection in monkeys. *J. Pathol.* **125:**131–138.

4. **Baskerville, A., S. P. Fisher-Hoch, G. H. Neild, and A. B. Dowsett.** 1985. Ultrastructural pathology of experimental Ebola haemorrhagic fever virus infection. *J. Pathol.* **147:**199–209.

5. **Bwaka, A., M.-J. Bonnet, P. Calain, R. Colebunders, A. Deroo, Y. Guimard, Katwiki, Kibadi, A. Kipasa, Kuvula, Mapanda, M. Massamba, Mupapa, T. Muyembe, Ndabere, C. J. Peters, P. E. Rollin, and E. van den Enden.** Ebola hemorrhagic fever in Kikwit, Zaire: clinical observations. *J. Infect. Dis.*, in press.

6. **Centers for Disease Control.** 1983. Ebola virus infection in imported primates—Virginia, 1989. *Morbid. Mortal. Weekly Rep.* **38:**831–832.

7. **Centers for Disease Control and Prevention.** 1995. Outbreak of Ebola viral hemorrhagic fever—Zaire, 1995. *Morbid. Mortal. Weekly Rep.* **44:**381–382.

8. **Centers for Disease Control and Prevention.** 1995. Update: management of patients with suspected viral hemorrhagic fever. *Morbid. Mortal. Weekly Rep.* **44:**475–479.

9. **Centers for Disease Control and Prevention.** 1996. Ebola-Reston virus infection among quarantined nonhuman primates—Texas, 1996. *Morbid. Mortal. Weekly Rep.* **45:**314–316.

10. **Dietrich, M., H. H. Schumacher, D. Peters, and J. Knobloch.** 1978. Human pathology of Ebola (Maridi) virus infection in the Sudan, p. 37–41. *In* S. R. Pattyn (ed.), *Ebola Virus Haemorrhagic Fever.* Elsevier/North-Holland Biomedical Press, Amsterdam.

11. **Dowell, S. F., R. Mukunu, T. G. Ksiezek, A. S. Khan, P. E. Rollin, C. J. Peters, and the E. H. F. Study Group.** 1997. Transmission of Ebola hemorrhagic fever: a study of risk factors in family members, Kikwit, Zaire, 1995. *J. Infect. Dis.*, in press.

12. **Ellis, D. S., D. I. H. Simpson, D. P. Francis, J. Knobloch, E. T. Bowen, P. Lolik, and I. M. Deng.** 1978. Ultrastructure of Ebola virus particles in human liver. *J. Clin. Pathol.* **31:**201–208.

13. **Emond, R. T. D., E. Brandon, E. T. W. Bowen, and G. Lloyd.** 1977. A case of Ebola virus infection. *Br. Med. J.* **2:**541–544.

14. **Fisher-Hoch, S. P., T. L. Brammer, S. G. Trappier, L. C. Hutwagner, B. B. Farrar, S. L. Ruo, B. G. Brown, L. M. Hermann, G. I. Perez-Oronoz, and C. S. Goldsmith.** 1992. Pathogenic potential of filoviruses: role of geographic origin of primate host and virus strain. *J. Infect. Dis.* **166:**753–763.

15. **Geisbert, T. W., P. B. Jahrling, M. A. Hanes, and P. M. Zack.** 1992. Association of Ebola-related Reston virus particles and antigen with tissue lesions of monkeys imported to the United States. *J. Comp. Pathol.* **106:**137–152.

16. George-Courbot, M.-C., A. Sanchez, C.-Y. Lu, S. Baize, E. Leroy, J. Lansout-Soukate, C. Tévi-Bénissan, A. J. Georges, S. G. Trappier, S. R. Zaki, R. Swanepoel, P. A. Leman, P. E. Rolin, C. J. Peters, S. T. Nichol, and T. G. Ksiazek. 1997. Isolation and phylogenetic characterization of Ebola viruses causing different outbreaks in Gabon. *Emerg. Infect. Dis.* **3:**59–62.

17. Georges, A. J., A. A. Renaut, E. Bertherat, S. Baize, E. Leroy, B. LeGuenno, J. Lepago, J. Amblard, S. Edzang, and M. C. Georges-Courbot. 1996. Recent Ebola virus outbreaks in Gabon from 1994 to 1996: epidemiologic and control issues, p. 47. *Proceedings of the International Colloquium on Ebola Virus Research*, September 4–7, Antwerp, Belgium.

18. Goldsmith, C. S., P. E. Rollin, X. H. Zhang, C. J. Peters, and S. R. Zaki. Ebola virus hemorrhagic fever, Zaire, 1995: an ultrastructural study. *Proceedings of the 55th Annual Meeting of the Microscopy Society of America*, in press.

19. Heymann, D. L., J. S. Weisfeld, P. A. Webb, K. M. Johnson, T. Cairns, and H. Berquist. 1980. Ebola hemorrhagic fever: Tandala, Zaire, 1977–1978. *J. Infect. Dis.* **142:**372–376.

20. International Study Team. 1978. Ebola haemorrhagic fever in Sudan, 1976. *Bull. W. H. O.* **56:**247–270.

21. Jaax, N. J., K. J. Davis, T. J. Geisbert, P. Vogel, G. P. Jaax, M. Topper, and P. B. Jahrling. 1996. Lethal experimental infection of rhesus monkeys with Ebola-Zaire (Mayinga) virus by the oral and conjunctival route of exposure. *Arch. Pathol. Lab. Med.* **120:**140–155.

22. Khan, A. S., T. F. Kweteminga, D. L. Heymann, B. LeGuenno, P. Nabeth, B. Kerstiens, Y. Freerackers, P. H. Kilmarx, G. R. Rodier, O. Nkuku, P. E. Rollin, A. Sanchez, S. R. Zaki, R. Swanepoel, O. Tomori, S. T. Nichol, C. J. Peters, J. J. Muyembe-Tamfum, and T. G. Ksiazek, for the Commission de Lutte Controle des Epidemies à Kikwit. The re-emergence of Ebola hemorrhagic fever, Zaire, 1995. *J. Infect. Dis.*, in press.

23. Kissling, R. E., F. A. Murphy, and B. E. Henderson. 1970. Marburg virus. *Ann. N.Y. Acad. Sci.* **174:**932–945.

24. Le Guenno, B., P. Formentry, M. Wyers, P. Gounon, F. Walker, and C. Boesch. 1995. Isolation and partial characterization of a new strain of Ebola virus. *Lancet* **345:**1271–1274.

25. Lloyd, E., S. R. Zaki, and P. E. Rollin. 1996. Long-term surveillance for Ebola in Zaire, p. 43. *Proceedings of the International Colloquium on Ebola Virus Research*, September 4–7, Antwerp, Belgium.

26. Murphy, F. A. 1978. Pathology of Ebola virus infection, p. 43–59. *In* S. R. Pattyn (ed.), *Ebola Virus Haemorrhagic Fever*. Elsevier/North-Holland Biomedical Press, Amsterdam.

27. Murphy, F. A. 1996. Virus taxonomy, p. 15–57. *In* B. N. Fields, D. M. Knipe, and P. M. Howley (ed.), *Field's Virology*. Lippincott-Raven, Philadelphia.

28. Murphy, F. A., D. I. H. Simpson, S. G. Whitfield, I. Zlotnik, and G. B. Carter. 1971. Marburg virus infection in monkeys. Ultrastructural studies. *Lab. Invest.* **24:**279–291.

29. Murphy, F. A., D. I. H. Simpson, S. G. Whitfield, I. Zlotnik, and G. B. Carter. 1972. Marburg virus infection in monkeys. Ultrastructural studies. *Med. Chir. Dig.* **1:**325–332.

30. Murphy, F. A., G. van der Groen, S. G. Whitfield, and J. V. Lange. 1978. Ebola and Marburg Virus morphology and taxonomy, p. 61–82. *In* S. R. Pattyn (ed.), *Ebola Virus Haemorrhagic Fever*. Elsevier/North-Holland Biomedical Press, Amersterdam.

31. Pereboeva, L. A., V. K. Tkachev, L. V. Kolesnikova, L. Y. Krendeleva, E. I. Ryabchikova, and M. P. Smolina. 1993. Ultrastructural changes of guinea pig organs in sequential passages of Ebola virus. *Vopr. Virusol.* **4:**179–182.

32. Peters, C. J. 1996. Emerging infections—Ebola and other filoviruses. *West. J. Med.* **164:**36–38.

33. Peters, C. J., A. Sanchez, P. E. Rollin, T. G. Ksiazek, and F. A. Murphy. 1996. Filoviridae: Marburg and Ebola viruses, p. 1161–1176. *In* B. N. Fields, D. M. Knipe, and P. M. Howley (ed.), *Field's Virology.* Lippincott-Raven, Philadelphia.

34. Rippey, J. J., N. J. Schepers, and J. H. S. Gear. 1984. The pathology of Marburg virus disease. *S. Afr. Med. J.* **66:**50–54.

35. Ryabchikova, E. I., S. G. Baranova, V. K. Tkachev, and A. A. Grazhdantseva. 1993. Morphological changes in Ebola virus infection in guinea pigs. *Vopr. Virusol.* **4:**176–179.

36. Sadek, R. F., A. S. Khan, P. H. Kilmarx, T. G. Ksiazek, and C. J. Peters. 1996. Outbreak of Ebola hemorrhagic fever, Zaire, 1995: a closer numerical look, p. 622–625. *In* 1996 *Proceedings of the Epidemiology Section of the American Statistical Association*, Chicago.

37. Swanepoel, R., P. A. Leman, F. J. Burt, N. A. Zachariades, L. E. Braack, T. G. Ksiazek, P. E. Rollin, S. R. Zaki, and C. J. Peters. 1996. Experimental inoculation of plants and animals with Ebola virus. *Emerg. Infect. Dis.* **2:**321–325.

38. World Health Organization. 1976. Ebola hemorrhagic fever in Sudan, 1976. *Bull. W. H. O.* **56:**247–270.

39. World Health Organization. 1978. Ebola haemorrhagic fever in Zaire, 1976. Report of an international commission. *Bull. W. H. O.* **56:**271–293.

40. World Health Organization. 1992. Viral hemorrhagic fever in imported monkeys. *Weekly Epidemiol. Rec.* **67:**142.

41. World Health Organization. 1995. Ebola hemorrhagic fever: confirmed case in Côte-d'Ivoire and suspect cases in Liberia. *Weekly Epidemiol. Rec.* **50:**359.

42. World Health Organization. 1996. Ebola hemorrhagic fever—Gabon. *Weekly Epidemiol. Rec.* **71:**320.

43. World Health Organization. 1996. Ebola hemorrhagic fever—South Africa. *Weekly Epidemiol. Rec.* **71:**359.

44. World Health Organization. 1996. Outbreak of Ebola hemorrhagic fever in Gabon officially declared over. *Weekly Epidemiol. Rec.* **71:**125–126.

45. World Health Organization. 1997. Ebola haemorrhagic fever—Gabon. *In* Emerging and other communicable diseases: disease outbreaks reported. (Newsletter online.) http://www.who.ch/programmes/emc/news.htm.

46. Zaki, S. R. Unpublished data.

47. Zaki, S. R., C. S. Goldsmith, P. W. Greer, L. M. Coffield, P. E. Rollin, P. Callain, A. S. Khan, T. G. Ksiazek, and C. J. Peters. Pathology of Ebola virus hemorrhagic fever, Kikwit, Zaire, 1995. *J. Infect. Dis,* in press.

48. Zaki, S. R., P. W. Greer, C. S. Goldsmith, L. M. Coffield, P. E. Rollin, P. Callain, A. S. Khan, T. G. Ksiazek, and C. J. Peters. 1996. Ebola virus hemorrhagic fever: pathologic, immunopathologic, and ultrastructural study. *Lab. Invest.* **74:**133A.

49. Zaki, S. R., and C. J. Peters. 1997. Viral hemorrhagic fevers, p. 347–364. *In* D. H. Connor, F. W. Chandler, D. A. Schwartz, H. J. Manz, and E. E. Lack (ed.), *Pathology of Infectious Diseases.* Appleton and Lange, Stamford, Conn.

Index